# LISTEN TO YOUR HORMONES

LISTEN TO YOUR **HORMONES**

# Sex, Love and Long life

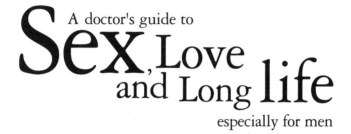

A doctor's guide to Sex, Love and Long life especially for men

ABRAHAM HARVEY KRYGER, M.D., D.M.D.

*WellnessMD Publications, Monterey, California ©2004*

ISBN 0-9748634-0-8

Printed in the United States of America

Published by WellnessMD Publications
1084 Cass Street, Monterey, California 93940
831 373-4406
Fax 831 373-4481
www.WellnessMD.com
www.sexloveandhormones.com
wellnessmd@earthlink.net

## What people are saying about *Listen to Your Hormones*

Absolutely essential information about hormones and the good life.

Andrew Van Goethem, English Professor, Japan

An insightful owner's manual for anyone with hormones.

Patrick Ian Cowan, Ph.D., Executive Director
New Hampshire Institute for Therapeutic Arts

Easy to understand, up-to-date, well researched.

Howard Wynne M.D., Assistant Clinical Professor
UCLA School of Medicine

Better than a prescription—this book puts you in charge of your own hormones.

Duncan McGillvary, Chief Executive Officer
Sunshine Healthcare Group, Phoenix

A quick guide out of the mumbo-jumbo of popular hype about hormones.

Scott L. Hershberger, Ph.D. Professor of Psychology
California State University, Long Beach

A hormone guidebook for everyone.

Dan Clary, pre-med student, University of Alabama

Read this if you care about your future.

Demetrios Perdikis, M.D., Mercerville, New Jersey

A treasure of facts and interesting explanations.

Patrick Knost, M.D., Family Medicine, Placerville, California

Everything you always wanted to know about your hormones but didn't know whom to ask.

David Prince, M.D., Internist, New York City.

A first step to great sex and long life.

Bob Flynn, Paramedic, Salinas, California, Fire Department

The complex universe of human hormones comes to life in this book.

Andre Guay, Endocrinologist, Harvard University

Dr. Kryger hammers home the key facts you need to know to manage your hormones effectively.

John Robbins, author, *The Food Revolution*

Highly recommended for anyone who wants better sex and a longer life.

Evelyn Waterman, Ph.D.
Psychotherapist, Santa Monica, California

I would often wonder where certain types of behavior would come from and never really associated behavior with hormones until reading this book. Dr.Kryger does a great job in explaining the various functions of hormones and how they affect our daily lives. He makes a very technical subject easy to understand without over-simplification. If you are using any hormone-altering therapy you will definitely want to read this book.

Jerry Johansen, VP, Research and Development
IntraLuminal Therapeutics, Inc., Carlsbad, California

Dr. Kryger's book is exactly what people (and their loved ones) need to read. I especially like the patient examples which add life and "a face" to this disorder which is usually suffered alone and in silence.

Leslie Lundt, MD. Psychiatrist, Boise, Idaho

*Listen to Your Hormones* is an important book for men who are suffering from hormone deficiencies that are adversely affecting their lives. Once diagnosed, male hypogonadism is an easily treated condition, the challenge is to accurately make a clinical diagnosis. Dr. Kryger's book clearly explains the signs, symptoms, causes, and effects of sex hormone deficiencies allowing his readers to initiate intelligent discussions with their health-care providers.

As a physician, I find it gratifying to care for well informed patients, and I am sure that this book will be responsible for many frank and open discussions between patients and their physicians. Hopefully, many of the thousands of hypogonadal men in America will have a higher quality of life once they are properly identified and treated. This book will make a significant contribution towards the accomplishment of that goal.

David Z. Prince, MD, FAAPMR
New York, Assistant Professor, Department of Rehabilitation Medicine
Clinical Instructor, Department of Internal Medicine

# Foreword

It has often been said that Rachel Carson launched the modern environmental movement more than thirty years ago with her seminal book *Silent Spring.* Her book detailed what was known then of the harmful effects on human health of pesticides and other toxic chemicals. She focused on pesticides, but she warned also of the ever growing plethora of untested chemicals that are increasingly concentrated in our bodies and environment. She focused on cancer, perhaps because she was suffering from it herself, but she warned also of birth defects, disrupted endocrine systems, sexual difficulties, and reproductive failures. *Silent Spring* opens with "The Fable For Tomorrow," and speaks of a farm where hens lay eggs that do not hatch, and farmers complain that they are unable to raise any pigs. The litters are small and the young survive only a few days.

Since Rachel Carson wrote *Silent Spring,* man-made chemicals have continued to spread across the planet, permeating every living creature and the most distant wilderness. Today, we are witnessing increases in birth defects, sexual abnormalities and reproductive failures in wildlife, and these are being traced with ever growing certainty to synthetic chemicals that mimic natural hormones, upsetting normal reproductive, sexual, and developmental processes.

Humans are not separate or immune. We are part of this planet as surely as the Florida alligators whose penises are one-third to one-half normal size. We are part of this planet as surely as the Beluga whales whose tissues are contaminated with toxic chemicals including DDT, PCBs, and mercury, and who suffer from malignant tumors, breast tumors, abdominal masses, ulcers of the mouth, esophagus, stomach and intestines, and some of whom have been born not only with testes and other normal male equipment, but also with a uterus and ovaries. We are part of this planet as surely as the panthers in Everglades National Park, who are experiencing an extraordinary level of sperm abnormalities, low sperm count, impaired immune response, and malfunctioning thyroid glands.

The man-made chemicals that are now disrupting the endocrine and reproductive systems of wild animals are also disturbing the species that has manufactured these compounds and introduced them into the environment. That's us. They are threatening our fertility, our intelligence, and our survival.

Even humans living in the most remote parts of the planet are effected. The Inuit people of Greenland are as far removed from the pollution of modern urban society as anyone on Earth. They are closer to the North Pole than they are to any city, factory or farm. Their language contains no word for contamination. If anyone would be spared the ravages of industrial ills, you might think it would be the Inuit. But even these remote and hardy people can no longer escape the chemical pollution that so effects our modern world.

A year-round ice sheet covers eighty-five percent of Greenland. In places, it is more than mile thick. There are very few trees, almost no grass, virtually no vegetable gardens or grain fields or fruit orchards. The Inuit depend almost entirely on the sea for their food. They eat as their ancestors have for tens of thousands of years. Only now they are perched atop the increasingly contaminated global food chain.

Recent exhaustive studies have found the bodies of Greenland's Inuit people (and other Arctic peoples) to contain some of the highest human concentrations of industrial chemicals and pesticides found anywhere on Earth. These levels are so extreme that the breast milk and tissues of some Greenlanders could be classified as hazardous waste. Hundreds of hazardous compounds are found in their blood, organs, and tissues.

The chemical contamination of the Inuit has occurred primarily through the whales, seals, fish, walruses and songbirds they eat. But the chemicals themselves originate in the cities of North America, Europe and Asia, and now permeate the lives and cells of all animals everywhere on Earth.

Whether we know it or not, you and I and the Inuit and the alligators are experiencing hazardous effects from exposure to endocrine-disrupting synthetic chemicals. These man-made compounds are scrambling the chemical messages that guide our development and sexuality. They are damaging our reproductive systems, altering the function of our nervous systems and brains, and impairing our immune systems.

In the landmark book *Our Stolen Future,* Theo Colborn and other experts on endocrine disrupting chemicals tell us of emerging problems:

> Synthetic chemicals can derail the normal expression of sexual characteristics of animals, in some cases masculinizing females and feminizing males… Exposure to hormonally active chemicals parentally or in adulthood increases vulnerability to hormone-

responsive cancers, such as malignancies in the breast, prostate, ovary, and uterus.

One of the most troubling consequences of the spread of hormone disrupting chemicals during the last half century has been a precipitous drop in male sperm counts. Perhaps the most comprehensive study of this worldwide phenomenon was published in the *British Medical Journal* in 1992. Researchers systematically reviewed the international scientific literature on semen analysis, and based their findings on sixty-one studies involving fifteen thousand healthy men from twenty countries and seven continents. (To be safe, the study excluded men sampled at fertility clinics who might have particularly low sperm counts.)

The findings were dramatic. Worldwide, between 1940 and 1990, the average number of sperm in a milliliter of male semen dropped 45 percent. At the same time, the volume of semen ejaculated dropped by 25 percent, making the actual drop in sperm count more than 50 percent. Meanwhile, the percentage of men with extremely low sperm count tripled.

Stunningly, if this downward trend has continued since 1990—and there is substantial evidence that it has—the average male born in 1975 has, at the age of thirty in 2005, a sperm count only one-fourth of the average male born in 1925.

For too long we have had elected officials whose priorities have reflected the short term interests of the chemical industry rather than the greater good of public health. The current system assumes that chemicals are innocent until proven guilty. But the burden of proof should work the opposite way. At this point, the evidence implicating hormonally active chemicals in human and animal health and reproductive damage has become overwhelming.

Fortunately, Dr. Kryger points out there are things you can do to defend and protect yourself and your family. There are ways you can greatly reduce your exposure and harm.

Eat low on the food chain. The most effective way to reduce your intake of toxic chemicals is to minimize your intake of meats, fish, dairy products and eggs—particularly those from modern factory farms. The Council on Environmental Quality states that meat and dairy products account for over 95 percent of the US population's intake of DDT. A study reported in the *New England Journal of Medicine* found that the breast milk of vegetarian mothers has less than two percent as much contamination as the breast milk of meat-eating mothers.

Decrease consumption of animal fat as much as possible. Eating less animal fat will greatly reduce exposure to hormone-disrupting chemicals. The EPA says that meats and cheeses are the major source of dioxin exposure in the US today.

Whenever possible, eat organic or pesticide-free produce and grains. Choose organic particularly with imported foods such as coffee, sugar, and bananas, because farmers in tropical countries often use much greater concentrations of toxic chemicals than are used in domestic food production. Supporting organic agriculture will reduce you and your family's exposure to toxic chemicals directly, by ensuring that residues aren't on or in the foods you eat, and indirectly, by helping to protect local water supplies.

Drink water that is clean and pure. If your water comes from a community source, find out what's in it. Find out if water officials are testing for hormone-disrupting chemicals, notably herbicides such as atrazine and dioxin. You may want to invest in a home water distillation or reverse osmosis system. Don't rely on inexpensive filters that are designed to remove chlorine and unpleasant tastes and odors, because they may not remove hormonally active synthetic chemicals. Bottled water is not necessarily an answer, because the standards it must meet are no higher than those for tap water.

If you are going to eat fish, be sure it's wild not farmed. Farmed fish has far greater levels of chemical contamination than wild fish. Avoid those types of fish that are highest in mercury and other forms of chemical contamination. (The highest mercury concentrations are found in large predatory species, particularly swordfish, king mackerel, shark, tilefish and opah. Medium to high levels are found in fresh and canned albacore tuna, red snapper, grouper, and orange ruffy. The safest fish, in terms of mercury, are salmon, shrimp, crab, light canned tuna, sea bass, herring, catfish and tilapia.)

If you are going to eat fish, watch for warnings about contamination. Public officials are concerned about lost license revenues and tourist dollars, and are reluctant to make these warnings unless the danger is dramatic. Children of mothers who ate even small amounts of Great Lakes fish while they were pregnant were born with smaller heads and reduced intelligence. Children who eat fish from Lake Ontario have been found to have reduced stress tolerance.

Don't heat or microwave food in plastic containers or with plastic wrap. Use glass or porcelain for microwave cooking. Hormone-disrupting chemicals can leach out of some plastics, particularly the softer ones.

Wash your hands often. Theo Colborn and her coauthors in *Our Stolen Future* tell us, "Many synthetic chemicals vaporize and then settle on indoor surfaces—kitchen counters, tables, furniture, clothes—where they can be readily picked up by those who touch them. In fact, indoor air experts now sample for contamination in buildings by wiping surfaces with special equipment."

Minimize your use of pesticides and household chemicals around the home. EPA researchers have found that products designed to kill fungus on fruits and vegetables can interfere with the synthesis of steroid hormones in animals (presumably including humans). Children and dogs living in homes that use pesticides in lawns and gardens have higher rates of cancer.

Listen to your hormones. This book by Abraham Kryger, M.D., contains a wealth of information, and provides practical ways that men can begin to rebalance their hormones and rebuild their health.

Recent research is making it increasingly clear that many middle-aged and older men could benefit from supplemental bio-identical testosterone. Dr. Kryger's book explains why, and introduces TestoCreme®, a compound that appears to have significant advantages over all the other testosterone products available today.

I am pleased to write the foreword for *Listen to Your Hormones.* It is an informative guide for the male who does not wish to remain a victim of pollution, but wants to understand his hormones and bring them back into a more natural and healthy functioning. The benefits of doing so can be extraordinary.

— John Robbins

John Robbins is the author of five international best-sellers, including *Diet for a New America,* and *The Food Revolution.* The founder of EarthSave International and Board Chairperson of Youth For Environmental Sanity (YES!), he also serves on the boards of many other nonprofit organizations working for a safer and healthier world. Widely recognized as one of the most eloquent spokespersons for a thriving, just, and sustainable future, he is the recipient of countless awards, including the Rachel Carson award, the Albert Schweitzer Humanitarian award, and the Peace Abbey's Courage of Conscience award. Further information about John Robbins and his work can be found at www.foodrevolution.org.

# Acknowledgments

It would be impossible to list the names of the many patients who have made this book possible by telling me their personal stories and innermost thoughts. The names of those mentioned sending emails or from interviews have been changed to protect their confidentiality. If any of them read this book, they might recognize themselves, but their stories are universal.

I give thanks to my wonderful mother, whose attention to detail and organizational sense taught me to focus on what is important. Guta Kryger—"Jean" as she liked to call herself—was a grand lady of eighty-three when she died. She had always looked about fifteen years younger than her age. I was fortunate enough to share her last few months and moments with her and I am forever grateful for that final gift.

From the bottom of my heart I want to thank my sons, Doctors Zol and Gil Kryger, for their insightful suggestions since they thoroughly understand how the human body operates. I pray that they will carry on the family tradition and create a dynasty of medical doctors.

I give thanks to my brilliant and helpful office manager, Cheri Gayman without whom this book could never have been completed. Her editing and insights were indispensable. Of course the advice and guidance I received from my high school friend, Joe Wiesenfeld, onetime scriptwriter and financial genius who received an Emmy for his Anne of Green Gables TV series, was immeasurable.

I was extremely fortunate to have Joyce Griffith as an editor. Joyce's decades of experience with medical doctor-writers made her invaluable as a guide. Her verification of my varied sources and constant corrections gave me great conviction. Her multiple edits of my many additions made it easier for my readers to digest the complex material in this book. Joyce really polished the manuscript and stopped me from using extraneous words. Thanks also to Lotte and Alan Marcus, Mike Kocsis, Steve Sisson, Bill Ahern, Rob Winninger, Larry Little, Leah Lehman, Bruce McFadden, Jason Grange, Bill O'Conner, Todd Berlin, and Frank Stark for their encouragement and assistance.

I am very grateful to Mat Squillante, a talented Monterey Bay graphic designer who gave his heart and soul to designing my cover and creating the illustrations which give clarity to the many difficult concepts outlined in my book. I am also thankful to Linda Griffith for her design concepts.

Special thanks to my fellow physicians who read my manuscript: Andre Guay, Adrian Dobbs, Norm Mazer, David Prince, Gene Shippen, Pat Lamb, Frank Stark, Larry Crapo, Wayne Meikle, Leslie Lundt, Jeanne Alexander, Mark Gordon, Demetrios Perdikis, Fritz Klein, Daniel Susott, and Howard Wynne. Many thanks also to those who read the earlier versions: my literary agent, Nancy Ellis; my first editor, Maria Owen; and my friends Robert Meyer, Chad Hawker, Jerry Johansen, Bob Flynn, Andrew Bending, Ken Saville, Lorne Balshine, Mike Falcon, Scott Hershberger, Mike Chandler, Mark Meeker, Michael Mintz and Scott Koenigsberg, who kept my spirits up over the two and a half years it took to write this book. A special kudos to Steven McOmber, whose intelligent comments, developed from years of scientific reading, helped to clarify my words, and special appreciation for Steven Bergman, photographer *extraordinaire.*

I honor those researchers who have done all the hard work and developed their unique concepts in genetics, environmental toxins, human sexuality, sleep disorders and neuropsychiatry that have provided the material to substantiate my theories. Jeff Bowles, John Manning, Dennis McFadden, Lisa Tenover, Steven Krimsky, Theo Colborn, Deborah Cadbury, Joe Thornton, Meir Kryger and Owen Wolkowitz, who are each great scientists and innovators in their own right.

A deep bow to John Robbins, who kindly wrote my foreword, and to Charles Patterson, Andrew Weil, and Paul Burwash for supporting a vegetarian or vegan lifestyle and organic farming advocacy. These gentlemen have increased my awareness and respect for all animals and the unique role they play in our food chain which keeps our world in balance. An exceptional individual, John Robbins has greatly contributed to the conscience of the world through his writings and work with EarthSave.

The development of a topical testosterone cream, used in my research with my patients, would not have been possible without the close association and talents of Dana Gordon, a superb compounding pharmacist, in Pacific Grove, California. The talented attorneys David Makous, James Ross and David Osborne were instrumental in protecting my intellectual property rights once this product, named TestoCreme®, was submitted for patent. I again thank all those individuals who have contributed from the bottom of my heart. I am grateful to the many others who have played a role anonymously in sustaining my research findings. You know who you are and again, I thank you all.

—Abraham Harvey Kryger, D.M.D., M.D.

## Dedication

The book is dedicated to my mother,
Guta Jean Kryger,
who inspired my thirst for knowledge and
told me never to stop learning.

# Contents

## Chapter Five



## Chapter Six



## Chapter Seven



## Chapter Eight

## Chapter Nine



## Chapter Ten



## Chapter Eleven

# Introduction

When I set out to write this book, I was frustrated by the incredible amount of information pointing out the risks of toxic pollutants that are creating hormone imbalances.

I was hearing too many stories of patients whose doctors ignored symptoms of hormonal imbalance, passing them off as part of the "normal" aging process. At the other extreme, I was seeing too many men so obsessed with their sexual performance that they were risking their reproductive and sexual capabilities by self-medicating with steroids and questionable nutritional supplements. I was ready to set up a podium with a speaker system powerful enough to blare my message from the West Coast to the rest of the United States of America. My message would be, "Doctors, patients, athletes, everybody—pay attention to your hormones!"

Once I started collecting research material in preparation for this book, my perspective softened somewhat. I began to see the complex intricacies of our hormonal system. I realized that many of my fellow physicians did not have the information they needed to make an accurate evaluation of their patients with hormone-related health problems. Instead of criticizing the way doctors deal with these conditions, I decided to base my book on the principle that doctors and their patients need to be more aware of the role hormones play in their lives. My role was not to condemn others but rather to point the way to new points of view based on sound medical research. New understandings, new paradigms, new ways to work with hormone supplements are just coming into public awareness. The more we learn about these new findings, the more intelligent we can be about the kinks and curves of our hormonal systems.

I wrote this book to help you, the regular guy, gain a more complete understanding of how your hormones work. The more you know, the more effectively you and your doctor can listen to your hormones. This book can teach you how to improve your sexual health. If you are having a problem with your sex life, it is probably because your hormones are out of balance. Restoring that balance will renew the sexual joy in your life, allowing you to "do it till you die."

In the first chapter of this book we will look at several of the distinguishing functions of testosterone in the male, including developing the penis, growing a beard, and enabling the penis to become erect in sexual intercourse.

Because of its power to create manliness, testosterone is the undisputed king of the hormones. It rules with total sovereignty. Like other hormones we will discuss in this book, testosterone is a steroid hormone produced by our body to perform vital tasks in regulating, stimulating, and controlling our body and our brain. The first four letters of the word come from the fact that the testicles produce it but its effects reach much higher levels of the human body.

Normally, compounds that travel throughout the blood stream do not easily cross the blood-brain barrier, which has evolved to prevent circulating poisons from entering the brain. This protective barrier has helped the human species survive. Fortunately, testosterone successfully crosses the barrier due to its ability to dissolve in fats, delivering signals that keep us sexually active and healthy. Of all the hormones circulating in our bodies, I believe testosterone has the most potential of helping each of us enjoy a more vibrant sex life and reap a whole set of other physical and emotional benefits in the process.

I will share my enthusiasm for this natural hormone with you throughout this book. All of my convictions are based on the considerable research of scientific studies published in reputable medical journals as well as my work as a physician. I will share stories from my patients, men and women who have found sexual fulfillment through adequate testosterone treatment.

Sex medicine is emerging as a new specialty. Physicians are beginning to become aware that the association between testosterone and other hormones can be tapped for treating difficulties in human sexuality. More doctors are taking advanced courses and studying new developments in this field to learn how to help people with sexual problems. Meanwhile, there are signs that the age of the medical manipulation of human sexuality in all its aspects has begun. Erection enhancers and drugs to stimulate sexual arousal are only the beginning. Melanocortins are a newly discovered group of sex hormones. It has recently been discovered that one of these hormones, melanocyte stimulating hormone, triggers sexual arousal in humans. In Chapter Ten we will discuss melanocyte stimulating hormone or alpha-MSH and the key role scientists now believe it plays in preparing us physically, emotionally, and mentally for the sex act.

My personal belief is that the role of testosterone as the key player in the behavior we call "love" will become more evident as research in sexual dysfunction progresses. Furthermore, I believe that sexual dysfunction may be the direct result of a hormone deficiency. To me it's not a big reach to believe that hormones are responsible for some of the emotional component of lovemaking. The process of bonding supplies the behavior humans need to be successful moms and dads for their children. The hormone oxytocin stimulates the mechanisms that help us adapt to our parental roles and assures bonding behavior. Apparently oxytocin unleashes a chemical that signals endorphins and dopamine receptors in the brain. These signals will be discussed in this book.

Hormones regulate every aspect of the sex act including readiness, initiation, erection, penetration, ejaculation and recovery. A problem in any of these areas can be traced to some imbalance or malfunction of the hormonal system. Several hormones and brain chemicals play an essential role in the interconnected feelings of sex, love and passion. Most of these biological compounds are closely interrelated. We have already mentioned oxytocin and testosterone.

Human beings have bonded to each other by falling in love since the beginning of time. Abundant evidence shows us that hormones are an essential component of most human reproductive functions, including feelings of love. Can hormones create love? The idea that "love hormones," can bring about the emotional sex-brain connection we call love may be somewhat of a stretch, but the role of hormones in sexual arousal, male erection and ejaculation has been proven with scientific tests. The first three chapters will show you how hormones work in both men and women.

A sexual problem should not automatically be assumed to be psychological in nature. With proper hormonal balance, sexual arousal, orgasms and passion can return your sex life to you. From my perspective, love and sex are complementary and essential for normal intimacy. Positive passion is essential for the enjoyment of life. Listening to your hormones will help you learn what you need to do to restore that passion for life!

This book is an attempt to make some of the physical aspects of enjoying the pleasures of sex a little clearer. Whether you're just curious or are struggling to achieve a higher level of satisfaction with your bodies and your sex life, why not learn everything you can to enjoy the sexual experience to the fullest?

In the final pages of this book I leave you with five valuable messages about our hormones. I hope these statements give you the core of what it takes to enjoy life to its fullest. At the same time, I trust you will realize that we haven't discovered all of the secrets of our hormones, how they work in our bodies and how to harness them for the healthiest results.

Consider this book as one doctor's invitation and instructive advice to help you improve your health and add years to your life. Use this book as a guide to understanding hormones and their effects on your lives. Use this book to educate yourself on how to "listen to your hormones."

# 1

# Your Hormones: Why You Can't Live Without Them

## Universal Power

Nothing in the universe exceeds the power of your hormones. From the instant you were conceived, your hormones have been driving your body and influencing your every thought. Without hormones you would never feel a longing for sex or a thousand other desires, and life, as we know it, could not exist.

Remember the surge that rammed through your body when you felt the first waves of love washing over you? You were electrified! Your heart beat faster, and you felt light-headed. A smothering set of new and bewildering emotions swept over you—just from touching the hand of someone you liked a lot. Hormonal impulses also spring forth at childbirth, instantly bonding the mother to her newborn baby. A burst of hormones emerges from the father to forge a permanent paternal relationship with the infant. Amazingly, the same hormone is responsible for this phenomenon in both sexes.

Hormones don't listen to our inhibitions but drive us to do things we never imagined ourselves doing. A passing glance or a faint scent arouses your hormones, triggering feelings that lead to a deep hunger for love. The sight of your child sliding off the bank into a raging river turns your muscles into steel as adrenaline empowers you to perform superhuman feats. You're drowsy at work because of too much melatonin—or you're up at midnight raiding the refrigerator because you don't have enough of this hormone.

What are these mysterious forces that rumble through your body and upset your naturally calm and logical way of viewing the world around you? If hormones can lead people to bizarre or criminal behavior, shouldn't we focus on eliminating their impact on human beings? Would life be easier without hormones? The simple fact is that you couldn't live without them. Hormones affect the way every cell and system in your body func-

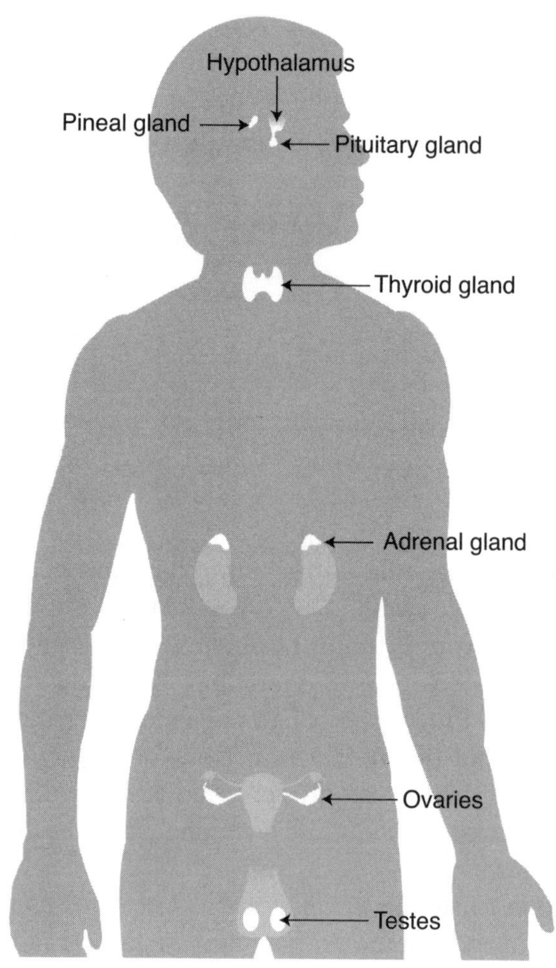


ENDOCRINE SYSTEM (male/female)

tions. They control your brain's ability to regulate everything you say, think, and do. They direct every bodily function, as well as your behavior.

Hormones are tiny molecules manufactured within your body according to strict codes set by your genes. Your body hosts eight miniature hormone-producing factories or "glands" located in strategic positions—the pituitary gland and the pineal gland in the brain, the thyroid gland in the throat, the thymus in the upper chest area, the adrenal gland and the pancreas near the kidneys, and the ovaries in the female and testes in the male. Some of these glands do double duty. For example, the pancreas, best known for the insulin hormone, also releases chemicals that help us digest our food. Vital organs—brain, lungs, heart, kidney, liver, skin and the digestive tract—also produce hormones, although that is not their primary function.

In amounts as tiny as a thousandth, a millionth, or a trillionth of a gram, hormones travel at lightning speed in your blood to reach targeted cells. After an immediate match, the hormones direct your body's organs to do their job.

Taken together, hormone-producing organs are known as the "endocrine system," and doctors who specialize in how hormones function and how to treat people with hormone problems are called endocrinologists.

Hormones enter your bloodstream directly from the secreting cells in the endocrine glands where they originate. For example, hormones from the pituitary gland in the brain bind to their receptors in the thyroid gland, triggering the immediate release of its hormones so they can reach every recess of the body in a heartbeat. If the pituitary senses that there is already too much thyroid hormone in the system, it cuts back its stimulation in a process of negative feedback.

Hormones operate an intricate command center more complex than the systems that control robots on Mars. Our hormones turn our genes off and on. They work like a power switch, signaling our genes to start up the processes that make specific proteins in the miniature protein factories inside our body's cells. Our hormones immediately circulate throughout our body, performing a fantastic set of signaling and triggering routines.

The pituitary and pineal glands plus the hypothalamus serve as the master control system deep within the brain. These glands govern the formation and release of many hormones. A short list would have to include melatonin, testosterone, estrogen, progesterone and dehydroepiandrosterone (DHEA). Others in this category trigger substances known as releasing

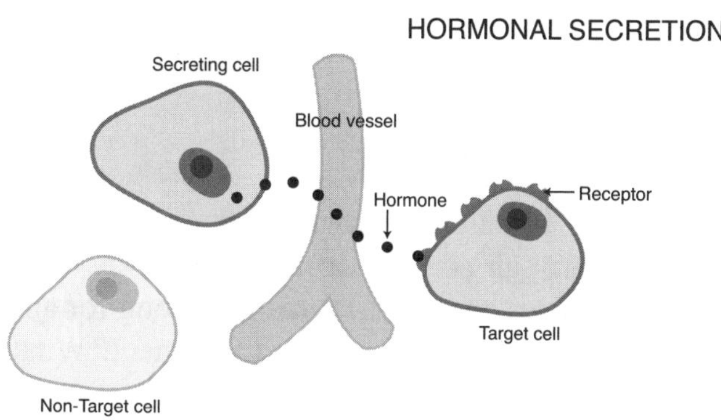

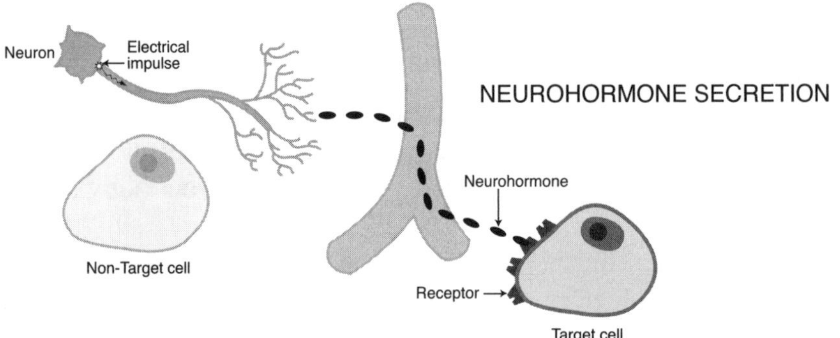


factors or neurohormones. This interesting class of hormones is produced in your brain's control center and serves as signaling, transmitting, and switching devices. While most other hormones originate in your endocrine glands and circulate in the blood to reach target cells, neurohormones come from specific brain cells we call neurons. They can travel to their destination in the blood, in the fluid of the brain and spinal column, or they may diffuse into the spaces between cells of the nervous system. Some neurohormones travel along nerves directly to the pituitary gland where they are stored and then released. Neurohormones are also called neurosteroids.

Whether you realize it or not, neurohormones affect the way your brain controls every system in your body, from moment to moment both day and night. They are not only responsible for the amazing changes that occur in your body as you grow from child to adult, but they also control hunger and thirst, breathing and blood pressure, perspiration and sleepiness together with thrills and chills. Neurohormones allow you to maintain a sense of well-being and determine most of your behavior from day to day. All of your body's hormones must function in perfect harmony in order for you to enjoy good health and normal sexual function, but the delicate balance of neurotransmitters and hormones can become disrupted for many reasons.

## Human Rhythms and Sex

Hormonal rhythms and genetics control our sexual behavior leading to the creation of new life through conception and pregnancy. As we grow into physical maturity, impulses and instincts make us long for an intimate relationship, guiding us on the path of sexual fulfillment. What drives these behaviors?

It all begins with our genetic code. Every living organism owns a unique set of genes made of DNA, the coded information or blueprint for life. Human chromosomes are coiled units of DNA with twenty-two identical pairs plus one set of sex chromosomes per person. They are located within the nucleus or center of the cell and determine the formation of every organ, tissue, and cell in your body.

Before you were born your body carried one X chromosome from your mother as well as an additional chromosome that could be either an X or a Y from your father. If the second chromosome happened to be a Y, you would be born as a male. An XX chromosome pair meant you would be a female. Early life forms did not contain any sex chromosomes because these organisms had no need for sexual reproduction. As animals evolved, the two X chromosomes mutated until eventually one of them developed in a way that caused the male and female sexes to emerge.

The Y chromosome therefore seems to be the result of a 300-million-year experiment. Some of the X chromosome's genes were deleted and new functions were added as the Y chromosome became more and more specialized in the developing mammals. The Y chromosome shrank and added the testes gene to produce and store sperm, and at that point males were created. The X chromosome has about two thousand genes, while the Y chromosome has only twenty-six. Evolution makes it clear that females evolved first and that males came from them—not the other way around.

Your sex chromosomes do far more than merely determine whether you will be male or female. The way you look, the color of your eyes and hair, and various physical and psychological features of each parent are passed on to you by your chromosomes. The level and functionality of your sex hormones and possibly your sexual preference are all under the domain of these powerful DNA molecules.

Hormones act as the on-off switch for genes, setting different production levels for the manufacturing of proteins. Some are secreted at a steady rate and others in spurts that repeat every few minutes or every twenty-four hours. Hormones that produce the menstrual cycle rise and fall during the month.

Nature's cycles are commonplace. Winter turns into spring, spring to summer; night becomes day. These changes in nature are known as biocycles, and our brains—and hormones—are set to follow them. The timing of life, known as chronobiosis, is present in every animal, insect and plant.

Flies also have a sleep-awake cycle, which is why you can sneak up on them while they're sitting on the ceiling or wall. They're sound asleep.

Circadian rhythms are twenty-four hour hormonal cycles based on light-dark sequences that are deeply embedded in our system. Chronobiology, a whole new way of studying and treating the body, has sprung from the science of the timing of life's cycles. Scientists specializing in this field have developed new time-specific drugs known as chronobiotics to restore hormone balance that has been disrupted.

You don't have to travel into space or descend deep into a mine for something to upset your ingrained cycle of day and night. In any situation where light and darkness do not vary on a predicable twenty-four hour basis, you will experience a disruption of your ingrained sense of the natural cycle of light in as little as three weeks.

Some night-shift workers complain of daytime fatigue because they have forced themselves to stay awake at night when their bodies want to sleep. Nurses on night shift, firemen, security guards, doctors, and police officers often work during the night and are able to adjust their circadian rhythms according to their schedules. Others are natural "night owls" and do not feel alert until midnight because their bodies have somehow developed biocycles for a reverse dark-light sequence. If they have a day job, people with this condition drag themselves through the day and lie awake at night. This results in too little sleep, which robs them of the energy to deal well with the next day's activities. The opposite effect occurs when people with a normal circadian rhythm must stay awake at night.

In animals, hormonal cycles determine the way seasonal changes trigger mating or territorial aggression. Mating hormones are released at peak levels, or, as we say, when the animals are "in heat" and ready to mate. Healthy humans, on the other hand, can mate any time they choose, without regard to nature's seasons or the time of day.

## Irritable Male Syndrome

"Irritable male syndrome" is a common condition that occurs in men when their male hormone level drops. This term is taken from the better known premenstrual syndrome that makes women irritable. Men afflicted with irritable male syndrome become grumpy, depressed, and lose self-esteem. Sexual desire declines. Interest in work and career diminishes. Living hardly seems worthwhile.

This problem involves a deficiency of the naturally occurring male sex hormones called androgens. By far the most important androgen is testosterone. Testosterone is a molecule that originates in both male and female sexual organs but circulates at different levels in men and women.

To learn more about testosterone in the lives of ordinary people, let's eavesdrop. Janelle, Russell's wife of several decades, is saying to him, "Russ, you aren't the same any more. After you come home at night all you want to do is sit in front of the TV. You used to like going places and doing things. I'm making an appointment for you to see Dr. Winter."

"Yes, dear," Russell agrees. He doesn't have the energy to argue with his wife any more.

Like Janelle, women are often the first to notice these symptoms in their men as well as the loss of sexual arousal, weight gain around the waist, and loss of strength and agility. Men tend to ignore these symptoms, chalking them up to old age.

Having scheduled an appointment, Janelle and Russell are sitting in Doctor Winter's office. "Russell just isn't the man he used to be," sighs his wife. "He mopes around the house and doesn't seem interested in meeting his sales quota at work. He used to be the top performer in his division. Now he's just hanging on." She looks around the room. "The worst of it," she says, her voice dropping to a whisper, "is that he doesn't seem to care for me any more. I mean he doesn't want to have sex." She sighs and fiddles with her purse. "I don't know what's gotten into him."

Russell listens patiently while Janelle describes his lack of get-up-and-go. "Russ doesn't play golf on Sundays any more, and I don't know when the last time was when he went fishing with his buddies. He makes it to work and back but then just sits around. After he goes to bed he tosses and turns and then gets up and makes himself a sandwich. He's gaining weight." She glances at Russell, who nods his head slightly. It takes less effort to go along. Then he hears the words that make no sense at all to him.

The doctor is speaking. "You have a classic case of Irritable Male Syndrome." Dr. Winter leans back, waiting for the impact of his words to settle in.

"What?" Russell protests weakly. "I'm always trying to please my wife. There's nothing irritable about me. I do the best I can."

Dr. Winter and Janelle exchange glances. "I'm sure you do," Dr. Winter says, "but we'll have to do more tests. My hunch is that a small dosage of testosterone could help restore your vigor, and you'll thank Janelle for doing something about it."

The doctor writes a prescription for testosterone and explains how the HRT, hormone replacement therapy program will work for Russell, who doesn't like the idea but knows he'll end up going along with it.

"Why can't my body just regulate itself?" he grumbles. "Isn't hormone replacement unnatural?"

After listening to the doctor's explanation, Russell walks out of the office convinced that testosterone will probably be beneficial for him. He may mention this to his buddies and if he does, the chances are high that he'll hear some misguided information that may give him second thoughts about hormone therapy because of the risks. He may be tempted to stop the whole therapy routine before it starts.

Like Russell, many men have a hard time accepting that anything is wrong with them especially when they have a marked testosterone deficiency. This is because in some men a deficiency might produce only modest changes at the beginning.

A man may be lacking in testosterone or other sex hormones without knowing it. If you are under the age of forty-five, the loss of morning erections could be the first sign that you have a hormonal deficiency. Unfortunately most men don't get motivated to do anything about this warning sign until they have lost the ability to have any erections at all!

Men experiencing problems due to low testosterone levels are often astounded by the benefits of a carefully managed testosterone replacement program. "I can't believe how such a microscopic bit of a natural body compound could make such a huge difference in my life," my patient Sean told me. "But here I am, proof positive. I'm my good-natured, hard-working self again."

Sean shared his experience with low testosterone levels. "Doc, I'm not a saint," Sean said. "I was a big drunk and a drug abuser when I was younger. Now I occasionally eat chocolate, ice cream, pizza, popcorn, and other junk. Sometimes I find myself smoking a cigarette or chewing tobacco, but that's rare."

Sean went on to describe a vigorous exercise program that he now follows, including stretching, weight training, and indoor running an hour or more at a time six days a week. But Sean isn't totally thrilled with his body. He still doesn't feel healthy. He knows he needs to lose a few pounds. He also feels he's not as sharp as he used to be. "I keep forgetting where I left my keys, or I lose my glasses," he says.

Lab tests confirmed that Sean had a testosterone deficiency, so I placed him on a hormone replacement program. Both he and I were pleased to see an improvement in his sense of well-being after he had been on the program for only a few weeks. This is very important. Testosterone not only increases lean body mass and improves memory but it creates the sense of well-being. How can a hormone make us feel so good? Testosterone releases potent endorphins that regulate our perception of pain, creating a state of euphoria, or feeling "high." Natural highs are important for the enjoyment of normal life and the creation of pleasure. There is nothing wrong with feeling naturally high.

Hormones enable us to achieve and maintain this sense of comfort and emotional satisfaction. In other words, they allow us to feel happy. Most men are satisfied with their testosterone levels as long as they have enough to enjoy a normal sex life. They don't even think about hormones. Should they develop a large belly, start losing their hair, or become aware of memory loss, they might consult a doctor.

Is testosterone the only hormone that makes men feel good? Can testosterone really allow a man to "do it till he dies?" Well yes, but there are other aspects of hormones that are just as important, especially for men.

## The Raw Power of Light

Although sexual desire can strike at any time, love tends to be something of a seasonal phenomenon. Lord Alfred Tennyson wrote, "In the Spring a young man's fancy lightly turns to thoughts of love." Tennyson was poetically expressing the observation that love seems to increase with the arrival of spring. He was scientifically correct. As the days get longer in spring, the additional light rejuvenates hormones and sets a series of titillating events in motion.

The evolutionary process has coordinated our bodily functions with the sun's energy so that we are physically dependent on light to function normally. Without light, life on this planet could not exist. In addition, light has special effects on our sexual performance because the sex act involves a harmonious symphony of many hormones, some of which are regulated by visible light.

This may sound like an advertisement—"Get more daylight in your life, and you will have healthier hormone levels and live a longer life"—

but bright light does help you enjoy improved moods, get more restful sleep, control your weight and, if you are getting old, develop a better memory. You may have seen articles in home improvement magazines about light boxes, skylights, indoor gardens, and full-spectrum light fixtures to bring more daylight and springtime indoors. These devices can help you absorb more health-giving light into your body. It works like this.

Intense visible light ends up in the brain after high-intensity light waves hit the retina at the back of the eyes. Light also works directly on the entire body. The sun's rays shining on your skin create "the sunshine vitamin," Vitamin D. To generate enough Vitamin D for optimal health, you need at least twenty minutes of exposure to the sun each day. Since this is not possible for everyone, particularly people living in northern climates during the winter, Vitamin D is added to your milk and your calcium supplements. Low Vitamin D levels are observed from November to April in most European countries and North America.

Humans cannot absorb calcium without Vitamin D, and the vitamin is essential for normal bone and prostate formation as well as the functioning of the nervous system. Very low levels can cause osteoporosis. Rickets and vitamin D deficiency may also be involved in multiple sclerosis. The hormone testosterone helps to transform vitamin D so that it can be utilized in the body to protect against prostate cancer development. I am sure you get the idea that adequate light is important both in creating energy and modifying our hormones.

How does light work in the body? It's complicated, but here's a little background.

Light begins as solar energy. Visible light from the sun stimulates the release of melatonin from the pineal gland, buried in the deep recesses of the brain behind the hypothalamus and near the pituitary gland. (See diagram on page 22) The pineal gland releases melatonin, ultimately inducing the release of regulating factors from the pituitary gland, which then trigger other hormones. The rhythm of melatonin synthesis is under the control of our biologic clock, located in the hypothalamus. This clock is exquisitely sensitive to light exposure in everyone, including people who are totally blind. I discuss this in more detail in the next chapter.

The sun resets your biologic clock each morning, modifying the rhythms of rest and activity as well as other important hormonal functions. The biologic clock in your brain perfectly coordinates your hormonal fluctuations. Consequently, bright light is essential for us to awaken in the morning. Darkness promotes sleep, and light wakes us up.

Light delivers energy that makes a big difference in your health and your sleep. In the darkness of night, while melatonin levels are peaking, your body is creating energy for the next day. While exercising, your body burns up the energy known as calories, and at night, during sleep, it recharges your batteries. This is why a good night's sleep is critical for optimum daily functioning.

The creation of energy from light involves a complex biochemical process that depends on other hormones besides melatonin. To assure that this vital process works smoothly, you need restful sleep plus adequate calorie intake during the day. Once you see how this works, you will be able to maintain your weight without dieting and sleep more soundly every night. You will find more on this subject in Chapter Nine.

## Hormones Are Not Sexist

Men produce about ten times as much testosterone as women, but the hormone is used by both sexes.

In men testosterone directs the development of male characteristics such as body and facial hair, a deep voice, sexual behavior and desire, and mature sperm. Normal testosterone levels guarantee the full development of a man's genitals from puberty to early adult life. Testosterone is so important in male sexual organ size that men with very low testosterone levels may experience shrinking of the testicles and penis. Testosterone also promotes the building of muscles and speeds up the healing process after an injury.

Testosterone has a powerful effect on the brain. When testosterone falls below critical levels, men suffer loss of memory as well as sexual desire. Sluggishness, increased weight around the waist and loss of strength are all negative results of low testosterone levels. Erectile dysfunction results in difficulty keeping an erection and we will discuss this further in Chapter Two.

From birth until about age twenty-three, men enjoy heightened levels of testosterone, usually reaching a peak during puberty and declining throughout the rest of their life cycle. The amount of testosterone in your body is carefully regulated by an intricate system of checks and balances. The regulating hormone called luteinizing hormone (LH) senses if there is too much testosterone and stimulates the production of sex hormones until you have just the right balance.

In response to our biologic clock, levels of all of our hormones rise and fall depending on the time of day. For example, the highest testosterone levels in men under forty normally occur during the early waking hours from 6 to 8 a.m. By early morning a man's internal clock has signaled the body go make more testosterone until it has reached its maximum level. The coming of daylight causes melatonin to decline and testosterone levels to decrease during the day, building up again during the night.

As men age, the peaks and valleys of hormone levels during the day become less pronounced, and the level of total testosterone in the body declines. Unfortunately, few men bother to find out what their normal testosterone levels are before they have a problem. Even if a man knows how much testosterone is circulating in his body, "ideal" levels vary so widely from one man to another that accurate treatment to adjust these levels is difficult.

Recent studies have confirmed that testosterone helps to prevent Alzheimer's Disease. Based on a considerable amount of scientific data, we now believe that testosterone modifies brain structures in both men and women, particularly the hippocampus, the part of the brain that is responsible for memory.

Testosterone also regulates the fluid in our joints and keeps them operating smoothly. Youngsters with arthritis have abnormally low levels of testosterone in the fluid of their joints. Older people with aches and pains in joints and ligaments that improve with exercise may also be deficient in testosterone. Other troublesome although less common effects of low levels of testosterone include inability to concentrate, diminished interest in daily activities, sleep disturbances, irritability, and depressed moods. It is a big mistake to let your testosterone levels drop so low that you begin experiencing symptoms such as these. Listen to your body and don't ignore warning signs of a hormone dysfunction that can be easily corrected if diagnosed early.

We need to think of the three primary sex hormones—testosterone, estrogen, and progesterone—as the heritage of the entire human species rather than favoring one sex or the other. Testosterone, for example, intensifies the all-important sense of well-being for all humans. Men and women respond equally to testosterone supplements with increased muscular growth and increased sexual desire.

Although women make a lot less testosterone than men do, the hormone plays a vital role in a woman's "ability to be aroused...and in her appetite for being sexual," according to Dr. Rosemary Basson, with the Center for Sexuality, Gender Identity and Reproductive Health in British Columbia. Dr. Basson points out that the hormone plays key roles in women's bodies. These include promoting bone growth, increasing bone density, stimulating the production of red blood cells, promoting muscle development, and improving moods and sex drive.

A woman with high testosterone levels is the owner of a firm body with high energy. She can be sexually aggressive and very attractive. Testosterone nurtures sexual desire and heightens a woman's sensitivity to sexual stimulation. The result is a deeper sense of physical gratification during sexual intercourse.

Testosterone therapy can help heighten sexual desire in women as it does in men. Although there is a slight risk of masculinizing side effects such as acne, facial hair, and a lowered voice in women who take too much testosterone, it is rare.

Women produce about one tenth the amount of testosterone as men and derive half of their testosterone from their ovaries and half from their adrenal glands. Their testosterone levels peak between the age of twenty and thirty, diminish by about fifty percent after menopause, but never disappear completely. The first indication that a woman may have a low testosterone level is usually a lack of sexual desire or erotic dreams.

For women experiencing menopause, levels of the androgen hormones, especially testosterone, drop. One researcher, Dr. Lorraine Dennerstein, a physician with the University of California at San Francisco, concluded from her studies that the primary drivers for a woman's libido are these androgens. Low dosages of a testosterone supplement—less than one or two milligrams a day—seem to improve sexual health for testosterone-deficient women without bringing on any masculine traits. Menopausal women appear to benefit from testosterone with increased energy and an improved sense of well-being.

Unfortunately, aging plus the exposure to high concentrations of phony or environmental estrogens eventually drive women's testosterone down just as it does in men. As their testosterone levels drop, previously youthful women begin aging more rapidly, often becoming overweight and more passive. Women with low testosterone develop heart disease sooner and lose their memory faster than women with normal levels.

Besides aging, other causes for the weakening of women's androgen levels include the use of birth control pills, the process of pregnancy and breast feeding, or the use of a popular class of antidepressants called serotonin re-uptake inhibitors or SRIs. Prozac®, Paxil®, Zoloft®, and Celexa® are four common SRIs that have been shown to cause a decreased libido in both sexes, as well as an inability to reach orgasm. As you may know, a delayed orgasm is not always a negative for women, but men are more likely to experience great frustration when orgasm fails to occur at the optimal moment.

While many of the same hormones function on an equal opportunity basis in both men and women, the truth is that when it comes to sex a woman doesn't think like a man. She doesn't see men the same way that men see women. A man sees woman as the perpetrator of the human race and is more interested in a woman's looks and other physical attributes than in the woman's thinking process or deep-seated emotions. This is why most men are able to enjoy sex with any woman if they are physically stimulated by the energy of their hormones. A woman, on the other hand, needs more than hormones to enjoy sex. She must be very interested in the man and feel her partner cares for her on an emotional level and not just for her body.

Because of our circadian rhythms (see page 10), for many people, sexual interest peaks in the morning because that is when hormones are at their height. For practical reasons, this is not always an ideal time to enjoy making love. The day is just beginning and the kids have to get off to school. We have to go to work or be on time for an appointment, and so on. Late evening is more convenient for sexual activity during an ideal niche in the daily schedule. It's quiet. The bed is soft and inviting. The kids are in bed. And it's dark. Time to snuggle and enjoy a repast of blissful sex.

"Honey," John says as he pulls off his socks and climbs between the sheets. "That was a lovely meal, but I'm stuffed."

"You're right," Martha murmurs, turning towards her man. "It was delicious. I loved the lemon dessert."

"You know," John, continues, "I had a beast of a day at work. I'd like to just settle in for a long winter's sleep. How about you?"

"Sure," Martha says with a sigh, turning off the light switch.

Two nights later John has a renewed zest for sex. Comfortable and not satiated with a big meal, he lures Martha to his side and gives her a big hug. With his hand on her back he guides her toward the bed. She kisses him, but knowing what is coming, she playfully struggles to free herself from his embrace. "Not tonight, John," she whispers. "I have a headache. I really do."

Couples like this are not sensitive to their sexual rhythms and as a result may become deeply frustrated simply because they are not in tune with their hormones. When one or both partners don't feel in the mood for sex, cuddling or kissing can often create arousal or simply satisfy the partner.

Our brain is sometimes called our most important sex organ because that's where sexual arousal begins. Women need intense emotional involvement with a man to be sexually stimulated by him. Whether her desire for sex begins in her head or in her heart, the reality is that a woman needs sufficient testosterone in order to feel sexually drawn to her lover. When diminished hormone levels return to normal, most people feel good and function normally. Martha and John are just two of millions of couples who need to pay attention to their hormone levels and natural cycles. They will come out winners when they work out a pattern of sexual fulfillment that will satisfy both of them.

You may assume from this example, that the loss of sex drive is a symptom of aging, but this condition is not necessarily inevitable. Talk to your doctor about your symptoms and ask him if your condition can be treated appropriately. Never hesitate to follow your doctor's recommendation to use hormones to restore normal functions. Whatever your age, you should retain a desire for sexual activity. If you are a man you should be able to achieve and maintain an erection for your sexual pleasure throughout your life. You should be able to "Do it till you die!"

# 2

# Hormones and Your Sex Life

## The Hormone of Darkness

Deep within the recesses of your brain rests the tiny pineal gland, home of the remarkable hormone, melatonin, the primary hormone regulator of your body's daily cycles. The word "melatonin" comes from the Greek word, *melas*, for "black." Melatonin may be our most important hormone since it starts the process of hormone regulation. The fact that melatonin is switched on by darkness and inhibited by light means that it responds directly to our environment. The interplay between melatonin and darkness gives rise to the hormone's title as the "hormone of darkness."

The pineal gland has been called the body's "third eye" because it connects us with the world of natural light. The pineal gland of animals also contains magnetic neurons that are sensitive to the Earth's magnetic field. Roughly the shape and size of a pine nut, the pineal gland has been the subject of study and speculation through the ages, credited by some for being the body's magical link between the physical and spiritual worlds. A hormone gland that can help us tell the time of day and pinpoints an animal's location in relation to the North Pole sounds pretty amazing.

How does this work? Twenty-four hours a day, steady as a metronome, specific cells in the hypothalamus move back and forth like the ticking of a built-in clock. When night sets in, melatonin takes on its sleep-inducing function. Our body is programmed to respond to the darkness by increasing the amount of melatonin. Melatonin reaches its peak between midnight and 2 a.m. when our brain has ten times as much melatonin as it does during the daytime.

How does melatonin compel us to fall asleep after midnight?

It's complicated, but I will try to explain. Two opposing systems help induce sleep—a wake-promoting center and a sleep-promoting center. Melatonin activates the sleep-promoting center. While you are asleep, your brain is at rest, dreaming and storing up energy for another day of activity. A chemical called histamine activates the wake-promoting center. In the early morning, daylight enters the eyes, even if they are closed, striking the retina and ending up deep within the brain where the timing mechanism kicks in to restore histamine levels to their daytime concentration.

In the routine day-to-night circadian rhythm, bursts of melatonin are released into our blood stream every thirty minutes. This rhythmic pattern is so strong that our brain keeps on following the twenty-four-hour cycle even if one cannot perceive light. So this capacity is retained even for blind people. Too much or too little melatonin can disrupt our body's natural response to these daily cycles of light and dark. Maybe you know someone who loves to munch at night or has problems going into a deep sleep. Inadequate levels of melatonin cause such problems. In that same manner, too little histamine in the morning creates fogginess and tiredness. This fact becomes very important when we discuss daytime sleepiness.

Since melatonin or histamine can change your circadian rhythms and affect your biologic clock, it should not surprise you to learn that these compounds can also help restore your hormonal balance if it goes out of kilter.

What happens if we damage this inner clock? Without a functional biological clock, you could not tell the difference between day and night. Disruptions in our circadian rhythms can disturb our entire life cycles. Melatonin is essential for normal sleep and wake cycles, particularly in the elderly. Yet as little as one milligram, a thousandth of a gram, of melatonin will induce natural sleep. Too much melatonin, on the other hand, can also make people fatigued, confused, depressed and psychotic.

Daytime sleepiness creates numerous problems: difficulty driving, poor concentration, memory loss and chronic fatigue. Multiple hormones, especially melatonin, are tuned so closely to normal patterns of light and darkness that any disruption of these cycles upsets their balance in the body.

We need balanced hormones plus abundant light for our minds to function normally. A lack of adequate lighting can throw our brains into a tizzy. Too much melatonin can aggravate depression. Too little histamine creates daytime fatigue. Any disruption of the natural circadian rhythm of our brains and bodies creates imbalance in our hormonal function.

Exposure to high-intensity natural daylight holds the potential to restore hormonal balance and banish depression from our lives. Adding high intensity, full-spectrum lighting in every room of our homes and workplaces promotes restful sleep and helps to eliminate daytime sleepiness. The benefits are unmistakable.

## How Do Hormone Deficiencies Cause Symptoms?

Melatonin generally follows a cycle with low melatonin during the day, skyrocketing to ten times the daily level at midnight. High melatonin levels in the early morning resulting from reversed daily circadian rhythms lead to a testosterone deficiency and sleepiness during the day. Testosterone supplementation can restore the negative effect of melatonin on the biologic rhythm in adults, and normal sleep patterns can usually be restored within three weeks.

Melatonin carries light signals traveling from the pineal gland by a pathway of neurons to the part of the hypothalamus we call the suprachiasmatic nucleus or SCN. Although the action of melatonin in the human body is not yet fully understood, we know that melatonin levels decrease with aging in much the same way as other hormones such as testosterone, oxytocin, vasopressin and growth hormone. Vasopressin, another light-sensitive hormone that keeps us from urinating during the night or during sexual arousal, originates in the suprachiasmatic nucleus.

Adolescence is the time of the greatest turmoil of all the hormones. Sleep cycles are altered because teenagers like to stay up late and then

HYPOTHALAMUS / PITUITARY

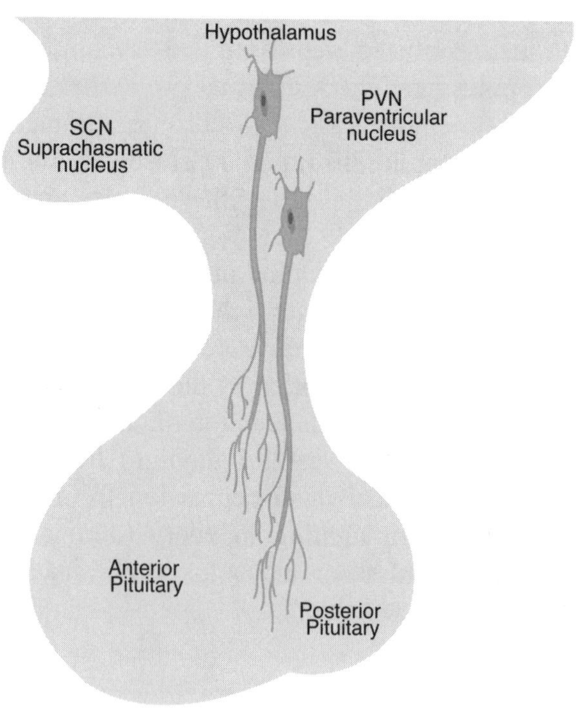

sleep in. Difficulty getting out of bed in the morning is a possible warning that depression might develop.

Circadian rhythm disturbances are common in various types of depression. If you've ever been depressed or been close to someone who was, you probably noticed changes in habits of eating and sleeping along with moods that swing to the lowest depths. Once something upsets the day-to-night cycle in a depressed person, he or she will have more difficulty functioning normally.

Low testosterone levels can cause higher blood levels of melatonin during the day and lower the levels at night, a reversal of the normal pattern—and a factor in many of the symptoms of depression. Lower-than-normal nighttime melatonin promotes wakefulness, stimulates the appetite, and disrupts the antidiuretic effects of vasopressin causing frequent urination.

Abnormal sleep patterns are a major symptom in depression, leading to increased weakness, a decrease of sexual drive as well as an abnormal appetite and daytime sleepiness. The deficiency of melatonin associated with aging correspondingly results in a reversal of sleep patterns. In spite of the fact that roughly fifty percent of the elderly have trouble sleeping, melatonin levels are rarely measured or supplemented.

Pilots and flight attendants who cross multiple time zones can also become subject to a shortage of certain brain hormones over time. Sometimes these frequent travelers, called "jet lag junkies," start to feel better at night and on overnight flights. Sometimes they stay awake the entire night and feel charged and energized the next day. As their sleep needs decrease, they become more and more tired, with mood shifts at highly inappropriate times. Deep within their brain, the flow of histamine and certain hormones has slowed or stopped.

One study indicates that jet lag from constant travel between time zones can disrupt the melatonin levels creating abnormal sleep cycles leading to depression, internalized anger, confusion and psychosis. Low histamine in the brain causes daytime sleepiness, as discussed earlier. This problem is being corrected with a new drug called Provigil®, from Cephalon, which increase brain histamine levels.

The human body maintains a balance of hormones through a complex system of regulating factors and feedback loops running from the pituitary to the hypothalamus and modulated by the pineal gland above the eyes.

What happens when stress causes the balance to go off?

Stress activates the hypothalamic-pituitary-adrenal or HPA axis, resulting in more cortisol (the "stress hormone") circulating through the body. (See page 58) Stress also arouses the sympathetic nervous system to release quantities of adrenaline and prepare the body for "fight or flight." Appropriate response to stress is essential for proper performance of tasks and positive social interactions. Exposure of the developing brain to severe or prolonged stress may result in an imbalanced system.

Sometimes the body may respond to stress inappropriately in a way that impairs growth and development and may account for hormonal and psychiatric disorders. The development and severity of these conditions can be negatively affected by genetics, exposure to harmful environmental factors or the timing of stress-producing events.

The principal hormones that deal with stress normally self-regulate, repairing problems much like a complex of computers, programmers, and repairmen. Signals travel by way of the neurotransmitters norepinephrine, dopamine and epinephrine. This highly effective self-monitoring arrangement helps prevent disorder in the coordination of the body.

## The Love Hormone: Is It Real?

Anthropologists suggest that nature embeds a constant state of sexual arousal in all humans following puberty in order to assure regular reproduction of the species. The feeling of readiness for sex is merely a simple reaction to our neurotransmitters. We now understand that many human behaviors may be spontaneously related to interactions between our hormones.

As a human being, you are continually responding to stimulants in your environment. Your resulting actions are known as behavior, and you do not have total control over the mechanics of your response. A change in your immediate environment sets in motion a series of actions or feelings and can run the gamut from kissing and sexual intercourse to depressive thinking or binge eating. An example of spontaneous response to influences in the environment is the fact that mating behavior increases in the spring when the weather begins to warm. This is because in springtime, higher levels of testosterone are present, and this triggers feelings of love.

Is there such a thing as a love hormone? If there is, which one is it? There is no question that the interplay among certain neurochemicals can create feelings of love, triggering a variety of sexually related behaviors.

In animals these behaviors include grooming, mounting and receptive posturing. In humans, love between the sexes prompts a wide variety of courting behavior. Once we fall in love, hormones take over. Difficult as it may be to accept, emotions and sexual behavior are mostly due to the circulation of specific hormones and not, as most of us have assumed, a direct result of our own wishes and desires. In other words, when we fall in love, we end up under some form of involuntary hormonal direction. Which hormones are involved?

Oxytocin and vasopressin are two hormones that play critical roles in sexual arousal and in the establishment of an intimate loving connection—including fathering, mothering, and pair bonding. These hormones originate in the hypothalamus, which sits in the center of the brain. The ecstatic hormonal cascade we call "falling in love" involves inspiring these hormones and others in a complicated process.

Oxytocin! The name sounds like a prescription medicine. What does it have to do with love?

Oxytocin is a neurohormone that is heavily involved in the sexual experience. A burst of oxytocin is released at the exact moment of ejaculation. Men and women also experience oxytocin-induced contractions at the moment of ejaculation. Women with high oxytocin levels seem to experience multiple orgasms and report greater orgasmic intensity than women with normal levels of this hormone. Oxytocin is obviously a hormone used by the body for lovemaking. A synthetic form of oxytocin once prescribed to encourage breast-feeding has recently been found to increase sexual desire and vaginal lubrication. At the moment of orgasm, ecstasy-like chemicals including endorphins make us feel "warm and cuddly." In other words, being in love really makes you feel "high."

Neurotransmitters such as epinephrine and norepinephrine regulate your moods, your appetite, your sleeping, dreaming, impulses, energy levels and perception of pain. Much like the feeling when you narrowly miss a crash on the highway or become angry enough to fight or run, the same feelings can terrify or motivate you. These responses of your sympathetic nervous system are considered involuntary, meaning you have no conscious control over them.

Of course you control many physical acts. Your muscles, for example, move your feet and hands because you will for them to move. We say that these muscles are under your voluntary control. By contrast, your body controls many functions without your conscious intervention. We classify these as the Autonomic Nervous System (ANS), which is also known as the visceral or automatic system. You might think of the ANS as a miniature universe within our bodies with its own brain and systems that run body functions without our being aware of their presence.

All of this is to set a background for the role of the sympathetic and parasympathetic systems, which are responsible for most of the physical and emotional activities we call "making love." The two systems together become the ANS. They oppose each other in some ways and support each other in other ways.

The sympathetic system, as mentioned earlier, comes into action when we are fearful or angry. Our pupils dilate, our heart beats faster, and our digestive system pauses while the problem is resolved. Whenever we feel panic or fear, sudden outpourings of adrenaline (epinephrine), discharged from the adrenal gland stimulate sympathetic receptors in our nervous system.

The parasympathetic system, by contrast, takes over certain functions when we sense that we are not under attack. These include a slower heart rate, smaller pupils, and stimulation of our salivary and digestive glands as well as normal breathing, eliminating, and sleeping. The neurotransmitter norepinephrine (NE) regulates most parasympathetic activities.

A balance between sympathetic (exciting) and parasympathetic (calming) responses is necessary to achieve equilibrium and general feelings of harmony.

Sexual arousal in men is a parasympathetic event that can be instantly suppressed by sympathetic action. In the real world this means that men with an erect penis made ready for penetration by the natural effects of sexual arousal can be stopped by a sensation of panic or other intense emotion. Interestingly, men and women experience profound differences during sexual arousal. The unconscious, or sympathetic, adrenaline-driven brain dampens arousal in men but stimulates arousal in women.

Sexual arousal also produces increases in concentrations of other hormones such as prolactin, vasopressin, luteinizing hormone (LH) and testosterone. The role of oxytocin depends on the presence of adequate levels of sex-steroid hormones such as testosterone. The three sex hormones plus thyroid, oxytocin, prolactin and human growth hormone modify the release of testosterone into the bloodstream. The hormone prolactin can halt testosterone's action, and both growth hormone and oxytocin can increase its activity. This interaction of hormones allows the body to regulate itself.

Multiple hormones flood the brain after an orgasm as the body's way of inducing feelings of "satisfaction." Hormones promote feelings of bonding, mutual attractiveness and a highly refined sense of appreciation of the "smell" of the sexual partner.

Like other behaviors we have thought of as fully instinctive, sexual attraction depends on the interactions between hormones and specific neurochemicals called pheromones that affect the "olfactory brain" (sense of smell). Pheromones are chemical triggers of sexuality that are detected by smell. Increasing the presence of female pheromones can boost testosterone levels by up to 150 percent in men, while male pheromones also increase testosterone levels in women.

Our sense of smell is so keen that we can actually sense the immune system of other humans. Women tend to seek out pheromones characteristic of the immune systems of their fathers. Men, on the other hand, prefer pheromones that provide a complementary immune system to their own. These "attractions" as we experience them are totally unconscious and lead to feelings of "love."

Complex regulating factors and feedback loops going from the pituitary gland to the hypothalamus and modulated by the adrenal glands above the kidneys maintain a balance of hormones in the human body. Thus we have a hypothalamic-pituitary-adrenal axis (HPA) much like a love triangle of interrelationships. Each gland affects and interacts with its target gland within the triangle.

Next time you think about having sex, take a moment to appreciate the way your hormones make sex an enjoyable activity that helps perpetuate the human race. Besides delivering satisfactory sexual performance, hormones allow us to achieve and maintain the sense of well-being that goes with a life of contentment.

## Sparking Your Sex Life

Your hormones are the sparks that make your sex life work. Hormones in your brain stimulate your sex organs and ready them for action. Hormones coursing through your body drive the intense pleasure you feel before, during, and after sexual intercourse.

Hormones trigger the complex process of creating a firm erection as well as the life-long challenge of maintaining the erection for maximum stimulation during the sex act. "The physiology of erection is like driving a car," according to Arthur Burnett, M.D., associate professor of urology at

Johns Hopkins. "You can't just turn the key and expect to go anywhere. You also need to hit and hold the accelerator."

Let's take a closer look at what is going on in a man's body during sexual intercourse. Because a limp penis cannot penetrate the vagina, the penis must become engorged with blood to be firm and complete the sexual act. A firm penis is therefore a vital component of healthy sexual functioning. The process of stiffening the penis for penetration is called erection.

Five steps must take place in order for erection, ejaculation, and orgasm to take place.

## Step 1. Arousal

Before the man senses sexual desire in his body, an image, smell, sound or thought stimulates his brain, creating a state of sexual arousal. In the animal world the chemicals that trigger these feelings from scents are called pheromones. Some research indicates that men as well as women are stimulated by pheromones, and merchants of perfumes and fragrances promise more and better pheromones in a wide array of "love scents" and other products, most of them of dubious value in seducing a man but are avidly purchased by women.

Whatever the source of stimulation, our brain immediately senses when we are ready for sexual activity. At that instant the hypothalamus triggers the release of melanocyte stimulating hormone, which discharges oxytocin and vasopressin. This hormone cascade sets off dopamine, triggering the male hormones, testosterone, and dihydrotestosterone (DHT). We will discuss melanocyte stimulating hormone, a multifunctional hormone, in greater detail in Chapter Ten.

Give your dopamine system credit for orchestrating the hormones your body needs to achieve erection or lubrication. Dopamine (also called the prolactin inhibiting factor or PIF) is a neurotransmitter, which means that it is able to bridge the gap ("synapse") between nerve cells and send signals from one neuron to another. The nerve cell receiving the message is called the receptor neuron, and dopamine sends its messages to special dopamine receptors in the hypothalamus deep inside the brain. These sig-

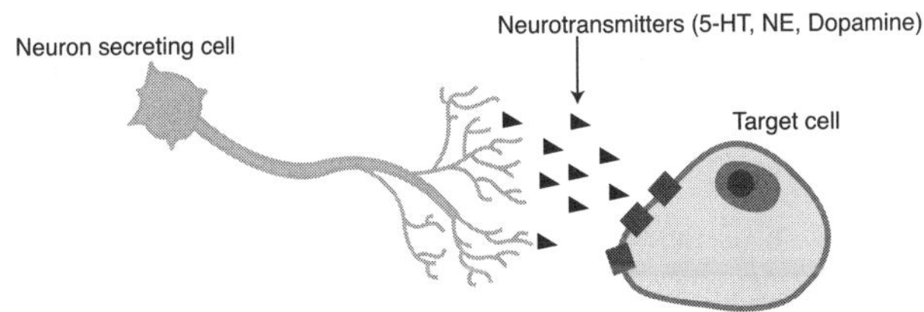


nals activate nerves in the penis that begin to change it from a flaccid to an erect state.

If the sex act is proceeding in an ideal manner, the woman's body responds to the stimulation in preparation for sexual intercourse. The same neurotransmitters that are working in the man in addition to adrenaline lubricate the vagina and swell the tissues to become receptive to penetration by the penis. Just as the "male" hormone testosterone stimulates the female, the "female" hormone estrogen is involved in setting up the male body for the sex act. Estrogen receptors in the brain must receive messages about the male's sexual thoughts in order for him to become fully aroused. Estrogen receptors are triggered by the conversion of testosterone in the brain to estradiol, the most active form of estrogen. Two other hormones, oxytocin and vasopressin, also play a role in delivering the message that the male or female is receptive to having sex.

## Step 2. Erection

Only when that special "horny" signal comes from the brain to the penis or clitoris will stimulation occur. Nerve endings in the penis and clitoris release nitric oxide gas that allows blood to flow into the organ. Testosterone regulates the amount of nitric oxide released. Nitric oxide changes the walls of the blood vessels, swelling the arteries so that blood can fill the spongy blood vessels in the two compartments running along the length of the penile shaft as well as the clitoris, which is really a miniature penis.

During the developing erection, the sex organs of both sexes become longer and thicker, usually doubling in length from the soft or non-aroused state. Approximately four tablespoons of blood are needed to create the erect penis, about eight times the normal blood volume of the penis. In the

MALE GENITALS

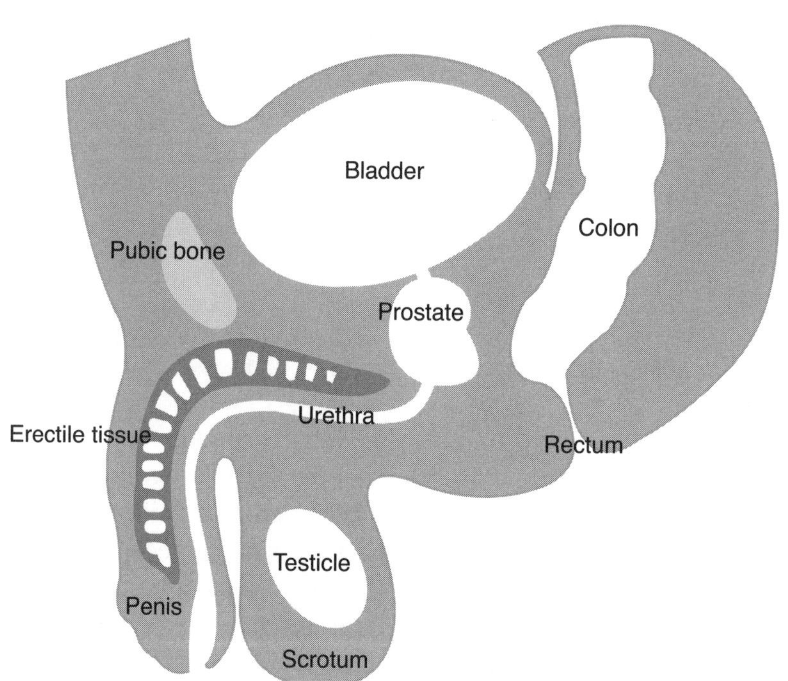


female the clitoris doubles its blood supply from one to two teaspoons. The neurotransmitter nitric oxide is intimately involved in this activity.

Viagra® (or sildenafil, by Pfizer), the first erection enhancer, was developed in recognition of nitric oxide's critical role in causing an erection. The chemical effect of sildenafil on erection was discovered by accident to increase the amount of nitric oxide in the penis. Few complications have been reported from men using sildenafil, and in pills of twenty-five to one hundred milligrams taken as needed, it is an effective treatment in men suffering from erectile dysfunction from an unknown cause.

**Step 3. Preparing the penis for ejaculation.** Tiny veins are squeezed shut by the inflow of arterial blood, trapping the blood in the penis and keeping it hard until ejaculation occurs. A man cannot urinate while the penis is erect because special receptors close off the bladder at its base. This protective mechanism requires the presence of biologic chemicals such as norepinephrine, nitric oxide, and adrenaline as well as the antidiuretic hormone (ADH) vasopressin.

We have now reached a critical point in the erection process. If the man becomes anxious at any time during the sex act, a flood of adrenaline immediately neutralizes his erection. Feelings of anxiety about sexual performance can therefore prevent an erection from occurring. Male erections occur only when the man is relaxed. A paradox is the fact that adrenaline, triggered by simple nervousness or feelings of fear, will cancel a man's erection—but stimulates a woman's desire.

## Step 4. Ejaculation and Lubrication

Triggered by oxytocin release in the brain, ejaculation is associated with genital contractions in the male and uterine contractions in the female. During this step the prostate gland, man's second most important sexual gland after the penis, fills up with prostate fluid. This fluid is added to secretions from the testicles and certain glands. These fluids accumulate within the prostate to produce semen, which provides a nutritive liquid so that sperm can swim toward the egg. Semen is ninety percent of the ejaculate.

As the ejaculate containing the sperm squirts from the penis, the release of the hormone oxytocin causes rhythmic contractions of the prostate as well as the anal sphincter and the muscles controlling the bladder.

In women oxytocin causes intense uterine contractions, increased moisture and lubrication of the vaginal walls, creating a flushed feeling in the neck, breasts and vaginal lips.

## Step 5. Orgasm

Sexual climax starts in the groin with a buildup of increased sensitivity of the penis and clitoris, which suddenly reaches the brain releasing a gush of neurotransmitters triggered by oxytocin. The mechanism is very similar in both sexes.

Orgasm occurs in the brain as well as the genitals. When news of this reaches the brain, intense pleasure results from the discharge of endorphins, dopamine and norepinephrine. The neurotransmitters engulf the receptors for oxytocin and produce feelings of profound eroticism and euphoria. In women multiple orgasms are related to the effects of oxytocin on the hypothalamus and pituitary.

This chemical flood soothes the brain with a natural morphine-like calmness, creating an associated "high" feeling. After the climax, dopamine levels drop, and the hormone prolactin kicks in and makes it impossible for another erection to take place for anywhere from one to eight hours. In women the prolactin acts for only thirty minutes, so women can achieve orgasm repeatedly depending on the length and intensity of the stimulation.

These five steps describe the process, in sequence that is required for a man and a woman to enjoy physically satisfying sex. If a man starts the day with a firm erection, he is normal. “Morning wood,” as some call early morning erections, is a welcome sign of the penis’s normal response to testosterone. Levels of this hormone usually peak between 6 and 8 a.m. and produce an erection. Because this occurs about the time most men wake up and have to urinate, some men think that needing to pee causes the erection. Not so. Morning erections result from the gradual buildup of testosterone during the night.

Erections are not always necessary for ejaculation to occur. For example, a man may be able to masturbate to completion without a firm erection. This is an early sign of a possible testosterone deficiency that can lead to erectile dysfunction (ED). Men who experience this should have their testosterone levels checked. Early morning samples of blood or saliva can be used to check the free or circulating hormone levels to diagnosis erectile dysfunction.

An energetic and enjoyable sex life is a major ingredient of life satisfaction, but some men cannot enjoy this pleasure because they cannot achieve or maintain a full erection. Often hormone imbalance is the cause for this problem.

Ron began having problems with erections at age 58, so he made an appointment with his HMO urologist. He wanted to know if it was normal for a man under sixty to have problems enjoying sex.

“I tested repeatedly with a low testosterone level,” he told me. “The clinic took an MRI because they thought there might be a problem in my brain. After that I saw a nurse practitioner, who prescribed a series of testosterone injections. Six months later, my testosterone levels tested consistently below two hundred.” (Normal total testosterone levels for adult males range from 300 to 1,100 ng/dl or nanograms per deciliter.)

At this point Ron was prescribed testosterone skin patches. When he called back for follow up, Ron’s nurse practitioner had gone on to another location, so a doctor told him by telephone that he should think about taking Viagra and recommended a consultation with an endocrinologist that belonged to the same HMO.

"This doctor proceeded to take me back to square one with a lecture on how risky it would be to use replacement hormone therapy, since my levels were not yet zero. I couldn't take Viagra because ten years earlier I had an abnormal EKG though I had never been on heart medication or treated for any heart problem."

After they showed him erection-inducing alternatives such as penis injections, he left the clinic. "My wife and I are extremely confused," he reported. You can imagine Ron's frustration.

He wondered if his HMO had treated him fairly or if the treatment the doctor had recommended was unacceptable.

As you may already know from your own experience, two negative characteristics of health maintenance organizations are the lack of consistent follow-up and decisions based on cost rather than the benefit to the patient. Skilled medical practitioners know that continuity of care is essential in order to diagnose and treat men with erection difficulties properly.

Bouncing a patient from one care provider to another, contradicting previous recommendations without consulting with the doctor who made them and regulating medicine according to financial concerns are not aspects of the type of medical practice doctors are taught in medical school. Many of us are going through a rude awakening to find good medical practices abolished wholesale under the HMO umbrella.

Most of us learned in medical school the importance of treating hormone deficiencies as vigorously as any disease. That means a diagnosis must be made and the best medicine selected. Viagra is recommended too often as a temporary solution for men with erectile dysfunction as if restoring erectile function is all that is needed.

Most men don't know they are hormonally deficient until they get tested, and the majority don't want to discuss it. What do you think happens when your hormone levels start to drop and your hormonal balance goes awry? What does that feel like? Look around you. Mid-life crises are affecting over forty million people in the US.

In spite of what you may have heard, sexual dysfunction crisis is not a normal part of aging. A normal human being should be able to enjoy an active sex life over the entire span of his or her life. Men and women should be able to do it until they die.

So what stops them? Low testosterone levels may be a factor in more cases of a lost sex life than we used to think. Most men who have low testosterone, known clinically as hypogonadism, first notice an increase in their waist size (a potbelly) plus a lack of motivation to get things done. Couple that with low energy and the absence of happiness and you have the makings of a mid-life crisis.

Lack of motivation dampens enthusiasm for hobbies as well as business ventures and sexual pleasure. Many men think they are just getting old and that there is nothing that can be done to correct the problem of losing their erections.

They couldn't be more mistaken. Just because your doctor tells you that your testosterone levels are normal doesn't mean that you have to put up with hormone-induced sexual problems. A man can have good sexual function if tests still show low levels of testosterone. Only when the circulating testosterone falls below minimal levels will erections disappear.

Circulating testosterone, or free testosterone, is only about two to four percent of the total testosterone, but it is the form of testosterone you need to remember because it is the main indicator of sexual ability in men and women. The drop in free testosterone usually occurs sometime in mid-life or in the early fifties and can be explained by the general decline of certain hormones during the aging process.

When a man has problems with sexual functioning, his wife is far more likely to bring concerns about sexual dysfunction to the doctor than is the husband.

Dale, a patient from Montana, hates discussing his sexual drive, but after encouragement from his wife decided to write to me.

"My sexual drive seems normal," he wrote, "not that I know what normal is. I don't have problems getting erect, maintaining and so forth. I wake up at least once a day with 'morning wood.' I never really paid that much attention to it because I probably only have sex once a week due to my wife's low desire. She suggested I write to you. I usually masturbate two to four times a week. I have felt a decline in sexual desire since my peak, but isn't that normal at age forty-six?"

Dale masturbates more frequently than he has sex with his wife. He blames his wife's lack of sex drive for his declining sexual desire and accepts the idea that familiarity has resulted in boredom in the marriage. Imagine his surprise when he learned that his free testosterone was that of an eighty-year-old man. No wonder he was feeling old.

Declining sexual desire is probably more common in men in their fifties and sixties, but it should be investigated whenever it occurs. Lack of sexual interest and fatigue are common complaints in men suffering clinical depression, and these are likely to be blamed on the aging process. Some men report the loss of early morning erections as their first symptom of testosterone deficiency.

More subtle signs of premature loss of testosterone include difficulty in finding the right word in a conversation, getting lost when driving in familiar areas, and a total lack of business motivation or sexual initiative.

Steve, another patient with erectile dysfunction (ED) complained of unusual symptoms. This man was not yet forty when he began suffering from ED.

"Doc," he wrote, "perhaps you can steer me in the right direction about my erectile dysfunction. I'm thirty-eight and my sex drive gradually has been diminishing since the age of about thirty-two. Recently it has become much worse. I am unable to have satisfying sex most of the time. I don't have as many morning erections as I use to and if I do they are not strong. My testicles often ache after ejaculation. I have seen a doctor although not for ED. My cholesterol is high, my blood pressure is normal. I don't smoke or drink, I'm not overweight and I have a good relationship with my wife. I do get exhausted easily, however, and need rest to calm my nerves. I believe I have a sensitive or overactive nervous system."

These physical symptoms are unusual for a man in his thirties, but anyone who thinks they have a problem with their nervous system will probably be handed a prescription for Prozac or tranquilizers to treat their problem. Steve, like many men suspects he may need testosterone without knowing his testosterone levels. A testosterone deficiency is a common cause of erectile dysfunction, and using a mood-boosting drug like Prozac or Paxil and not admitting that the difficulty is with hormones only makes the problem worse.

Silence creates a difficult situation for both doctors and their patients. Doctors depend on patients to tell them what is wrong yet they seldom ask about their sexual performance. Men are not alone in keeping their sexual problems secret. Most women tell their hairdressers more than they tell their gynecologists. Women like to discuss sexual problems with other women but seldom with their husbands and rarely with a physician.

Young adults and teenagers, the highest risk group for sexually transmitted disease, hardly ever discuss sexual problems with their physicians. Teenagers prefer to discuss sex with their friends, but they usually end up bragging and exaggerating more than telling the truth.

Doctors know that men are especially reluctant to talk about their sexual problems and should take the initiative to discuss this subject with their patients.

## Erectile Dysfunction and What to Do About It

For most men ED (erectile dysfunction) refers to "inadequate" erections, meaning they are unable to achieve or maintain an erection sufficient for satisfactory sexual performance. Erectile function is dependent on the penis receiving its full dose of blood on a daily basis. If for some reason, erections do not develop during the night while the man is in REM or deep sleep, then eventually these tissues will scar and shrink, causing erectile dysfunction.

An inadequate production of nitric oxide does not allow the blood vessels in the penis to fill with blood, resulting in anything from an impaired erection to complete impotence. The penis needs to become filled with blood on a daily basis in order to prevent scarring and ED. The saying, "If you don't use it, you will lose it" is definitely true in this condition!

As I mentioned earlier, normal erections start with sexual drive (libido) and sexual thoughts in the brain. The stimulation of either the androgen or estrogen receptors triggers sexual arousal in men and women. A rapid rush of neurotransmitters, propelling blood into either the penis or vagina, instantly follows the mental stimulation.

At the instant of sexual arousal, men develop an erection, and women feel their clitoris grow both in length and diameter. Once the erection is firm, penetration and ejaculation are possible, sometimes within sixty seconds. The penis should stay firm for as long as arousal is present or until ejaculation occurs. During foreplay, the woman's vaginal muscles relax, the clitoris swells, and the vagina becomes engorged and lubricated. The period of excitation is slower for women, who reach orgasm fifteen to twenty minutes after foreplay while men usually ejaculate within a few minutes of penetration. Timing for sex can be mismatched if both partners expect to achieve orgasm at exactly the same time during sexual intercourse.

Erectile dysfunction (ED) is usually due to inadequate blood volume filling up the spongy penile tissues. A non-erect penis contains about eight cubic centimeters of blood compared to a fully erect penis engorged with sixty-two cubic centimeters of blood. That's eight times the normal volume of penile blood! Any process that decreases blood volume to the penis or does not keep the blood within the penis will obviously result in unsatisfactory erections. Men with ED caused by a hormone disorder should be treated appropriately—first with hormone replacement, followed by nitric oxide enhancers such as Viagra®, Cialis® (Lilly/ICOS), and Levitra® (Bayer) and then by dopamine stimulants such as the antidepressant bupropion (Wellbutrin® from Galaxo®).

Impotence, the most common sexual disorder, is the total inability to get an erection. The risk of this condition increases in men as they age, but three out of four men are too embarrassed to discuss their sexual concerns with their doctor. This is nonsense. The doctor isn't going to point a finger of blame at the patient. In the vast majority of cases—85 percent or more—the cause is a physical problem. Psychological weakness is highly unlikely to be the cause of this problem. Still, if there is an emotional component, getting professional advice is the quickest way to restore normal functioning.

The causes of ED range from the effects of certain drugs and depression to psychological impotence. The use of antidepressants can prevent normal sexual function because they suppress oxytocin activity. Discontinuing the medication can reverse this effect. For adult men, with every year of age, the risk of ED increases by 10 percent. ED is associated with changes in liver function, obesity, drug and alcohol abuse, zinc deficiency, many over-the-counter medications, diabetes, heart disease, lower urinary tract symptoms, heavy smoking, and depression.

When the cause of ED is unknown, Viagra, Levitra or Cialis are highly effective. They increase the response of the penis to sexual stimulation by enhancing the amount of nitric oxide in the organ. One big problem with Viagra is that it doesn't work unless there is already enough testosterone on board. No libido equals no sexual drive!

Libido is an instinctual, creative emotion, and the loss of libido is perhaps one of the first signs of a potential sexual problem. The common definition for libido is "the instinctual craving or drive behind all human activities." Sigmund Freud said that libido is the energy all animals have to fulfill the goals of their lives. Aside from the sayings of wise people, we almost always think of libido in sexual terms. "My libido (sex drive) is low," complains a middle-aged woman, meaning sex has lost its appeal.

You can find "libido enhancers" for sale on the web and elsewhere without a prescription. Many are Viagra-like products made in India or China. Regardless of their composition, without adequate available testosterone erection enhancers have absolutely no effect. Hormones play a definite role in creating libido. They regulate how energetic we feel tackling the challenges we face from day to day, including the attainment of a good sex life.

Lawrence Hakim, chief urologist at the Cleveland Clinic, points out in his book, *The Couple's Disease,* that about thirteen percent of the thirty million men affected with sexual dysfunction are treated, but less than five percent of those affected with a loss of libido actually seek help.

I think a major reason for the gap between what we need and what we seek is that we are so tuned into the cacophony of messages bombarding us at every turn that we don't take the time to sit quietly and listen to our bodies. The thirty-six hormones that operate our nervous system have something important to say to us about how we can help them work for our ultimate happiness.

We often lack harmony because our bodies have been subjected to a variety of punishments—some inflicted on ourselves by not enough exercise or lack of good nutrition; others are inherited from our grandparents of generations past, and still others merged into our systems from a tainted environment. It's time for us to sit up and take notice. Our hormones have something to say to us about joyfulness in living. It's time for us to listen to our hormones.

## Erections and Viagra®: Does it Work for Everybody?

Though we know a lot about sexual urges that are driven by our hormones, sexual problems are still far too common in our society. One out of three American men and women has some type of sexual dysfunction. Viagra-like erection enhancers are often promoted as the best solution for sexual dysfunction, but the plain fact is that these drugs cannot generate the human sex drive.

The world of male sexual performance changed forever in March of 1998 when the Food and Drug Administration (FDA) approved the prescription sale of Viagra by Pfizer Pharmaceuticals. The drug made history as the first medicine that would enable a man to achieve an erection and maintain it throughout the act of sexual intercourse. Viagra has freed millions of men in more than ninety countries from the disappointment of ED (erectile dysfunction). Worldwide, sales of the drug approach one billion dollars per year.

From the jokes and comments made about Viagra, you would think it's a magic pill that brings sexual fulfillment to all men. Viagra has become a household name associated with sexual arousal. Pop a Viagra in your mouth and enjoy blissful sex.

Pfizer makes no such claims about its popular drug, warning men who take it that a dose of Viagra will not enhance sexual desire. Without sexual stimulation, a man who has taken Viagra as prescribed will feel no effect whatsoever. Viagra is nothing more than an erection-enhancing drug that works in only seven out of ten men who try it. Because of high demand for the drug, Viagra is being prescribed to men with low libido before their testosterone levels are measured. In otherwise normal men who complain that they do not respond sexually the way they did in the past, hormone levels are seldom checked. Sadly, in today's society, the focus is usually on function and not feelings.

Viagra has another benefit besides making it possible for men with sexual dysfunction to experience an erection. The drug cuts recovery time following sexual intercourse by about half. A firm erection with a shortened recovery time—no wonder Viagra is so popular!

Some urologists prescribe Viagra to their patients before and after prostate surgery to ensure the return of normal erections. The effects of Viagra are so powerful that some men use it before every sexual encounter.

However, giving a man an erection enhancer is not the answer to restoring his virility. Men need sexual arousal in their brain for their penis to become erect regardless of their dose of Viagra. The right balance of sex hormones, the correct amount of testosterone and estrogen are essential for normal sexual function.

Most men associate erections with sex drive and see their prowess at attaining erections as a sign of their sexual power. Medically speaking, they are wrong. Researchers have found that men can achieve an erection chemically without any sexual drive or arousal whatsoever. Drugs that block actions of the sympathetic nervous system can be injected directly into the penis, permitting an erection to occur—if nitric oxide (NO) is present. This vital gas, produced within our blood vessel walls, causes relaxation, permitting an erection once sexual arousal has been achieved. Medications like Viagra can induce an erection in men with a less-than-normal sexual drive, but the effect is only a result of the release of nitric oxide in the blood vessels of the penis.

The use of Viagra has become so common that doctors often write a prescription for the drug at the patient's request without bothering to determine the cause of the man's erectile problem. For almost two thousand years, understanding the underlying mechanisms that make erections possible—and assure that our population will survive in the future—have eluded us. Only now are we conducting studies and reaching science-based conclusions that explain both the neurological and physiological characteristics of penile erection.

Not everything about Viagra is wonderful. Men who depend on Viagra regularly to maintain erections can become psychologically dependent and become impotent without it. Also, as we have noted, Viagra works only about seven out of ten times, and is merely an erection enhancer.

New drugs have appeared on the market to compete with Viagra, promising to deliver an erect penis faster with fewer side effects. Two of these new erection-enabling drugs are Cialis and Levitra.

Even women with female sexual arousal disorder are being given Viagra rather than testosterone. The use of Viagra for women is an off-label or alternative use, and if the hormones of these women were to be studied, I suspect it would be found that what these women really need is testosterone. Testosterone is, I believe, a far more effective stimulant of sex drive than Viagra.

Testosterone restores erectile response to stimulation of pelvic nerves in castrated animals. Testosterone is also essential for a full firm response in the erect penis, according to studies by André Guay, professor of Endocrinology at the Center for Sexual Function, the Lehey Clinic at Harvard.

Studies in Germany by Dr. Becker seem to indicate that during sexual excitement, levels of testosterone increase many times over in the penis itself and that men with ED had levels that were twenty-seven percent lower than in normal men. Dr. Guay's research in men with hypogonadism showed that raising testosterone had a positive effect on sexual function but as testosterone levels decreased so did the response to Viagra. For men, testosterone is vital in achieving an erection. A man with low testosterone may produce an erection with the assistance of Viagra, but without sexual arousal, nothing much will happen once the penis hardens. It takes testosterone to stimulate a man's sex drive to complete the sexual act.

Patients who tried Viagra and did not like the results are rare, but Todd is one man who took Viagra twice and decided it was not for him. "I would not take this medicine again," Todd said. "My reaction was a bad headache with sinus pressure and a warm sensation in my ears." He was disappointed with Viagra's effect on his erection. "With manual stimulation after taking Viagra I became erect," he said, "but without continual stimulation my erection immediately started to go down. I was not able to achieve orgasm through intercourse even though I remained hard, and when I finally reached orgasm with manual and oral stimulation it felt like nothing at all."

Although his testosterone levels seemed adequate, and he was able to masturbate successfully, Todd was unhappy because, he said, "I was unable to achieve orgasm performing vaginal intercourse. The erection from Viagra usually lasted for over an hour until I was exhausted and no longer interested in continuing because of lack of sensation, or because my partner had enough."

Todd would probably be much happier using testosterone therapy to help improve his erections, and the combination of testosterone and Viagra could give him an optimal sexual experience.

Unlike Todd, many men who are impotent find a whole new outlook on life with Viagra. Their sexual performance improves to such a degree that they are willing to put up with the relatively minor side effects. Viagra has brought sex out of the closet and all but replaced the use of injectable prostaglandins that were used in the past to give rise to a firm erection.

One reason for Viagra's popularity is the fact that, in general, Americans like taking pills a lot better than using creams, patches, or injections. The penile prostaglandin insert (Muse® by Vivus) was the least popular of all types of treatment designed to enhance the sexual experience, even though it worked 85 percent of the time. Another factor in the success of Pfizer's Viagra is the large number of men who are affected to some degree by sexual dysfunction and are willing to try a pill to solve their problem.

But there's something even better than Viagra.

## Testosterone, a Safe and Natural Aphrodisiac

If you want more love making in your sex and are looking for a way to add spice to your sex life, consider the benefits of testosterone. This naturally occurring hormone is like a wonder drug that can give you more energy and a sense of well being—and reduce your body fat while increasing your muscle mass—whether you are a man or a woman. Used in a hormone replacement therapy program (HRT) as prescribed by your doctor, testosterone is also good for your heart and may help prevent heart disease.

Unlike Viagra, testosterone can increase erections within twenty-four hours of administration without sexual stimulation. Testosterone is safe for men with heart disease; regardless of the medication they use and has a sixty-year track record of medical use to increase sexual desire or potency for both sexes. By contrast, Viagra is simply a treatment for erection difficulties in men.

The word "aphrodisiac" comes from the name, Aphrodite, the goddess of love and beauty in Greek mythology, and means "arousing or increasing sexual desire or potency." From jasmine to onions, from Yohimbine to Spanish Fly, sex-enhancing substances have been popular throughout the ages. Ancient documents tell us that aphrodisiacs are as old as civilization—and as varied as human nature. Aristotle mentioned Cantharides, a formula extracted from the powder of dried blister beetles and applied to the penis to irritate and stimulate it to action. The mandrake, a plant from the potato family, has been used as a sexual stimulant since Old Testament days. Some attempts at heightening sexual pleasure border on the bizarre such as the habit of a Chinese emperor who is said to have kept a herd of deer so he could drink their blood to increase his sexual prowess.

If you're like just about everybody else, you'd love to be able to enjoy sex more, but before you can have great sex, your sex hormones must be working in your brain. The essential hormone that makes it possible for you to experience powerful sexual desire is testosterone. It's your body's own natural aphrodisiac. The testosterone hormone stimulates sexual desire in either sex without irritation or dangerous side effects.

The ability of testosterone to improve sexual desire was first noted in the 1940s. As the years rolled by, more evidence accumulated about the multiple benefits of testosterone therapy. In 2001 Malcolm Carruthers, MD, a British physician, observed in his book, *The Testosterone Revolution*, that men with higher testosterone levels possess a superior degree of business motivation as well as a more robust sex drive than do professionals with less testosterone in their systems. Among his patients in London, Dr. Carruthers found that actors and prosecuting attorneys had the highest testosterone levels and the strongest sexual drive. The increased drive to succeed in business, stimulated by testosterone, seemed to ensure improved function in both the boardroom and the bedroom.

"Hmm," you may be thinking, "Dr. Kryger really believes in testosterone replacement therapy."

You would be absolutely right. Of all the hormones circulating in our bodies, I believe testosterone has the greatest potential for helping each of us enjoy a more vibrant sex life and reap a whole set of other physical and emotional benefits in the process. I will share my enthusiasm for this natural hormone with you throughout this book.

In my clinic I encourage my patients to have their hormone levels tested as part of their annual exam. That way, as soon as problems arise, I can determine if correcting their hormonal deficiencies could be part of the solution.

Is it possible to find out your own testosterone levels? Yes! Testosterone can be easily measured in saliva. Accurate determination of a subnormal testosterone may require more than one test. Saliva, a secretion of the salivary glands, contains only free or circulating testosterone and can therefore be used as a highly effective screening test. A low reading of free salivary testosterone indicates that a man or woman may be suffering from inadequate testosterone.

Knowing your total testosterone levels will not always predict your sexual function or give your doctor a complete hormone profile. Saliva tests measure only the small quantity of free testosterone—about one to four percent of the total testosterone—that circulates in the bloodstream. The rest is bound to proteins in the blood stream and is mostly used as a storage form of testosterone.

Restoring testosterone to levels that are normal or slightly above normal can be beneficial for men and women. An above-normal level gives a person an opportunity to feel what it is like to have the testosterone of a younger man or woman. Studies at Johns Hopkins Medical Center investigating the use of testosterone supplementation in men with normal hormone levels, have found no harm resulting from above-normal testosterone readings for a short period of time.

Low testosterone levels should always be interpreted in the context of symptoms and not by numbers alone. While some men can have totally normal sexual function with very low levels of total testosterone, others lose their erectile function when levels are in the normal range. The normal range for serum total testosterone varies by as much as 400 percent at different ages in a man's life.

An important mechanism in the interplay of sexual hormones is the conversion of free testosterone to DHT. (See diagram on page 122.) Dihydrotestosterone (DHT) is considered to be a powerful form of testosterone because it regulates sexual libido in both sexes and promotes sexual arousal as well as erectile function. DHT is also the hormone that actually causes adolescents to develop beard and body hair, a deeper voice and enlarged genitals—traits we call secondary sexual characteristics. This process is genetically controlled and is considered essential for normal sexual function in men or women.

Men probably have low DHT levels for one of two reasons: they don't produce enough of the enzyme that converts testosterone to DHT, or else some factor is blocking its activity. DHT gels are being developed to restore normal sexual functioning without serious side effects. Tests to measure DHT levels are still in the experimental stages as this book is being prepared for printing, and two slightly varied forms of DHT have been recently identified. Because the information about DHT is so new, doctors seldom consider DHT in their evaluation of sexual dysfunction.

The patient and the doctor may agree that there is sexual dysfunction caused or made worse by a hormonal deficiency, but the recovery to a normal sex life is not always an easy one. I am constantly amazed at what some patients go through to get help for an obvious testosterone deficiency.

Meribeth came to see me about her fifty-six-year-old husband, Jason, who had been receiving testosterone injections from their family doctor. When Jason was forty-seven he experienced complete erectile dysfunction (ED) and was found to have very low testosterone levels of 130 ng/dl. His doctor gave him monthly injections of testosterone, but they seemed to work no longer than ten days following the shots.

The couple moved several times, and every time Jason switched doctors, he received the same prescription for treatment. "We think that the amount he is currently getting is far less than originally prescribed because they have no effect at all, when used in conjunction with Viagra," Meribeth told me. "We feel this has been a waste of time and money." She went on to say that Jason's current physician wouldn't increase the dose. "He says it can cause prostate cancer," she said. "We went through another disruption in his treatment for over six months when he didn't receive any injections because the drug was unavailable."

After triple bypass surgery, Jason was placed on Lipitor®. He complained of pain in his muscles, and the dosage was cut in half. Now Jason's wife is getting desperate, wondering if Jason's problem with Lipitor is related to the lack of testosterone in his body. He has all the symptoms of low testosterone levels. Where can she go to find real help for her husband?

Meribeth is not alone in her futile search for a doctor who will deal knowledgeably with Jason's problems. Too many doctors are turning a deaf ear to the signals their patients' hormones are sending. Why? They, too, need to "listen" carefully to the evidence showing how beneficial a simple but adequate testosterone therapy program can be to men like Jason.

Until the start of the new century, the standard of care for testosterone replacement has been the use of injections of synthetic testosterone. The treatment has shown immediate and marked results. A single testosterone injection generates a temporary feeling of well-being, greater strength and the return of sexual arousal. Unfortunately, these benefits are short-lived. An injection delivers a high dose of testosterone at first and then subsides over several days, leading to side effects such as hair loss, liver damage, high cholesterol, unstable moods, and acne.

Enlargement of the prostate, accelerated progression of a hidden or undiagnosed prostate cancer, increased thickening of the blood due to an increase in red blood cells and a variety of liver changes can also occur with the injection of synthetic testosterone. Definite health problems in older men are associated with testosterone delivery by injection into the large muscles of the body. So, although testosterone injections represent one of the older and cheaper techniques for delivering the hormone, today the preferred delivery system for testosterone is timed-release, natural testosterone preparations applied directly to the skin as patches, creams and gels. These methods work well and involve fewer side effects than injections.

Columbia Laboratories recently received FDA approval for a new topical medication named Striant™ that delivers testosterone from "oral" patches shaped like tablets. When applied twice a day to the area of the gum under the upper lip, Striant releases testosterone for more than twelve hours.

When testosterone was originally synthesized, it was used to treat a common heart complaint called angina, a pressing pain in the central chest caused by low oxygen levels in the heart. In a recent study, men with angina reported less pain after taking a low dose of topical testosterone. ("Topical" simply means that it is applied directly to the skin.) It was a single blind, placebo study, in which the men did not know what they were taking but the doctors did.

The Latin word, "placebo," by the way, means "I shall please." The term, "the placebo effect," refers to the ability of neutral substances to create good feelings because the person taking them believes they are powerful. Scientists today estimate that the placebo effect produces over forty percent of the results observed with some drugs. In a clinical placebo controlled study, one group of people being tested receives a neutral substance or placebo while the others receive the substance being studied. The majority of the patients taking testosterone in this study experienced less pain and improved blood flow to the heart compared with the placebo group. In these clinical trials, the testosterone was applied directly to the skin and absorbed directly into the blood stream in a method called "transdermal delivery."

Topical testosterone is a relative newcomer to the field of hormone replacement therapy. It has been widely observed that men using the topical testosterone preparation reported an incredible feeling of well-being. Not surprisingly, new topical testosterone products have been approved for the U.S. market since the new millennium. This is not exactly breakthrough science, since in Europe transdermal hormone creams and gels have been used for decades.

Pharmacists who are able to prepare topical or transdermal products such as these are called "compounding pharmacists." They follow techniques for mixing natural hormones with chemicals that enhance their absorption through the skin, a new and effective form of hormone delivery. Compounding pharmacists across the country have been making these products prescribed by a doctor for many years, although the FDA (Food and Drug Administration) does not approve them for marketing to the public. Instead, the FDA allows compounding pharmacists to fill a prescription for any form of an FDA-approved product used for a doctor's own patients. Hormone preparations for transdermal use provide a relatively inexpensive solution to the problems reported with oral or injectable hormones.

Women with sexual dysfunction have also been treated successfully with testosterone in a cream form as an alternate strategy for treating loss of sexual pleasure. Psychiatrist Susan Raiko states in her book, *The Hormone of Desire,* that the addition of a pea-sized amount of topical testosterone cream applied to the mucous membrane of the genitals effectively saturates the local skin receptors with testosterone. For some women, applying the testosterone directly to the clitoris, the female equivalent of the male penis, enhanced sexual sensation and desire all the more.

Today treatments with topical testosterone gels have entered mainstream medicine. Finally, doctors recognize that inadequate hormone levels disrupt essential sexual outcomes such as vaginal lubrication in women, erectile function in men and sexual interest in both men and women. For a successful outcome, dosage requirements must be monitored, and a trained physician must supervise the course of treatment.

With the recent release of a testosterone gel, Testim® by Auxillium in 2003, options for safe treatment with low potency testosterone have expanded. No man or woman lacking an adequate supply of this vital hormone should be denied the benefits and the restoration of normal sexual vigor. More information on Testim® is provided in Chapter Eight.

## How Estrogen Affects Male Sexual Function

Estrogen is so closely linked in our minds to feminine qualities that we are not surprised to learn that a company making bicycling apparel for women calls their product line, Estrogen or that the "Estrogen Files" are a cyber sitcom led by a cast of women.

One of the most powerful hormones in the human body, estrogen produces an extensive array of effects in women. It stimulates the ovaries to produce mature eggs. It signals the endometrium, the lining of the uterus, to proliferate in preparation to receive a fertilized egg. Estrogen acts upon many other parts of the body as well, including the brain, breasts, kidneys, liver, blood vessels, and bones. Estrogen also regulates the proper functioning of other hormones.

Estrogen is not a single hormone but a trio of hormones, working together to perform a complex network of tasks. We have already spent some time discussing estradiol, the most biologically active of these three hormones (page 29). The other two are estrone and estriol. In a healthy young adult female, the typical mix of these hormones is ten to twenty percent estrone, ten to twenty percent estradiol, and sixty to eighty percent estriol. This ratio is not accidental. Mother Nature sorted through the possibilities over the millennia and came up with this optimal hormonal balance for women. All three estrogen types are called "conjugated estrogens."

Estrogen is essential for normal female sexuality, but it can become a dangerous compound if its levels get too high. The link between estradiol and breast cancer is well documented, although some medical researchers believe that *both* estradiol and estrone can lead to a higher risk of breast cancer, if very high levels are experienced over a long period of time. An excess of estradiol has also been shown to decrease the action of either testosterone or DHT in women and men. Estrogen has also been implicated in causing endometriosis and sex organ cancers in both sexes when tested in other mammals.

In women, an estrogen deficiency can result in the loss of sexual thoughts, vaginal dryness, memory loss and decreased fertility. To counter these bad effects, one out of five post-menopause women are taking some kind of an estrogen supplement as part of their post-menopause HRT. Close monitoring is essential if women are using an estrogen supplement alone without progesterone. As important as "the female hormone" is to women, estrogen also plays a vital role in the body chemistry of men. Men produce only small amounts of estrogen in their testicles, but enough to help men create a healthy libido, support sperm production, protect hair and skin, and strengthen their bones.

An amazing way the testosterone hormone works for us is by producing estrogen. Testosterone is, in fact, the primary source of estrogen in our body, coming to us by the interaction of enzymes and cells in our brain as well as via the testicles of men and the ovaries of women. An enzyme complex called aromatase is responsible for the conversion of testosterone to the form of estrogen known as estradiol. This essential role of aromatase is not always desired.

Athletes and others who take testosterone to beef up their physical prowess and don't want any of their testosterone diverted to a form of estrogen sometimes use anti-aromatase drugs that interfere with the formation of estradiol. This is not a good idea if men want to retain their sexual arousal function and not lose their hair.

Estradiol has good and bad effects. On the positive side, estradiol positively improves memory by stimulating nerve cell growth and survival in the brain. This reaction occurs in both sexes and was formerly believed to delay the onset of senility and memory losses such as we observe with Alzheimer's. Estrogen also keeps skin and hair soft and prevents balding in men. The negative effects of estradiol include activating cancer cells and worsening the effects of autoimmune diseases such as rheumatoid arthritis or rare diseases such as lupus erythematosis, scleroderma or Sjogren's Syndrome.

As we men grow older, our testosterone levels drop, but our estradiol levels tend to stay more or less constant. The resulting change in the ratio between testosterone and estradiol causes an apparent excess of the "active" estrogen. Eugene Shippen discusses the phenomenon called estrogen dominance in his book, *The Testosterone Syndrome.* He believes that estradiol is actually the "primary active estrogen in all women." Estradiol also acts as an anti-androgen, working in opposition to male hormones and interfering with the beneficial effects of testosterone. The relationship between testosterone and estrogen is universal in other animals as well as in humans. When testosterone goes up, estrogen usually goes down and the other way around.

Too much estrogen can be extremely harmful. Excess estrogen levels among men are so prevalent today that the estrogen levels of men at age fifty-four are higher than those of the average woman at age fifty-nine, according to current studies. This might help men keep their hair, but they are losing their prostates over it.

Where does all this estrogen come from? A variety of sources including normal aging, increased body fat, high pesticide residues, nutritional deficiencies, and the use of certain prescription medication can be blamed for an excess of estrogen. Too much alcohol intake may cause men to experience levels of estrogen that are too high for good health. High levels of estrogen in men can cause reduced levels of testosterone, fatigue, loss of muscle tone, increased body fat, loss of libido and sexual dysfunction along with an enlarged prostate.

Men who are listening to their hormones need to pay special attention to their body's estrogen levels. Because of the teeter-totter relationship between many hormones, low testosterone levels are associated with higher-than-normal estrogen levels. Any man with symptoms of low testosterone or undergoing testosterone replacement therapy should ask his doctor for ways to reduce these levels to a safe range if tests indicate the presence of excessive estrogen.

## Remembering the Mother of All Hormones

Progesterone is one of several female sex hormones known as progestins. Other female sex hormones include estrogen and testosterone. The most important progestin, progesterone is made from cholesterol and is produced in the ovaries, testicles, and in the adrenal gland. When the body breaks down progesterone, it becomes either testosterone or estrogen. The metabolic breakdown of progesterone also contributes to the production of many other hormones we will discuss throughout this book, including cortisol, aldosterone, estradiol, DHEA, and testosterone. This is why progesterone can be thought of as the "mother of all hormones."

Progesterone is the forgotten hormone because it is hardly ever considered in male hormone replacement therapy. Progesterone can be made from the conversion of cholesterol to pregnenolone in the adrenal gland, and it can also be produced in the brain. When cells in a woman's ovary produce progesterone during the monthly release of the egg cell, it prepares the lining of the uterus to absorb and protect the fertilized egg. This commonly known action takes place in the body whereas progesterone in the brain is able to mimic many of the actions of neurotransmitters that regulate sleep, moods, appetite and deep sleep breathing. Because of these capabilities, progesterone is actually considered a neurosteroid when it is produced in the brain.

To put this in proper perspective, I would like to review the role of progesterone in women. Pregnenolone produces many different hormones, and one of its production pathways leads to the formation of the hormone, progesterone ("pro," meaning "for," and "gesteron" meaning "gestation" or "pregnancy"). A woman needs a good supply of progesterone in order to be fertile. Often called the "pregnancy hormone," progesterone is known for its role in protecting the health of a pregnant woman. To carry out its helpful role, progesterone skyrockets during pregnancy to a thousand times normal levels.

Natural progesterone taken by mouth is rapidly absorbed by the body. By the time it reaches the liver, most of it is no longer active so few benefits are received. To deal with this problem, researchers developed synthetic progesterone products that are not absorbed as rapidly and thus assure the delivery of adequate progesterone.

One of the first things we learn about hormones when we study them is how intricately they are connected. Changes in the level of one hormone affect the levels of other hormones. In men, for example, a deficiency in either testosterone or progesterone can create a deficiency in other hormones and vice versa.

Males and females normally secrete one to five milligrams of progesterone daily. This level rises higher in women during the egg-releasing stage of the menstrual cycle about ten days to about one week before menstruation. This monthly cycle repeats itself if the egg is not fertilized or implanted into the uterus. Progesterone levels rise and then fall just before bleeding signals the start of a woman's menstrual cycle. This premenstrual time is called the progesterone withdrawal phase. For some women it is an extremely anxious, nervous time. Some women report symptoms of depression such as shedding tears and feeling low self-esteem.

Other problems during the premenstrual time of month range from mild to severe cramps and from a slight sense of sadness to wild emotional swings that can drive them to violence. The well-publicized pre-menstrual

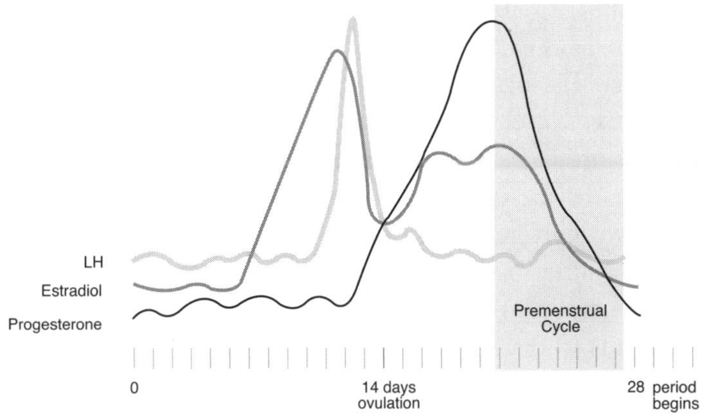


FEMALE HORMONE CYCLE

syndrome, or PMS, has been used as a defense for murder in the UK. Fortunately, not all women suffer PMS to such a degree. In its milder forms, PMS is more common in women with irregular menstrual cycles, little exercise, endometriosis and a family history of miscarriages. The premenstrual signs signal women that their period is coming.

Today there are about ten different brands of synthetic progesterone or progestins on the market but only one natural progsterone, Prometrium® (Solvay). Next to estrogen, progestins are the second most common hormone women use. You have probably heard of Provera®, a synthetic progesterone manufactured by Wyeth. Women complain of increased breast tenderness, bloating of the abdomen and extremities, and ever-changing moods when progestins such as Provera are used premenstrually. These symptoms are almost identical to those of patients with a deficiency of natural progesterone.

I do not recommend the use of synthetic progesterone because too much progesterone can be harmful. An excess of this hormone in the body can create unusual symptoms by competing with another hormone known as aldosterone, the salt-regulating hormone. Aldosterone comes from the adrenal gland and affects the functioning of the kidney. Too much progesterone or small amounts of synthetic progestins can prevent the kidneys from excreting salt, leading to fluid retention. When men or women crave salt, it is usually because their body levels of salt are low. An oversupply of progesterone could be the reason. Physical and emotional symptoms, including cravings for salt and sugar, may be triggered by excessive progesterone in both women and men.

Progesterone supplements can prevent premenstrual cravings for sweets in women who experience huge drops in progesterone levels before their period starts. Taking natural progesterone in small doses of ten to one hundred milligrams per day safely boosts low premenstrual levels. Recently, progesterone has been added to estrogen replacement therapy for its role in decreasing the cancer-causing effects of estradiol on the uterus.

Treatment with progesterone may help protect against both prostate and breast cancers. Another benefit to women with a uterus who take progesterone is that when the hormone is added to a woman's estrogen replacement treatment, it seems to cancel some of the negative effects of estrogen taken alone. Progesterone also affects our rate and depth of breathing.

Athletes from China at the Olympics have already turned to progesterone supplements to improve their breathing while running. The benefit came from the fact that progesterone reduces carbon dioxide levels in the blood and lungs. Next time you huff and puff when walking up a hill, consider the fact that a progesterone deficiency might be the cause of your shortness of breath.

The ability of progesterone to stimulate breathing has been known for years, leading to a theory that this hormone protects pregnant women and young women from disordered breathing and snoring during sleep, according to Dr. Meir Kryger, a national sleep expert.

Progesterone, in its role as a neurohormone, acts like a tranquilizer on the brain promoting sleep. You may have heard a person stop breathing temporarily while sleeping. About nine percent of adult women and twenty-four percent of adult men have this problem, called sleep apnea. A shortage of oxygen or excess of carbon dioxide causes this condition, which can be life threatening. Both estrogen and progesterone seem to protect from this type of sleep-disordered breathing. Progesterone treatment has also brought positive results to men who snore—much to the relief of their sleep partners. Another neurosteroid role of progesterone is in regulating body temperature. Cold hands and cold feet may be due in part to a progesterone deficiency. An added benefit is that natural progesterone helps protect arteries from thickening as a result of Type II diabetes and may help regulate cholesterol levels.

Like most hormones, progesterone levels drop with age. Some of the negative results of this "natural" decline could be overcome with appropriate use of progesterone supplements. Considering all of the beneficial factors, I believe that therapy with progesterone, the mother of all hormones, can prove an effective tool as a vaginal gel or capsule to help men and women maintain and restore their hormonal balance.

## Sexual Function and the Suckling Hormone

Pigs and some other animals can prolong intercourse for hours after ejaculation. What stops humans from ejaculating repeatedly? The answer is prolactin, another hormone from the pituitary gland. Prolactin is also responsible for the suckling reflex. When an infant suckles at its mother's breast, prolactin is secreted. This allows a woman to produce milk from her breast.

Nursing women have naturally increased levels of prolactin, ("pro," meaning "for the purpose of" and "lactic" for "milk"). The production of prolactin brings in the breast milk and works to prevent another pregnancy from occurring immediately. Prolactin also causes women to feel less sexual desire after giving birth. In addition, it is secreted as dopamine levels drop following ejaculation in order to bring about the refractory period to prevent another erection from occurring immediately. Prolactin inhibits sexual desire in both men and women, and breast-feeding can act as a type of birth control for the first year of a baby's life.

In women, abnormally high levels of prolactin have been associated with the ending of their menstrual periods, infertility, and decreased sexual activity. In men, prolactin has been considered detrimental to sexual function. When estrogen rises, so does prolactin, working to impair testosterone secretion and its triggering control mechanism, luteinizing hormone (LH). High prolactin can lead to a total loss of libido—with consequences that can be embarrassing.

Scientists have found that prolactin is essential for creating the refractory period after ejaculation. Without this mandatory period of sexual inactivity, men could not rest adequately after orgasm to recover in time for their next sexual experience. Erectile dysfunction has been described in men with abnormally high—and unusually low—levels of prolactin. This suggests that there is more to prolactin than the simple blocking of continuous erections.

Prolactin increases during stress when dopamine levels are lowest, leading researchers to conclude that stress or depression could be one reason for sexual dysfunction. At one time, too much prolactin from the presence of a prolactin-secreting brain tumor was thought to be a rare cause of male sexual dysfunction. Brain scans were often used to aid in the diagnosis. For many years if a man complained about his sexual drive, the idea was that there must be something wrong with his brain. Some doctors—and even some wives—still think this way today. More information about the interaction of prolactin and other hormones follows in Chapter Five.

# 3

# Submerged in Sadness

## The SAD Disease

By now you realize that humans and animals depend on light for health and normal development When the interrelationship between hormones and visible light is disrupted, problems surface. In Scandinavian countries low light levels cause the "winter blues" or Seasonal Affective Disorder (SAD). Seasonal disorders also occur in many parts of North America and northern Europe when the intensity of the sun decreases in wintertime.

People with SAD face depression every autumn or winter because it is a chronobiotic mood disorder such as those we discussed in Chapter One. Seasonal Affective Disorder results from a pineal gland that is not functioning properly. For victims of SAD, the darkness of winter brings more sleepiness, adds pounds, and heightens cravings for carbohydrates.

The farther you live from the equator, the more likely you are to suffer from SAD. People living in Scandinavia and in the northern latitudes of the US and Canada have the highest rates of this disorder. High solar light areas around the equator where you can travel to escape SAD include such vacation spots as the tropics of Africa, the Caribbean, Mexico, Israel, Australia, the South Pacific and others. In these locations you can enjoy adequate natural light year round, which protects your brain from SAD. These are great places to visit during the winter to help keep hormones in balance, especially if you suffer from SAD.

A long trip to a sun-drenched vacation site is not the only way to correct SAD. A new drug has recently been approved for treating jet lag and shift workers: Provigil® (or modafinil, by Cephalon), which stimulates brain histamine. This and other drugs show promise in helping people cope with long dark nights that can lead to symptoms of SAD.

## The Absence of Happiness

Steve holds down an executive position at a major financial services company. His career is secure, his family intact, his wife accommodating, his home comfortable, but Steve seems incapable of enjoying his good fortune.

At the office he goes through the motions and covers the details. At the end of the day he goes home feeling tired and sad. He doesn't eat much, goes to bed early, and says almost nothing to his wife and five-year-old daughter. Is Steve just sad, or is he depressed?

Steve is showing symptoms of "anhedonia," the medical term for the "absence of happiness" an identifying characteristic of depression. As a depressed person, Steve is a victim of the most common mood-related disorder in the world, and his life is on hold unless he can get a grip on his problem and overcome it.

We all get up on the wrong side of the bed from time to time, but we snap out of it. Not so with people who are suffering from the condition known as clinical depression. For these people sad feelings linger for weeks, months, even years. An event such as a parking ticket or sharp words by the boss may trigger the sadness, but severely depressed people continue to be weighed down by a sense of doom and despair long after the event has faded from memory.

Worldwide, depression is the fourth leading cause of disability, according to the World Health Organization (WHO), and is increasing at a rapid rate. In Western countries, one out of three people have endured at least one episode of depression and one out of five of people so affected have chronic, recurring depression.

One study estimated the total annual cost of depression to the US economy at over $43 billion—a depressing amount of money in an economy that depends on workers who can focus on getting the job done. Depression costs more than all other chronic diseases combined, including heart disease, HIV/AIDS and other infections. This amount is more than one third of the US trillion dollar national health care budgets.

Older people are hit hardest by clinical depression. One out of four Americans over the age of sixty-five suffers from the condition. Young Americans are not exempt. One out of 33 children and one out of eight adolescents suffers from clinical depression. The tragedy is that thousands of depressed children and teenagers are overlooked by our schools and families and are left to suffer on their own without adequate diagnosis or treatment. Especially likely to fall through the cracks are youngsters with bipolar depression (also known as a "manic-depressive personality"), who experience rapid mood swings from elation to despair.

At any age, depression brings about physical problems and drains people's sexual vitality and energy. Depressed people are more likely to experience substance abuse, financial losses, divorce, and suicide. They can make others uncomfortable by seeming to complain about everything and experiencing problems in every organ of their body.

If an individual has a medical problem, depression can make it worse. Heart disease and other chronic conditions such as asthma, diabetes, arthritis, and cancer are more severe in depressed people. Depression may initiate these problems directly or merely lead to unhealthy behaviors with serious consequences.

Classic symptoms of clinical depression include sleeping too much or too little and trouble controlling one's appetite and finances. This is not the same as failing to balance your checkbook. Ultimately, depressed people develop serious work-related problems, frustrating friendships and failed sexual relationships.

Screenwriters know that laughing at our emotional hang-ups is a sure way to keep the audience engaged. That's why we've laughed for years at the foibles of the racist Archie Bunker, the dim-witted Barney Fife, the sex-obsessed Sam Malone, and dozens of other characters.

Our humor often stabs at the darkness of despair. Raymond, the main character in the highest rated TV comedy show of 2003, says, "You know what the amazing thing is…that I can function at all." And we keep laughing. Serious drama expands beyond humor to deal with the tragedies of suicide, addictions, and despair. We'd much rather watch or read about depressed people than deal with the cause of depression in our own lives.

Most depressed people do not understand that an imbalance in their brain chemistry is almost certainly the cause of their depression. Instead, they assume they're depressed because they didn't deal effectively with stress in their lives. They feel the depression is their fault. People with a strong religious orientation are likely to feel guilty for giving in to depression. Even doctors, who should know that depression is a treatable medical condition, may go along with the idea that self-discipline is the best way to cure depression.

Not realizing that there is a biological cause of depression, friends of depressed people often assume they can help with a "pep talk" or positive reinforcement to boost self-esteem. Partners of depressed people often have the fantasy that if the other person would only stop complaining, everything would be all right. This shortsighted strategy never works. It only ends up raising the frustration level for all concerned.

To combat the lack of understanding about depression, pharmaceutical companies and mental health organizations sponsor mass media campaigns to educate the public. Their efforts are commendable because without proper information, too many parents, teachers, and health care providers fail to recognize the symptoms of depression or assume that depression is easily overcome with the exercise of a little will power.

Diane shared with me the reality of depression and its effect on her life."I have been unhappy and extremely irritable for a long time now," she wrote. "I have no patience with friends and family. I have little or no interest in any of the things or people that used to interest me. I feel like crying entirely too often, and I do cry over ridiculous things. My appetite has decreased. I'm having a difficult time getting a good night's sleep. I've tried to ignore these symptoms for too long. I feel embarrassed to admit that I have a problem, though there's no doubt in my mind that I do. I feel sorry for my family. They have to deal with my moodiness and inattentiveness. I can see that it is affecting their behavior as well. When I had a flat tire three days ago, I began crying and became terrified that I wouldn't be able to stop. Over a flat tire! That was the last straw, as they say. Please give me some advice. I need it."

For Dianne and others like her, depression sucks the joy from life. The depressed person, seeing no hope for change, may consider suicide as the only option that makes sense.

What does depression have to do with hormones?

Our adrenal glands release several hormones. One of these, cortisol or cortisone, also known as "the stress hormone," is secreted whenever we feel anxious or stressed. This hormone helps our bodies cope with an emergency, but if the levels get too high cortisol can become destructive. Throughout the day levels of cortisone increase and subside in a predictable rhythmic pattern called the "cortisol cycle." The normal cortisol cycle peaks at about 8 a.m. and again at about 4 p.m. When you woke up this morning, the process of waking up triggered a surge of cortisol that boosted you out of bed. Most people suffering from depression receive their first burst of cortisol about 3 o'clock in the morning. No wonder they usually feel worse when it's time to get up, with increased anxiety and mood disturbances followed by negative moods in the evening.

Evidence suggests that the corticotropin-releasing factor (CRF) from the pituitary gland is involved in regulating our cortisol levels so that we can cope with stress in our daily lives. However, unremitting stress, such as divorce or the death of a loved one, can result in an overactive response from this cortisol-regulating hormone.

People who are severely depressed tend to have a higher concentration of CRF in their spinal fluid, and many of these people have more CRF-producing brain cells. Research studies link the production of additional corticotropin-releasing factor by the brain with chronic stress. Today we are looking at blocking drugs that show promise of bringing relief to depressed persons. It could be that these drugs will be more effective than many of today's medicines that are aimed at increasing the action of the "happy" neurotransmitters, dopamine and norepinephrine.

These neurotransmitters are special chemicals in the brain that make it possible for nerve cells to "talk" to each other. Too few—or too many—of them can cause depression or make it worse. How we deal with stress is related to the way our brains are "wired" but these sensitive neurotransmitters, fluctuate according to our hormone levels, which are altered by stress.

The good news today is that the vast majority of depressed persons can find complete relief with new medications, talk therapy, or a combination. New developments in the use of hormones to treat depression promise treatments that exceed our capabilities today and promise more effective ways of dealing with this illness tomorrow.

## Hormone Dysfunction during Depression

All of our hormones are affected by stress, but as I mentioned a few paragraphs ago, the hormone that gets most of the attention for being associated with stress is cortisol, also known as "the stress hormone." Here's how cortisol works.

During times of stress cortisol converts proteins to glucose. The resulting burst of glucose gives us energy to deal with the stressful situation. Divorce, death of a loved one, retirement, or financial losses carry a heavy load of stress that can override the regulating mechanism for cortisol. Constant stress can eventually produce very high cortisol levels that lead to confusion, dizziness, memory loss and a weakened immune system.

Dehydroepiandrosterone (DHEA), another adrenal hormone, has a very different developmental history. Its levels increase rapidly during childhood, reaching a peak in youth, and then decline thereafter in both the blood and the brain. DHEA, in contrast to cortisol, has brain protective actions, reducing the toxic actions of cortisol on the brain. DHEA levels are reduced in major depressive disorders in both adolescents and adults.

DHEA may thus have a beneficial role in the treatment of depression. This is an example of how two hormones with directly opposite effects can help the body regulate itself.

Cortisol responds to the day-night cycle we call the circadian rhythm. Levels of cortisol normally peak between 7 and 8 a.m. when we're getting out of bed to face the day. Bright light early in the morning signals the sudden release of brain histamine, which activates cortisol. High cortisol levels can suppress both brain and tissue histamines. At night the hormone, melatonin, responds to darkness and reverses the effect of cortisol. This push-me, pull-you action of melatonin, DHEA and cortisol is typical of the way most hormones interact with each other.

What happens when hormones become imbalanced? Bright computer or television screens or partying into the late night hours can delay melatonin from reaching its usual nighttime peak. This prevents melatonin from disabling cortisol's effect so we can awaken clear-headed the next morning. A life style with carousing or work extending into the early hours of the morning therefore causes a delayed release of melatonin so that cortisol will be activated at night instead of during the day. After a few days, the sleep-wake cycles automatically adjust. People who continue with nighttime work or play will develop a pattern of waking up in the middle of the night regardless of when they go to bed. The next day they will feel exhausted all day long. In these situations, Provigil® or modafinil can again be used therapeutically to increase brain histamine, increasing wakefulness for the sleep-deprived.

For those whose schedules require them to sleep during daytime hours, cortisol levels can be held constant by shutting out light with heavy blinds or wearing blinders. This reinforces the melatonin response to darkness and allows us to sleep during the day. Unfortunately, when we wake up at night after sleeping during daylight hours, we miss the cortisol boost that is triggered by light and feel lousy, confused, and disoriented. Night after night of poor sleep can bring on mood disorders like depression.

People who are depressed wake up with abnormally low cortisol levels that slowly creep up as the day progresses until the stress diminishes. This is why depressed patients usually say they feel terrible in the morning but might improve as the day goes on. Unfortunately constant, unremitting stress in the long run upsets the normal cortisol cycle, reversing its circadian pattern, so that the highest cortisol levels are reached during the night, completely putting a stop to deep sleep and creating more fatigue. This vicious cycle of poor sleep and daytime fatigue permanently disturbs the timing of peak cortisol levels, which is crucial for normal mental functioning.

Above normal levels of cortisol during sexual intercourse can suppress erections by decreasing testosterone levels. One of the serious biochemical consequences of depression is a steady increase in cortisol, and a decrease in DHEA, which occurs as stress levels build. Too little cortisol is also harmful. Some new studies show that cortisol levels are low in people who suffer from a condition known as post-traumatic stress disorder after being exposed to a frightening situation. In these cases poor sleep, daytime anger explosiveness and depression can result.

How can you tell if you have too much or too little cortisol?

Tests on saliva collected at different times of the day have proven to be a sensitive indicator of an abnormal cortisol/DHEA pattern. Measuring cortisol levels in morning saliva can be very useful as a screening test for depression. If treated early, such cortisol deficiencies can be corrected with DHEA supplemental therapy for a few months and stop the depression from worsening.

Another unique approach to depression treatment that works for many patients with dangerously high cortisol levels is testosterone supplementation. Medical research suggests that testosterone has positive effects on mood, and that raising testosterone to normal levels will suppress the production of excess cortisol, reducing the chances of depression. DHEA supplementation in women has been found to increase testosterone levels. In clinical surveys, patients diagnosed with depression and associated hormonal imbalances who were treated with testosterone reported that they not only felt better but also had more energy, better sexual function and improved moods. Could testosterone therapy offer a new treatment for depression?

Two research papers using testosterone to treat depression showed conflicting results. In a Columbia University six-week study the researcher could not find any statistical difference between the depression of patients with very low total testosterone who were given weekly testosterone injections and those who received peanut oil placebo injections. He did notice, however, that sexual function improved with testosterone. In another more recent eight-week study at McLean Hospital involving men with low or borderline testosterone, a significant improvement in unresponsive depression was observed and linked to an increase in the levels of circulating free testosterone using transdermal testosterone gels.

These studies provide evidence confirming that low levels of testosterone can cause negative moods and reduce mental acuity, conditions we see commonly in aging persons as their testosterone levels dwindle.

## The Sad Days of Menopause

The hormone problems that cause men to feel depressed fade in comparison with those that women endure. Women become depressed about three times as often as men and are more than twice as likely to suffer bipolar depression with wild mood swings. Scientists believe that women suffer more from depression than men because a larger portion of their brains is devoted to recognizing and processing emotions. Think about the roller coaster of hormones in a woman's life. She is constantly adjusting to hormone fluctuations. From menstruation and pregnancy to childbirth and menopause, she confronts an array of hormone-driven activities. Some women cannot achieve a perfect balance of all hormones during these natural but chaotic phases of life. As a result they suffer from deficiencies in the key chemicals needed for the brain to function optimally, and this can lead to clinical depression.

For example, a woman whose testosterone levels drop while her estrogen levels are rapidly fluctuating is probably going to suffer from some type of depression. This frequently occurs in a condition called post partum depression—becoming depressed soon after giving birth to a baby. With this type of depression the new mother's mood might shift rapidly from elation to despair primarily because of dramatic changes in her hormones. She now has a classic case of what is known as bipolar depression, with chaotic mood swings from high to low.

Women who are clinically depressed, a condition also known as unipolar depression, are likely to complain of fatigue, distress, increased appetite and excessive sleepiness. Severely depressed women often have trouble getting out of bed in the morning or experience difficulty falling asleep at night. Normally, sexual dreams are an indication of a woman's erotic desire. An "early warning sign" of depression could be fewer dreams of this nature. Women whose testosterone and DHEA is waning report fewer erotic dreams.

Jan, a young mother, wrote to me presenting a classic example of a person who feels "stressed out" but is really depressed.

"I am thirty-one," she wrote, "and have a highly stressed life." Jan described her situation: three small children, a husband who travels for work, barely any support system, and a mom who lives out of town. “I feel worried, anxious, and a lot of the time like I am not doing it ‘good enough,’ she continued. “I have a hard time getting the appropriate sleep I need, and feel miserable and ‘mad at the world’ in the morning because I didn’t sleep as well as I should have.”

Sometimes the stress level is better and sometimes worse. “But,” she observed, “I do snap out of it, and I am OK with the kids and stuff. I just feel overwhelmed a lot and can’t get my head straight. I take time-outs quite often for myself, but don’t get as many as I should. I wish I could just go with the flow more, and handle things better.”

I could tell that Jan was worried. I could almost hear her anxious voice when I read her plea, “Can you recommend a mild medication that can help with my anxiousness, and my feeling like I want to cry but usually can’t even if I tried? I feel I only need something to take the edge off.”

Many women like Jan feel distressed most of the time. Their predominant symptom is anxiety, common in both unipolar and bipolar depression. Although they may be on the edges of clinical depression, they may think all they need is a tranquilizer—something to “take the edge off.” They have no idea that they are seriously depressed. Treating anxiety with calming drugs may work for a short while, but it only masks the problem. If the feelings persist longer than six months, they are probably due to clinical depression, not just stress.

Women who have gone through menopause and feel depressed can cheer up with good news about dehydroepiandrosterone, the DHEA steroid. Scientists have learned that menopausal women are deficient in several hormones—and that when they are treated with DHEA, they are likely to notice improvement in their sense of well-being. Apparently DHEA has a positive effect on the central nervous system. In addition, post-menopausal women can enjoy higher levels of testosterone following a program of taking DHEA supplements. Higher levels of these male hormones or androgens, make women feel better—much the same effect they have on men.

Joyce is fifty-two and went through menopause five years before writing to me. “My libido and sexual arousal and responsiveness are now practically non-existent,” she wrote. “I wake up every day with hot flashes and pain in my joints. I could probably not do anything sexual even if I wanted to. I love my husband, and he loves me. We both miss the closeness of the wonderful physical relationship we once had.”

Joyce's experience is a classic menopausal reaction, and it closely follows the changes that take place in men as well during the time we call mid-life crisis. Men may blame their discomfort on retirement or problems at work, but anyone with constant pain or hot flashes would feel depressed.

As I mentioned earlier, the reason women seem to suffer from depression more than men may be that they talk about their feelings more. This is good for them because the earlier depression is recognized, the sooner it can be diagnosed and treated.

Men, on the other hand, apparently want to bolster their invincibility and do not like to complain to their doctors about anything as personal as their emotions. When they feel depressed, men often turn to self-medicating with alcohol or drugs only to slide into a deeper depression.

In desperation men too often take their own lives when they can no longer deal with the overwhelming feelings of despair. Four times as many men as women commit suicide, according to data analyzed by the American Association of Suicidology, an organization dedicated to preventing suicide in the US. The association also notes that every year nearly thirty thousand people decide to commit suicide in the US and succeed in their attempt. For every suicide there are from eight to twenty-five attempts that do not result in death.

Locked in depression, people of both sexes feel as if their life is slipping away and that they have nothing to look forward to but the inevitability of death. It's a dismal picture. However, more evidence is emerging that this hopeless state may be reversed with hormone supplementation. This point is important for women and the men that love them. Keep in mind that depression is predominantly a disease of mental imbalance linked to a shortage of the specific chemicals known as neurotransmitters, particularly serotonin, dopamine, and norepinephrine.

Medications to counter the effects of depression have existed for over thirty years, but they don't work for everyone. Newer medicines are capable of increasing the levels of both serotonin and norepinephrine. These dual-action antidepressants cause fewer side effects and produce a better therapeutic effect than older chemical compounds.

They aren't cheap. The newer antidepressants are the single largest item in the total US pharmacy budget, but the costs of not treating depression are much greater! Unfortunately, it sometimes comes down to a choice between poverty and sanity.

Depression co-exists with other health problems. For example, a patient who is hospitalized for any reason ranging from heart disease to cancer has an incidence of depression of twenty to forty-two percent. Most patients with diseases of the central nervous system are depressed, for example—

| | |
|---|---|
| Epilepsy | 55.0% |
| Parkinson's | 51.0% |
| Cushing's (or abnormally high cortisol levels) | 83.0% |
| Multiple sclerosis | 55.0% |
| Alzheimer's | 11.0% |

Most depressed people have no inkling that a chemical imbalance could be the cause of their depression. They find the cause for their sadness in the problems of their lives such as feeling uncontrollable sadness after breaking up with a girlfriend or a boyfriend, crying all the time to mourn the death of someone dear to them, or not wanting to get out of bed because they hate school or their job. It's not uncommon for depressed persons to despair and feel "crazy" or "out of control," although the root of the problem is a chemical imbalance. Today the "nervous breakdowns" some folks used to dread can be treated with appropriate medications.

Depression is far more severe and intense than a bad mood. Physicians need to stop rushing through clinical consultations with their patients and take the time to spot early signs of depression. Diagnosis is the most important aspect of this disorder since it cannot be treated until it has been diagnosed. The doctor's index of suspicion should rise whenever patients complain repeatedly of not feeling right or experiencing rapid mood swings.

If a person responds quickly to a new antidepressant drug, but the medicine loses its effectiveness a short time later, chances are that the person has bipolar depression. Another sign of this type of depression is the patient who marries more than three times or one who returns to a doctor's office more than a dozen times in a year but is not on a long-term treatment program requiring such frequent visits. A person with a close relative (parent, grandparent, sibling) who has a mood disorder is much more likely to be a victim of depression than someone without family members who have been diagnosed with clinical depression or have experienced depressive feelings in childhood or adolescence.

Hormones are valuable in counteracting the disruption of the circadian rhythms (see page 23) that occur with depression. Depression and sexual dysfunction relate to each other in a time-dependent fashion. In other words, one can lead to the other. Additionally, the intensity of depression and sexual desire can vary depending on the time of day, week, or month. Like a roller coaster ride, depression is not always downhill.

Constant stress takes its toll on the regulating system in the brain. The memory terminal of the hippocampus, located between the hypothalamus and the pituitary gland, begins to malfunction after a few months of constant stress. Stress may be unavoidable in today's world. But for someone with depressed relatives, prolonged stress can lead to dementia or severe loss of memory. Regaining control in our life can help us cope with stress, but medication is often necessary.

The irony of depression is that those who suffer the most from its effects may be the least aware of its presence in their lives. If the disease has caused the person—usually a man—to lose his ability to experience pleasure, he will also be lacking the insight to realize that he has a problem. You can't help a person who thinks nothing is wrong.

## Mid-life Crisis and Male Andropause

Andropause is the medical name of a syndrome in aging men consisting of all of the consequences of aging as well as other physical, sexual and psychological symptoms. Men going through andropause suffer from weakness, fatigue, reduced muscle and bone mass, sexual dysfunction, depression, anxiety, irritability, insomnia, and memory impairment. Sounds terrible, doesn't it?

As we just discussed, menopause occurs in most women between forty and sixty years of age when a loss of menstrual periods announces the change. In men, the process of hormone depletion is long and complex with fluctuations in testosterone over many decades. Andropause, in other words, is a prolonged process with decades of suffering.

Only recently have researchers begun to focus on the "male menopause." This term loosely applies to the mid-life crisis that men reach in their late fifties or early sixties. Many doctors do not believe in the male menopause or "andropause," but the word first appeared in the medical literature as far back as 1952 when it was defined as "the natural cessation of the sexual function in older men."

Notice two points in this definition: (1) andropause was considered "natural" and (2) it was assumed that sexual function should cease at a certain point in a man's life. Neither of these assumptions is true.

Men and women adjust to increasing depression and sexual dysfunction associated with advancing years in vastly different ways. Women, for example, go through "the change" rather abruptly, while for aging men the decline in hormones is slow and hardly noticeable over time. The slow course and unpredictability of andropause contribute to its lack of recognition and its dismissal as nothing but a sign of "normal" aging.

Think about that the next time you hear an acquaintance being described as a "grumpy old man." Consider the possibility that he is not grumpy at all—just depressed.

Hormones may play a significant role in the mid-life crisis of men. Let's take a closer look at how this works.

As time goes by, hormone deficiencies generally cause failing memories, more irritability and fatigue—symptoms similar to depression. The development of arteriosclerosis, varicose veins, thinning of the skin, high blood pressure and increasing cholesterol levels are also physical signs of aging.

There's more! Some of the obvious signs of andropause: include: progressive aging of the face, development of a potbelly, loss of pubic hair, shrinking of sexual organs, balding, increased ear hair, and loss of muscle and skin tone. These occur in most men as they age.

Over the years several hormones, especially testosterone, become depleted, leading to a deficiency. The good news is that just as women with menopausal symptoms respond to treatment with hormones, males going through andropause can also be treated effectively.

The so-called natural aging process results in both ejaculatory and urinary problems in many men due to low testosterone. As men progress through their fifties and sixties, their andropause is commonly associated with a decrease in sexual motivation and the deterioration of their general condition. Should men accept this as part of "normal aging"?

I don't think so. These men are only manifesting early warning signs of a more serious problem. With gruesome consequences testosterone deficiency diseases are showing up in men as young as thirty to forty.

Alarming statistics from recent research suggest that men who become impotent—unable to develop an erection—die about twenty years earlier than other men, usually from heart disease. A study in 1988 by the well-known hormone researcher Conrad Swartz confirmed the fact that total testosterone levels are much lower in men with severe heart disease than in healthy men. Total serum testosterone levels were found to be one hundred points lower in patients who had suffered a heart attack than in those who had not. Once a man becomes totally impotent (no erections), he loses his drive for life. Subsequently or simultaneously, he loses his libido, his muscle mass, his mental acuity fades and depression sets in.

At forty years of age, roughly one-third of the male population is unable to achieve an erection at will. By eighty years, three out of four men are impotent. The only encouraging detail here is that one out of four men in his eighties or older is not impotent. Many men live out their lives to an old age without ever losing their sexual ability. If andropause were "natural" every man would experience its effects.

While andropause is not synonymous with impotence, it is usually associated with loss of libido and sexual function. Problems related to andropause may be caused by a deficiency of multiple hormones including growth hormone, DHEA, thyroxine, melatonin, and oxytocin as well as the primary male androgens, testosterone, androstenedione and DHT. The good news is that men can retain potency and enjoy good sex up to twice a week into their nineties despite dropping hormone levels.

We need to pay more attention to two troubling facts about male sexuality: (1) more and more men are living into their nineties or beyond and (2) in developed countries fertility rates for men of all ages are declining.

A program of testosterone supplementation portioned out in individually adjusted amounts will increase sexual drive and function in most men. Testosterone replacement therapy will break down fat, provide more lean body mass, improve insulin sensitivity, enhance anti-clotting action, and expand blood vessels to reduce blood pressure. These sound like important responses.

Even so, despite enormous medical progress during the past few decades, the final years of life in the US are still accompanied by increasing ill health, depression and disability. This does not have to happen to you if you listen to your hormones and find a doctor to help you keep them balanced.

## Depression and Sexual Dysfunction

Sexual dysfunction refers to a lack of sexual desire or difficulty in achieving arousal, climax, or ejaculation. Depressed people tend to avoid sex because they cannot perform the sex act in a normal manner and because they lack sexual drive. Anxiety about sexual performance can cause sexual dysfunction, although in most cases there is a physical problem.

Sexual indications of depression include failure to achieve erections and the lack of interest in someone who has been a sexual partner. Loss of early morning erections should be seen as an early warning sign of depression in men. These men may be experiencing very low testosterone levels and a lack of sexual fantasy because of their depression. Doctors should be concerned because men with these problems are at risk for much more serious conditions than simply the lack of erections.

You may be familiar with symptoms of depression as they affect sexual dysfunction. Or, if you or someone you know has never been severely depressed, the facts about such mood disorders may elicit a yawn and a shrug. So some people are depressed. So what? So some men have trouble getting it up. What else is new? So some women are sexually frigid. Maybe they just don't love their husband. Maybe he's a jerk.

Excuses abound, and we try not to think about it. The truth is that depression is a disease of denial, and the reality is that too many people are suffering from the condition.

One reason millions suffer from depression is that many depressed patients are not diagnosed appropriately. Though sexual dysfunction is a dependable "warning sign" of impending depression, these warnings are easily ignored by busy physicians and by patients in denial. Patients with depression are simply told that they need to see a marriage counselor or take a vacation. By the time depression advances to the latter stages, involving a loss of any interest in sex, love or even in life, it is too late. Suicide is a real threat.

Physicians should stop dodging the issue and start listening carefully to their patients when they complain of "feeling hopeless" or "isolated," and not wanting to do the things they used to enjoy. When patients describe the sudden onset of a lower sex drive or unstable moods over which they have no control, a red flag should go up. These patients are trying to give us a clue to their future diagnosis. They could be suffering from clinical depression, as well as a loss of libido.

Does depression cause sexual dysfunction or is it the other way around? To solve the dilemma of which comes first, we should pay attention to those patients who are not depressed but only have sexual dysfunction as their primary problem. I remember talking to Michael, a math teacher in Chicago, regarding his sexual dysfunction.

Michael's testosterone fell in a few months from 550 to 270, and his energy and sexual drive also fell to low levels. He was deeply disappointed when his urologist and personal physician put him off, both of them assuring him that his condition was either his unfortunate lot in life or just part of the aging process.

At forty-one, Michael was physically active, playing full court basketball and running without undue fatigue for long periods of time. His only health problem was high blood pressure, but he was taking twenty milligrams of Lotrel, an anti-hypertensive, every morning to hold that in check. His identical twin brother also had a problem with blood pressure.

Michael's level of testosterone was definitely below the normal range, and he was still fairly young. Did he get treated? No. His doctor didn't ask about his family history, although the fact that Michael's twin brother has high blood pressure could have been a clue to the hereditary basis for his problem. His doctor should also know that hypertension is a valid predictor of early heart disease. The cause of Michael's high blood pressure should be diagnosed well before he is handed a prescription for a bottle of blood pressure pills.

If Michael's situation is typical, the doctor's next step will be to add more medication without considering the possibility that Michael may have a hidden testosterone deficiency. The more medications the doctor adds to his treatment plan without a correct diagnosis, the greater the likelihood that Michael's sexual problems will increase. Sometimes physicians continue to add more blood pressure medications when a single agent doesn't work, overlooking testosterone deficiency or an inherited problem as the cause.

What should Michael do if he continues to suffer from low testosterone with no help from his urologist or his general internist? Should he see another doctor? What if he can't find anyone on his health plan who believes that testosterone may be playing a role in his hypertension?

The scenario is not that far-fetched. Michael will probably give up in frustration and take matters into his own hands. He might consult the Internet and order a testosterone preparation that is available without a doctor's prescription. Michael could end up with a totally ineffective and counterfeit testosterone product or, worse, a more dangerous oral anabolic steroid.

Unsupervised prescription sales over the Internet are all too prevalent and lay the groundwork for a tragedy waiting to happen. I believe in free speech and support the marvelous power of the Web, but I do believe that this part of the World Wide Web needs regulating.

In spite of adequate exercise, Mike reported a drop in his testosterone level and a discouragingly low sex drive. Testosterone therapy would probably help Michael lower his blood pressure. Too many doctors treat symptoms instead of searching for the root cause of the disorder. The reasoning is often that a thorough investigation would take too much time or cost too much money.

Without an adequate diagnosis and an understanding doctor, men in Michael's shoes often give up on doctors and opt for the dangerous route of self-medication. They do not understand that the real reason for their problem has not been determined. Trying to solve the problem without finding its cause means taking more and more medication to treat the signs and symptoms without addressing the underlying cause.

A correct diagnosis makes all the difference!

## The Secret to Treating Depression Successfully

Depression is not a simple disease, and the first step in treating this complex disorder is to sort out the type of depression we are dealing with so that the doctor can implement a successful treatment plan. A doctor who recognizes the role that hormones play in depression would prescribe a combination of an antidepressant plus a thyroid hormone, for example, to correct an unresponsive depression. The improvement in patients with other hormonal therapies using DHEA, testosterone, or cortisol supports this approach for many patients.

In 2000 a California researcher, Alan Michaels, discovered that elderly people with depression are often deficient in the hormone DHEA. Although low levels of practically any hormone will produce some depression in either sex, Owen Wolkowitz, a psychiatrist at the University of California at San Francisco has successfully treated depression in people who did not respond to other therapy with high doses of pharmaceutical-grade DHEA.

Over-activation of the adrenal system immediately elevates levels of cortisol, the stress hormone, bringing on symptoms of depression that are often accompanied by pain and distress in the abdomen. High cortisol levels overpower the nervous system, and the entire human organism becomes unbalanced.

Lower total testosterone and DHEA levels are also common in depressed persons, resulting in sexual dysfunction such as premature ejaculation or the inability to maintain an erection long enough for a woman to experience orgasm. These hormones can sometimes be used effectively instead of anti-depressants.

While DHEA or testosterone works for some depressed patients, nearly nine out of ten people respond well to one of the newer dual-action antidepressant medications. Occasionally no antidepressant works because of differences between people and the various types of depression. In these cases a combination of medications including lithium may be helpful. Dr. Leslie Lundt, a psychiatrist in Boise, Idaho, has been using Provigil in combination with antidepressants to induce rapid remission of depression.

You may wonder how doctors can find the right antidepressant. Sometimes patients feel as if it is simply a "trial-and-error" process. This is wrong. We do not treat a major mental disorder by guesswork. The first step in treating any type of depression is for the individual suffering from its effects to take ownership of the problem. If a person believes, instead, that some life circumstance is dictating his or her moods, it will be next to impossible to change that person's mind and get them to take their medication.

Depressed people tend to take one of two positions: they believe they have a physical problem and the doctor does not know what it is, or they are convinced that they are fine and that everyone around them is sick. This is denial at its deepest level.

Once the doctor and patient focus on the depression and eliminate other important issues as the root of the person's problem, they can work together to achieve total relief from the disease. Recovery and the correction of hormone imbalance should be the goal. Remission of depression means a return to normal functioning, not simply a positive response to taking certain drugs. The goal in all types of depression therapy is total relief from all symptoms.

As the physical symptoms of depression—sleeplessness, lack of sexual arousal, and abnormal cortisol levels—wane, the person's healthy mental capabilities return. People who do not achieve remission are three times as likely to suffer a relapse, three times as likely to become depressed again, and just as likely as before to attempt suicide. Those who become involved in substance abuse are more likely to experience a worsening outcome than those who take their non-addictive antidepressants as prescribed.

The good news is that depression is one of the most treatable illnesses in medicine. Nearly all patients with depression begin to feel better after taking their first medications. But not all antidepressants are equally effective in terms of overall rate of response. Certain SRIs such as Paxil and Zoloft (see page 18) are short-acting and when stopped abruptly cause symptoms of withdrawal such as anxiety, headache, dizziness, and severe depression. This condition is called "discontinuation syndrome." Others, like Prozac, stay in the system for weeks after stopping the meds.

If the doctor's prescription doesn't work, patients sometimes turn to over-the-counter (OTC) remedies. So-called "natural antidepressant therapies" such as St. John's Wort, valerian root and SAM-E are popular. Because they can buy these without a doctor's order, some people take all three! Many people seek out these three drugs because they lift their depression and make them feel better. They may be "natural" drugs from an herbal perspective, but they contain compounds that can act like drugs in the human system.

St. John's Wort or hypericum is prescribed as a serotonin stimulant in Germany. It relieves depression in some people, but in combination with SRIs it can create too much serotonin, a condition called the "serotonin syndrome." A potentially lethal overdose of serotonin (5-HT) is associated with vomiting, loss of orientation, and possibly death.

Even over-the-counter hormones like melatonin, DHEA and androstenedione that anyone can buy without a prescription can help ease depression, but because of their close relationship to the functioning of other hormones circulating in our bodies, we should not play games using these drugs. Just because you can buy them at the drug store doesn't mean they're good for you or that they will work the way the advertisers claim.

My plea is, "Don't try to treat your own depression." Depression is a complicated disorder involving your brain, your chemical make-up, your hormonal system and your sense of who you are. The disease has so many facets that a physician must diagnose it correctly before any treatment is given. After the diagnosis is made, hormones and neurotransmitter levels must first be restored to a balanced state. Finally, a brief course of intense psychotherapy is essential to train the once depressed person to recognize triggers and personality quirks that encourage depression-associated behavior and thinking.

We now know that hormonal and brain systems work differently in men and women in response to the same emotional experience. Obviously, it is important to consider the unique and changing biology of males and females when planning treatment for depression and stress-related illness. Read more about differences between the brains of males and females in Chapter Seven.

Thanks to miraculous advances in pharmacology, the branch of medicine that deals with the treatment of disease by using drugs or medications, a new life in a very real sense is available to those suffering from depression. Of course, the right prescription does no good unless the patient stays on the medication program. It's a big temptation to stop taking medicines especially after they begin working and the person starts to feel great.

Listening to your hormones is more important than knowing all the facts and stories about mental diseases. A prevention-oriented mid-life check up and a hormone screening can make the difference between health and future problems or disease. Hormone balancing is an important tool for preventive medicine physicians. Added to the age-old essentials of good health—proper diet, regular exercise, and adequate sleep—a visit to the family physician when something goes wrong can help you keep right side up when it comes to a depression-free life. If a hormonal imbalance is the problem, new hormone delivery systems are available to help suffers obtain relief.

## Testosterone Hormone Gels

We know that levels of free testosterone increase with the use of testosterone gels. These gels are a quick and easy way for men to apply testosterone replacement medication. Some men, however, do not do well with alcohol-based gels, possibly because of the low potency of the testosterone.

"I have been on AndroGel for about a year and a half now due to secondary hypogonadism," Richard wrote to me from Chicago. "Before AndroGel, my T level was 210. After starting AndroGel at 5 milligrams per day, the level went to 755. Six months ago it was down to 505, and my most recent test just last week it had dropped to 415. I'm starting to feel some of the old symptoms of low T—foggy thinking, low energy, and low sex drive. Has anyone else had this problem of AndroGel becoming less effective? My doc says my T levels are still within the normal range."

Richard's problems may be due to inadequate hormone replacement. Some men require ten milligrams of AndroGel per day for full testosterone replacement therapy. His doctor should be careful about monitoring results and adjusting the dose of hormones. Correcting low hormone levels can prevent suffering from decreased libido, erectile dysfunction or a lack of orgasms, but it isn't always possible to restore the balance of hormones with a standard dose of hormone supplement. Other hormones such as progesterone, melatonin, and DHEA might be required.

Out of desperation men suffering from erection or orgasmic problems sometimes turn to alcohol or street drugs to medicate their problems. When properly administered, supplemental testosterone could make these men feel great without depending on dangerous drugs or tempting alcoholism.

Men who receive restorative testosterone therapy often describe feeling of heightened motivation, excitement, inspiration, and passion. Other benefits frequently reported include a sense of confidence, freedom from fatigue, and powerful, aggressive, but positive moods.

Now please don't get me wrong. I don't want you to rush out and start using hormones so you can feel this way immediately. Not everyone responds to hormone replacement therapy in the same way because people have different hormone and biochemical requirements.

In my practice I see more patients with depression and hormone imbalances than those with vitamin deficiencies. As a matter of fact, testosterone deficiency has become such a common condition that it is no longer an exception but the rule. Because of my experience with my patients, I recommend that every man over forty should have his hormone levels tested. See the next chapter for more details.

Joe wrote to me, giving a classic description of the devastating consequences of testosterone deficiency in men.

"I was just reading some testimonials on your site and it seemed like I was reading about myself. I'm tired of getting responses that I'm normal when I know there has been a huge change in my life. I feel like my virility has gone downhill. My sex life has been terrible. I have weak erections and lose them quickly. I have had these symptoms for at least a year now. I know it's not diabetes because I've been tested for that three times along with my testosterone levels, measured between 320 and 340."

Joe is starting to feel desperate. "My weight has ballooned from 175 to 245 pounds in a year and a half," he continued. "I know it's not a mental thing because I had the physical symptoms and then gained weight. I don't feel like a 29-year-old man but more like one in his eighties who can't get it up and whose virility has disappeared. This has depressed me so much that I don't go anywhere and have no energy and motivation to work out like I used to. I'm too tired to exercise. I hope you can help me. I would be happy to drive to your office from Orange County."

Poor Joe. He's not yet thirty and is complaining of having a terrible sex life, weak erections—a loss of his virility. Why does Joe feel like an old man? Joe's testosterone level sits in the low normal range for his age, so any medical doctor would tell him the problem is not his testosterone, but more likely a family problem or too much stress. Are his doctors correct?

If Joe were in his sixties or seventies, nobody would be surprised by his low normal testosterone levels, which drop about one hundred points for each decade of life. A young man like Joe should not have sexual dysfunction if he has a normal testosterone level. Nevertheless Joe knows that his performance is far from his normal experience only a few years earlier. Something is not right. In Joe's case—and he has plenty of company—total testosterone levels do not always provide a useful measure of his sexual ability. Joe's doctor needs to consider his bioavailable testosterone and free testosterone as a more accurate indicator of hormonal function.

At least Joe has been listening to his hormones. Doctors who only measure their patients' total testosterone levels are using the accepted standards but fail to notice men who could benefit from treatment.

Reports from the Massachusetts Male Aging Study found that free testosterone was a more accurate measure than total testosterone. The study showed that while free testosterone drops by 1.4 percent and SHBG increases by 1.2 percent per year, the total testosterone in aging men does not show a marked decrease. Dr. Guay points out that the total testosterone decreases only about 0.4 percent each year, and this is not reflecting the true state of testosterone deficiency. When free testosterone, which is normally 11-35 picograms per milliliter, drops below 7.4 picograms per milliliter he adds, there is no response to Viagra. (A picogram is one trillionth of a gram.)

After asking him several times, George persuaded his doctor to test his free testosterone levels. "He pronounced me normal," he said, "but I had still all the signs of low testosterone levels—depression, lack of concentration, low libido, and even enlarged breasts. Finally, I demanded to see an endocrinologist who gave me a proper diagnosis of hypogonadism (deficient testosterone levels). He gave me an injection of testosterone, and

I began to feel much better immediately. My smile returned and so did my sexual desires. I was so happy I was persistent about my problem."

All was not well, however, after this. George's endocrinologist subsequently switched him to a five gram packet of AndroGel daily, and George did not react well. "I have been 'drunk' ever since," he told me. "I've had lots of side effects, but the main one is that I feel drunk, dazed, and depressed most of the time. My eyes stay red and people think I am impaired."

When George reported these side effects to his endocrinologist, the doctor tested his blood levels and found that his testosterone levels were higher than before but were still low normal. He suggested 10 grams of the AndroGel a day. "I did so and am as drunk and dazed as before, and my eyes are redder than ever," George said.

George was fed up. "What can I do?" he wondered. Part of his thyroid gland had been removed surgically, but his thyroxine level was normal. "Should I be taking a thyroid supplement and DHEA in addition to the AndroGel?" he asked. "Or should I give up this doctor and have you recommend another physician—perhaps one who is trained in the use of the testosterone cream you wrote about on the web that was successful in treating the university professor?"

Obviously at this point George is not happy with AndroGel. Furthermore, he does not trust the first doctor who missed the diagnosis. He wants to know what else he can do. George's problem is not unique. Some men simply cannot tolerate the skin reactions resulting from treatment with AndroGel for their testosterone deficiency. The alcohol base of the gels dissolves the testosterone needed for transdermal delivery. George could try applying the AndroGel to areas away from his face, but the fumes might still affect him. AndroGel studies at UCLA indicate that larger volumes are needed to reach the required levels of testosterone. It also does not seem to depend on whether the compound is applied to one site or several sites but large body areas must be coated with gel.

What is going on? Why do so many men suddenly need hormone gels? Testosterone deficiency is increasing rapidly as depression spreads around the world. Could there be a connection between the two?

## Dopamine: Hormonal Rescue from Depression and Attention Deficit Disorder

Some patients treated with antidepressants have what is called a "flat affect" and display no emotion at all. They may perform their job and might even put on a happy face, but they do not feel totally alive and seem unable to maintain relationships with others. They often feel over-medicated but may simply be out of balance. They experience "anhedonia," the absence of happiness, which is not always responsive to antidepressant therapy. Here's what may be going on.

A neurotransmitter named dopamine is essential for feeling pleasure and arousal. A person who does not have enough dopamine can experience chronic fatigue, loss of libido, and a stimulated appetite. In addition, a lack of dopamine interferes with a person's ability to concentrate and is sometimes associated with novelty-seeking behavior. Low dopamine levels are common in anhedonia and addictive behavior as well as in depression and attention deficit disorder (ADD). Caffeine or nicotine is often used for dopamine supplementation in those with attention deficit disorder.

Too much dopamine is also dangerous and can produce weight loss, hallucinations, aggressive behavior, and increased libido. In schizophrenics—mental patients who hallucinate by hearing voices or seeing things—dopamine deluges their brain. The excess dopamine creates actual images or voices called hallucinations that do not exist except in their own minds.

Dopamine is stimulated by nicotine use, one reason that depressed people and those who need to increase their ability to focus tend to be heavy cigarette smokers. The momentary pleasure they derive from nicotine in the cigarette is short lived, and another puff is soon needed. Caffeine, speed, cocaine and methamphetamine are also powerful dopamine stimulants that are habit-forming. By revving up the brain's dopamine production they banish any lingering wisps of anhedonia and create feelings of being all-powerful without the need of food or sleep. Of course after days of sleep deprivation, other hormones suffer, and the addict "crashes."

Dopamine aids concentration, suppresses appetite and creates insomnia. Anyone who has tried a few cups of strong coffee at night knows this well. The problem is that after the mind has been stimulated for hours or days, levels of dopamine diminish, and feelings of depression and worthlessness take over. This cycle drives a "speed addict" to continue to abuse drugs. The stress builds up, cortisol levels climb and before long the "junky" can no longer get high using the drug. Depression has set in!

Problems occur when the person doesn't have enough dopamine in his or her body. Dopamine deficiency may account for a number of psychiatric disorders. Patients suffering from excessive fears and debilitating depression affect not only themselves but also the caregiver or spouse. Depression is not contagious, but caregivers often become depressed when they are involved with a loved one who is depressed or mentally ill—and may go on to develop full-blown clinical depression themselves.

"I have been caring for a son who has been diagnosed with bipolar depression with schizophrenic tendencies," Lisa wrote to me from Canada.

Besides being her son's sole support system, Lisa had to cope with legal issues that dragged on throughout an entire year. "His illness is so up and down and unpredictable," she said in her letter. "He has a therapist and psychiatrist, but I have been the one everybody has depended on to aid him. I will do it until the day I die."

Now Lisa is wondering about herself. "Lately, I cannot function like I normally do," she wrote. "I normally keep a spotless house, have dinner on the table, am busy with lots of activities and friends. Now I look for any excuse NOT to be with my friends, I leave laundry in the dryer for days, I don't clean, I don't eat right, I can't sleep and I'm extremely edgy and moody."

Lisa thinks she may be depressed. "I have learned a lot about mental illness," she said. "I never felt it could hit me. I was the strongest. I was always up, the life of the party. Not any more. I can't tell you the last time I have really enjoyed myself. I'm worried because I can't do anything about it. I can try to make a list of things to do around the house and even though I know they need to be done, and even though it is my nature to do these things without prompting, I just don't do any of them. I don't know how to explain that. I don't see sunshine anymore. I used to love the sun, but now I can't seem to find it even when it's shining above me."

Lisa has other problems in addition to depression. She feels she is not getting enough sunshine, which may be a metaphor for her lack of joy. Lisa is caring for her son who has a serious mental disease that causes him to have huge mood swings and hallucinations. Lisa is probably suffering from "situational depression" or "burnout," which many caregivers experience when dealing with loved ones who are seriously ill.

Burnout taxes the victim emotionally and physically until the person simply shuts down. Caregivers with this problem may stop eating, stop sleeping and develop that flat emotional state, anhedonia. This type of depression is also common in children dealing with aging parents, frequently leading to chain smoking or drug abuse.

Lisa's problem was probably caused by a deficiency in dopamine. What medication can she take? Only one antidepressant at this time, Wellbutrin, will increase norepinephrine, the precursor of dopamine.

## Chemical Meltdown

What happens when brain chemicals are so messed up that self-destruction seems to be the only solution? Total hormonal deterioration, a chemical meltdown of sorts, can lead to avoidance behaviors, irrational fears and dissociative personality. A letter I received from a flight attendant in Australia tells what happens when chemical meltdown occurs.

"Dear doctor," Alex wrote. "I have feelings of emptiness and uselessness, although I am told how capable and intelligent I am. " 'You're so beautiful; you have a great body, you're so lucky to have accomplished more than others.' I hear this all the time. I recently lost my job with an airline (one of only two in Australia) after it went broke. Thousands lost their jobs, and my relationship with a great guy, who lives on the other side of the country, ended because it was no longer easy for me to visit him on my flights with my job.

"I had to rent my house out as I couldn't afford the mortgage repayments, and now I'm living with my mother, I went to France to try and work on the mega-yachts but stayed only three weeks as my head wasn't there. I cried every night, came back to Perth and have been depressed ever since. I have no self worth and constantly think of ending it all. I don't see anything positive in my future. I am aging and people can't believe my age. I can't seem to shake off these feelings."

Alex blames old age and the loss of her job as a cause of her depression. She has no idea that her feelings might be related to a chemical meltdown in her brain. The angrier she becomes, the more her brain function degenerates, and the more her cortisol level increases from the constant stress. This translates to still more anger aimed at herself.

Studies show that anger turned inward can lead to high blood pressure, irregular heart rates, and suicide. The impulse for suicide may be sudden and illogically considered. If Alex's depression remains untreated, this young lady may be at risk for suicide or other chronic diseases associated with depression.

The loss of her job might have triggered Alex's depressive disorder. She may have become stressed out because of the loss of her lover and the broken relationship. Each of these factors might be the reason she uses to explain her sadness, and she is correct in realizing that something is wrong. The decisive conditions creating her misery are the imbalance of her brain chemicals or her hormonal chaos and not her job or boyfriend problems. She is not listening to her hormones.

If she did listen, what might she hear? She would hear herself saying, "I have no self worth and constantly think of ending it all." Then she would know, if she listened to herself, that this is not a normal human reaction to stress. The real tragedy would be if Alex never told anyone else about her feelings, threatened suicide and was ignored. Suicidal threats must be taken seriously, yet they are often ignored.

To function normally, your brain depends on a good supply of all its mood-altering chemicals. Either a deficiency or excess of hormones and neurotransmitters or inadequate light can lead to depression, heart attacks, mental stress, and premature death. Left untreated, depression can become so serious that the mind decides that "ending it all" is the only solution. A person who feels life is no longer worth living is in great danger!

Tragically, suicide still occurs in eleven to fifteen percent of depressed patients, mostly elderly men. Hearing George's story, which is more serious than Alex's, will give you a picture of what is going on.

"I have lost interest in my wife, my job, my life," George says. "They said I was depressed, but nothing has helped. I took all the antidepressants and still felt bad. I feel like there is no hope left for me. I may as well just drown my sorrows in a bottle. Now the doctor says I am just getting old. I am only fifty-five years old. Is this normal?"

No doubt about it. George is in the depths of severe or extreme depression. He may have unipolar depression with a constant sense of despair and hopelessness. Or he may have what is called "bipolar depression" with moods that seesaw between mania, an extremely excited state, or hypomania, a state that causes him to feel agitated and anxious.

People with bipolar (manic-depressive) depression frequently experience disruption of their normal day-night rhythm. The combination of the circadian disruption and the unbridled passion of a manic episode can be deadly. Sufferers of this type of depression commit suicide three times as frequently as those with unipolar depression.

Many men like George fail to improve with standard antidepressant therapy because it is not effective with the bipolar variant of depression. This disorder is often associated with alcohol abuse or the use of illicit drugs and a strong family history with several close relatives suffering from the same type of depression.

George probably didn't tell his doctor that he was not responding to medication because, like most men, he doesn't like to talk about anything personal to his doctor. However, without help from his doctor, George's mental state may deteriorate, and he may end up hurting himself and self-medicating with alcohol. In other words, George may suffer and then drink to ease his pain—the opposite of the common holiday celebration when people treat themselves with alcohol and then suffer from a hangover.

Out of desperation, many depressed people turn to mood-altering drugs such as cocaine, speed or "uppers," and Valium®, sleeping pills and marijuana, or downers"—all for sale on most big city streets. Some resort to legal mind-altering drugs such as alcohol, nicotine or caffeine—anything to make them feel better.

Depression runs rampant in seventy-five percent of all drug abusers, including alcoholics. Even patients who have had their symptoms medically treated sometimes continue to abuse narcotics, downers, tranquilizers, or sleeping pills. When they visit their doctors, their depression has not disappeared, but they won't confide in their physician to reveal that they are self-medicating.

Without a doubt depression is more common than we used to think. The hidden diagnosis should be pursued aggressively if a person is constantly complaining and seems to be suffering from some unknown or undiagnosed disease.

Regardless of the cause, all types of depression—from "dysthymia" (constant sadness) to major depressive disorder and bipolar disorder—respond to antidepressants or mood stabilizers, or both, in combination with other therapies such as appropriate hormone replacement.

Antidepressants have therapeutic value in many other conditions associated with depression. Pain disorders such as chronic pain syndrome, migraine headaches, and fibromyalgia respond well to antidepressants. Irritable bowel syndrome, chronic fatigue syndrome, and premenstrual syndrome are groups of symptoms that can be successfully treated with antidepressants.

Listening to our hormones is good preventive medicine. By taking time out to treat ourselves as well as we treat others and by reducing stress before it becomes unmanageable, we may be able to prevent the onset of a major mood disorder. By increasing exercise before the pain of inactivity sets in or by seeing an understanding physician or psychologist when we start to experience emotional problems, we may be able to avert the disruption of our neurochemicals.

Hormonal therapy, which should be prescribed by a doctor, has turned into a tangled mess over which we have no control. According to Theo Colborn, senior scientist at the World Wildlife Fund, "we are neutering the population—we are making females more masculine and we are making males more feminine....We've uncovered a new series of subtle effects, which probably take place during embryonic and fetal development and which have long-term effects that keep an individual from reaching his or her full development."

We do not always have control over the disruption of our hormones. Hormones can get mixed up despite well-intentioned hormone therapy prescribed by a doctor. Other factors, over which we have little or no control, can lurk in our environment.

In the next chapter we'll look at what this has done to us.

# 4

# Tangled Hormones

## Hormones Can Get Mixed Up

An incredibly complex set of commands and interactions known as the genetic code governs our genes and makes life possible, healthy, and satisfying. Each of us possesses an estimated 66,000 genes, the architects of the human body. Our genes set our hormones in motion, and hormones, in turn, drive our emotions, our sexual responses, our height and weight, the length of our lives, and many other characteristics When things go wrong, our hormones immediately synchronize their strengths to combat the challenge. Usually they win.

As remarkable as our ability to recover from disease and injury may be, it is nevertheless true that a flaw or injury to even one strand of the genetic structure can have repercussions for a lifetime and even into future generations. Sometimes, our hormones become tangled, sometimes our genes fail to produce essential proteins but without a precise balance of hormones, we cannot survive for any length of time.

## Cancer from Estrogen

Estrogen, the "female hormone," crossed the line from helpful to harmful on January 1, 2001, when the National Institute of Environmental Health added estrogen to the list of chemicals known to cause cancer.

This ominous listing came after studies showed that women who take estrogen supplements to cope with their menopause problems have a slightly higher risk of heart disease, dementia, and breast cancer, as well as a stronger risk of uterine cancer than those who do not.

Estrogen is present in men as well as women, and excess estrogen can cause sexual dysfunction, prostate cancer, and even breast cancer in men. Current evidence indicates that many tumors, especially in the breast, feed on estrogen. The mechanism that causes this is not fully understood, but we do know that a specific enzyme called aromatase helps produce estrogen and that estrogen, in turn, stimulates the multiplication of cells, making tumors grow. Pharmaceutical companies are jumping on the anti-estrogen bandwagon by developing estrogen blockers like Tamoxifen® and Arimidex® for treating breast cancers and preventing their recurrence. Other drugs that interfere with the cancer-inducing properties of estrogen (Faslodex™ or fulvestrant) are being developed, and not a minute too soon because currently from sixty to seventy-five percent of all breast cancers are estrogen dependent.

High levels of estrogen can have serious negative effects in men, including testicular cancer, undescended testicles, low sperm counts, shrinking sex organs and the inevitable sexual dysfunction. Breast cancer was reported in three males who underwent sex-change surgery to become females and received prolonged treatment with estrogen. Primary breast cancer also develops occasionally in the breast of men with prostate cancer treated with estrogen to suppress testosterone.

Don't men need estrogen?

Yes, they do. Estrogen plays an important role in a man's physical development and is a vital hormone for both men and women. Our concern is not for the estrogen your body produces naturally. We are looking at artificial substances like dioxin that mimic the chemical actions of estrogen. We call these estrogen-like compounds "environmental estrogens." For years they have been shrugged off as not powerful enough to cause serious problems. The problem with dioxin-type estrogen mimics is that differences in their composition are not properly regulated by the body's hormone feedback systems.

Straying into the human system from polluted air and water, these estrogens have been found in humans in concentrations measured in parts per million or parts per billion. At such microscopic levels, they were once considered safe. Now we know that environmental estrogens are active at extremely low concentrations measured in parts per trillion. This means that the risk of harmful symptoms from this type of estrogen is thousands to millions of times greater than we used to think.

Though estrogen produced outside the human body is a proven carcinogen, medical researchers have agreed that the benefits of estrogen therapy far outweigh the risks. Estrogen therapy for women with a deficiency continues despite evidence that estrogen supplements could be responsible for increased cancer of the sexual organs. Estradiol is the form of estrogen that has been linked most directly to higher risk of cancer in the sexual organs. Nevertheless, it is the only active ingredient in FDA-approved female hormone supplements.

You may have heard that estrogen supplements reduce the risk of age-related senility or heart attacks, but evidence was lacking. We do know from recent research that there is a hormone that protects women's hearts, but it is testosterone, not estrogen. Appropriate levels of this "male" hormone also reduced the risk of heart disease, Alzheimer's and age-related senility among women.

The good news about estrogen therapy is that doctors can protect women against some of the negative effects of estrogen by adding natural progesterone or testosterone to the hormone replacement therapy program. The addition of these hormones can also cancel the higher risk of breast and uterine cancer associated with estrogen therapy.

It is easy to assume that for women, estrogen is more important than testosterone. This assumption is not totally accurate. Androstenedione, a testosterone precursor, is at least as important for women as well as men. This hormone becomes estrone, the primary estrogen, and has regulatory powers over female reproduction as well as male sperm formation. It is also able to bypass conversion to estrone and form testosterone directly. Studies suggest, however, that androstenedione—once sold over the counter for bodybuilders—converts to excess estrogen rather than more testosterone as desired. Consequently, young boys who are looking for muscles end up with breasts instead.

When estrogen levels increase beyond acceptable limits, the ratio of testosterone to estrogen is tipped. Changes in the interrelationship of these hormones stimulate the growth and transformation of malignant cells. This is a dangerous situation with serious consequences ranging from cancer to a heightened risk of certain autoimmune diseases in which the body attacks its own tissues. The production of higher than normal estrogen levels in either sex leads to blood clots, unwanted breast development, heart attacks, and cancer along with depression, aggression, moodiness and violent tempers.

For more than three decades, doctors have debated whether estrogen replacement therapy using estradiol alone is more effective than full hormone replacement therapy as well as testosterone and progesterone. While the battle about ERT versus HRT raged, pharmaceutical companies rigorously promoted horse-based estrogens as the standard of care. The name as well as the ingredients of Premarin®, probably the most popular of these estrogens, is derived from pregnant mare's urine (PREgnant MAre's urINe).

Horse urine may soon be replaced in new hormone replacement medications by natural estrogen and natural progesterone—which have fewer side effects such as dementia, cancer, heart disease and stroke. These products will be on the market soon and are already available to all pharmacists at a low cost for compounding into gels and creams.

Why would doctors prescribe synthetic estrogens when natural estrogens are available? The answer is both financial and promotional. The perception has been that Premarin has been used for so long that it must be safe and effective. This same reasoning is also used by the pharmaceutical company which made a combination estrogen-testosterone pill, known as Estratest® (Solvay, Belgium) for women.

Experts have long debated the safety of estrogen replacement with Premarin alone, and recent studies question its effectiveness after decades of traditional use. Unopposed, estrogen can cause cancer in the sexual organs of both men and women. Progesterone naturally opposes the action of growth stimulation by estrogen in women just as testosterone opposes estrogen excess in men.

Provera® (medroxyprogesterone), a man-made progesterone, has been blamed for causing breast cancer and multiple side effects with replacement therapy. Since companies can't obtain a patent for natural hormones, there was no competitive advantage in marketing them to women. As a result, pharmaceuticals focused on substituting synthetic hormones that could be patent protected for twenty years.

For the past twenty-five years it was assumed that women had the benefits of life-enhancing hormone treatments which were both safe and effective. New research from the Women's Health Initiative (WHI) puts traditional hormone replacement therapy in a very bad light. After long-term studies lasting over a quarter of a century involving thousands of women, news reports indicated that equine (horse) estrogens and synthetic progestins did not protect women against heart disease but actually increased the risk of breast cancer and heart attacks.

Evidence is still inconsistent about any relationship between the use of HRT and the risk of breast cancer after more than fifty years of use and numerous studies. The absence of convincing evidence is reassuring because it implies that any risk of breast cancer from hormone replacement therapy is small. HRT lasting less than five years seems to confer no increased risk of breast cancer. By contrast, women using hormone replacement therapy for ten to fifteen years seem to have a somewhat higher risk of breast cancer.

Doctors today have several options in treating women with hormonal replacement. Estrogens are currently available in transdermal patches, vaginal rings and oral tablets. Soon a new gel form of estrogen will be released. Natural therapies are also competing for the estrogen market.

Phytoestrogens are plant-based compounds that can bind to the estrogen receptor, blocking excess estrogen activity and stopping the occurrence of hot flashes, decreasing bone loss and reducing the risk of breast cancer in some women. Phytoestrogens are extracted from soybeans and sold as "isoflavones," which seem safer and more natural than some pharmaceutical agents. Japanese women, who generally have one sixth the incidence of breast cancer as Western women, eat large quantities of soy in their diet. Soy is a natural blocker of environmental estrogen.

Women around the world have been using the potentially dangerous synthetic hormones Premarin® and Provera® (now combined as Prempro®) for menopausal symptoms for almost three decades. This is unfortunate, since some women can get relief by using safe and natural menopause treatment with bioidentical hormones instead of synthetic hormones.

In the shift from synthetic estrogens, new non-synthetic testosterone patches and natural estrogen gels for women are in the works and will soon receive FDA approval. The future looks bright for a safer, more effective hormone treatment using bioidentical hormones in a form that can be safely applied directly to the skin for both men and women.

## Toxic Products and Their Effects on Children

The difference between "toxic" and "intoxicating" is that a "toxic" substance is harmful, while an "intoxicating" one is addictive. Pesticides are an example of toxic items. They are deadly to the pests we bombard, but we probably won't get hooked on swallowing pesticides. They are toxic, but not intoxicating.

Intoxicating substances create insatiable desires for more of the substance and can damage hormones. The most common intoxicants in our culture are illegal drugs and some legal drugs such as alcohol and caffeine. Any mind-altering medicine or herb can become intoxicating, including prescription drugs.

The intoxicating effects of drugs are harmful to pregnant women and children, but even more so to the embryo because it is at the most delicate life stage. When the cells in mother's womb are multiplying and joining together, the developing form is extremely sensitive to drugs, alcohol and other harmful substances.

The emerging endocrine system distributes hormones throughout the fetus, playing a vital role in the baby's normal development. At this vulnerable stage of life, tiny amounts of toxic compounds can easily disrupt hormones. Possible consequences include improperly formed male and female genital organs, infertility, cancer, and a dozen other health problems. It may be years before you suffer the consequences of pre-birth exposure to these substances, but they leave their mark.

We need to consider the embryo when we talk to the public about the growth and development of the child. Theo Colborn, noted author and expert on ways that hormones are disrupted, points out that the federal government's new Children's Health Initiative talks about the child from the day it is born through puberty but doesn't mention prenatal exposure to toxins—apparently because of possible association with the abortion issue.

This is unfortunate, Colborn stated, because of the embryo's susceptibility to exposure to toxins. The unborn baby is incapable of defending itself against these substances, spelling tragedy for the growing child. "During embryonic and fetal development, the brain isn't developed thus far, so you've got an individual that has no feedback mechanism to protect itself. The fetus is still growing new tissue, constructing its nervous system, constructing elements of its immune system and the reproductive tract." As an adult, Colborn says, "when all your organs are formed and fully functioning, it takes a lot more to blow them away."

Most chemicals that are toxic to insects are weakly estrogenic. This means they mimic the action of estrogen in the human body to some extent. Too much of this effect upsets the normal ratio between testosterone and estrogen in the system. Common products such as insect spray, weed killer, PVC pipe, plastic wrap, furniture finishes, and baby bottles contain low amounts of toxic chemicals. For years we assumed that the level of toxicity in these items was so low that it had very little effect on human health.

Now we're having second thoughts.

By studying all of these substances collectively, we find that the way these chemical mixtures interact with the estrogen receptor and the androgen receptor may have profound biological implications.

In the US we release more than sixty million pounds of chemicals into our water, air, and soil every year. These chemicals can disturb our physiology, including our endocrine systems, and lead to cancer, poorly functioning ovaries, reduced sperm count, and lower fertility rates. Babies born after being exposed in the womb to these chemicals have a higher probability of birth defects and low birth weight.

The hazards of insecticides were first made known to the public in Rachel Carson's *Silent Spring,* written in 1962. A writer for the US Fish and Wildlife Service, Carson was disturbed by the nation's widespread use of chemical pesticides. After resigning from her government career in 1952, she became the world's first environmentalist. Carson theorized that humans are a vulnerable part of the ecosystem and are threatened by the increasing use of harmful substances in the environment. Her work influenced environmental policy, leading eventually to the total ban of DDT in the US in 1972. DDT, or dichlorodiphenyltrichloroethane, was the most widely used insecticide until that time.

Unfortunately, chemicals like DDT take many years, perhaps even centuries, to degrade. So persistent is DDT in the environment that the bodies of penguins in Antarctica, seals in the Arctic oceans, and frogs living at very high altitudes in remote regions, are found to contain DDT.

In 2001 a comprehensive study of heavily industrialized communities found that residents of these communities were experiencing an increase in reproductive and developmental defects. Environmental toxins were produced in high volume by the factories in the areas studied.

Eight years prior to that study, a research project reported in the prestigious British medical journal, *Lancet,* examined the effects of excess estrogen on sperm. Their study suggested a cause-and-effect relationship between estrogenic chemicals and declines in human sperm counts. In addition, exposure of pregnant women to these chemicals was linked to higher rates of cancer and malformations of the penis and testicles in their male babies.

Another study by French and Argentinean researchers added further evidence to the case against environmental toxins. Argentinean men who had attended an infertility clinic between 1995 and 1998 were quizzed about their lifestyle, medical history, occupation and exposure to pesticides. The scientists concluded that being exposed to pesticides might have been a factor in the men's inability to have children. Men exposed to these chemicals were more likely to have sperm levels well below the minimum limit for male fertility. They also had higher levels of female sex hormones in their system than men who had not come into contact with the chemicals.

Adding to the load of toxic waste in our bodies is our growing dependence on intoxicating drugs. Over thirty-six million Americans regularly use the two most powerful legal drugs known to mankind—nicotine and alcohol. Habitual use of these and other household drugs contributes dramatically to sexual dysfunction in Americans. A dangerous stew results when drugs and pesticides mingle in the human body. The combination can disrupt the sensitive hormonal balance of entire populations.

## Alcohol, Nicotine and Testosterone

Tobacco and alcohol abuse have a negative effect on sperm levels, libido and overall health. Cigarettes often act as a "gateway drug" leading to the abuse of other drugs. The longer people use alcohol, marijuana or nicotine, the lower their levels of testosterone fall and the higher the levels of estrogen rise.

People resist giving up drug habits that are so harmful to their hormones, minds and bodies because addiction is stronger than common sense. Health wins no prizes in the minds of those who are unhappy, stressed out or depressed, relying on the chemical reactions of drugs to get them through the day.

Besides damaged sperm, the consequences of drug abuse include a weakened immune system, and a heightened risk of heart disease, stroke and cancer. Prolonged reliance on drugs can result in lung or liver disease and enlarged breast tissue in men. Unfortunately, many health problems associated with drug use do not become obvious until later in life when it is too late to reverse their effects.

Not long ago cigarette companies were claiming that their products were safe and that users were responsible for choosing to become dependent. Losing their first class action suit was a wake-up call. Their defense faded away following strong language by the Surgeon General's report in 1999 stating that, "...nicotine is one of the most addictive substances known to man." People who stop using nicotine experience severe withdrawal symptoms including cravings like a rat gnawing at the stomach, irritability, anxiety, difficulty concentrating, increased appetite, and sleep disturbances.

Lung cancer and emphysema are well known health problems associated with heavy cigarette smoking. Tar and other pollutants in the smoke of cigarettes can initiate these illnesses. The real culprit, however, is nicotine, the powerful, habit-forming drug that can create dependence after only a few exposures. We are just beginning to realize the devastating effects of this poison on our society. The nicotine in five cigarettes is sufficient to paralyze and kill almost any insect. Toxins in nicotine and other pesticides threaten our hormonal balance and the normal sexual function of our citizens.

Prolonged use of popular drugs such as alcohol, marijuana and nicotine decrease testosterone and DHT levels. Certain high blood pressure pills, fungicidal medications, acid suppressors, and over-the-counter pain pills also lower testosterone levels. Studies show that smoking is the number one cause of ED, erectile dysfunction, in the Western world.

Most smokers never imagine the consequences of their habit on their sex life. They are lulled into a sense of complacency and a deceptive belief that "it won't happen to me." The alarming fact is that nicotine has the potential of rendering entire segments of our population infertile. We need to wake up, listen to our hormones and stop pretending that smoking doesn't affect our sexual performance and reproductive abilities.

Depression is another major factor relating to the loss of sexual drive and arousal.

David, a young man in South Carolina, blames his depression and low sex drive on low testosterone. "I have been experiencing symptoms such as fatigue, lack of motivation, severe depression, loss of sensation throughout my entire body, memory loss, difficulty concentrating, visual acuity, and especially loss of male sexual features such as strong voice, body strength, motor function controls, warm comfortable sensations, feeling of sexual arousal, etc.," he wrote in an email message to me.

He has suffered from depression for a year and a half. "I believe my testosterone levels are low," David continued. "I can't even get interested in girlfriends." For David, a diagnosis of low testosterone levels would be a relief. "I'm hoping my levels are low because I know there is a treatment for this," he said. "It is hard to believe it could be a hormone problem since I am only nineteen, but anything is possible."

Is it really possible that David has low testosterone levels at the tender age of nineteen? David's physical symptoms could very well be caused by other factors like depression or an inadequate diet or some hereditary condition. Very few young men that young experience testosterone deficiency unless they abuse alcohol, marijuana and nicotine during their formative years.

David doesn't seem to know what's causing his difficulty. In his correspondence with me, he didn't see any connection between his problem and his habit of smoking two packs a day plus his heavy use of alcohol, (one to two six-packs of beer each day.)

I suspect that David's problem is connected to nicotine and alcohol dependence. It has been pointed out that cigarettes are the only product legally manufactured and advertised in the United States that, when used as directed, will cause death and disease. The rate of addiction among regular cigarette smokers aged twenty-four and younger is rising though the overall popularity of smoking has dropped. Younger smokers have a stronger tendency to become addicted than those who are older.

The risk of cell damage from smoking and other environmental hazards in the early stages of life is apparently greater in males than in females. Reduced numbers of sperm produced, lower quality of sperm and less capacity of the sperm to penetrate or fertilize the egg are signs of damaged sperm cells caused by environmental toxins. Sperm with DNA damage have a lower fertilization rate and may be the cause of the delay in impregnation routinely seen in smokers.

There is more bad news! Drinking more than four cups of coffee added to smoking more than one pack of cigarettes will increase the number of dead sperm and decrease sperm motility. Smoking can also damage blood-clotting factors called platelets.

What about cigar smoking? Many people assume that cigar smoking doesn't pose a significant health risk since cigar smoke isn't usually inhaled to the same degree as cigarette smoke. Lung disease may not be as common among cigar smokers, but they are likely to encounter circulatory or heart-related health problems from toxins that are absorbed through the lining of the mouth. Carlos Iribarren, at Kaiser Permanente in Oakland, California underscored the dangers of cigar smoking, in a 1998 study. The overall death rate among cigar smokers was found to be twenty-five percent higher than for non-smokers.

The perils of smoking are drawing the attention of our country's leaders as never before. For the first time our government's "top doctor," Surgeon General Richard H. Carmona, has said publicly that he supports the banning of all tobacco products. Nicotine accelerates tolerance, physical dependence, and withdrawal symptoms more quickly than any other drug known to man. Nicotine exposure can lead to shrinking of the testicles, impaired sperm formation, poor semen quality, including decreases in sperm density and a lower count of total and living sperm.

What about the combination of alcohol and nicotine? For many sixty-year-old men, former abuse of alcohol and nicotine has a much greater impact on their sexual function than the aging process. Drinkers and smokers also have a tendency to develop higher blood pressure. The combination of nicotine, alcohol, and anti-hypertensive medications leads to the loss of erections.

When Shakespeare said, "Drink increaseth the desire and decreaseth the performance," he didn't realize how right he was. In men, a moderate amount of alcohol is considered to be about one ounce of pure alcohol per day. That is the equivalent of two beers, two glasses of wine or two shots of whisky. For women, half that amount is considered moderate consumption because women are more sensitive to alcohol than men.

The wine industry spends major chunks of their advertising budget promoting the consumption of wine as a way to reduce the risk of heart disease. The popular press has echoed their claims, giving considerable attention to the favorable effects of alcohol on the heart. To date, however, there are no controlled trials to prove this beneficial effect. There is some evidence that certain antioxidants in grape juice may be protective of the heart. As far as sexual health is concerned, however, studies indicate that past heavy drinking is definitely associated with a reduction in testosterone levels over time.

Men in their middle ages or older are unknowingly affected by alcohol-induced hypogonadism, a condition marked by impaired production of testosterone. Most physicians do not stress the relationship of these drug habits to their patients' hormones. Men develop greater tolerance to alcohol or other drugs over time but may not notice a problem with erections until their intake of alcohol becomes excessive.

Lobbyists and international corporations defend the legality of the two most abused drugs in our society—alcohol and tobacco. The American government has chosen to yield to financial and political pressures to protect industries that are damaging the health of the American public. It is time for our government leaders to stop talking about lofty goals for tomorrow's society and start listening to the symptoms of poor health and loss of reproductive vitality among the people of this country.

The sad reality is that the love Americans have for drugs will not disappear on its own. Rich and poor alike will continue to abuse their health by using excessive amounts of illegal and hazardous legal drugs for their intoxicating effects.

Drunk drivers are still the leading cause of death on the road. Drinking and smoking are popular with our youth, at parties and bars as well as at home and on the street. In states where smoking is permitted in bars, cigarettes and alcohol are social lubricants. A cigarette or a glass of whisky is a prop for people who are nervous about what to do with their hands.

In spite of that, there is a simple and effective way to eliminate the effect of dangerous toxins in tobacco and alcohol—avoid smoking and drinking altogether. This is not easy in a society where the use of these products is not only legal but actively promoted. Our government considers the economic losses measured by lost jobs and revenues as too great to risk crippling the industries that deliver these poisonous substances to our citizens.

Our hormones are warning us that testosterone is only the first victim of our nonchalance about the use and abuse of legalized drugs in the United States. Let's listen to these warnings and take steps to curtail the delivery of toxic products to the mothers, fathers, and the future generations of our culture.

## Dioxin, the Most Toxic Substance Known to Man

Did you know that the most toxic substance in the world is used to make credit cards? The manufacturing of vinyl is the leading source of dioxin in the US environment, and dioxin wins all the awards as the most deadly substance on the planet. First making its debut in the American consciousness as the herbicide "Agent Orange" used in the Vietnam war, dioxin is toxic at a dilution of less than five parts per trillion. It has been proven to *cause* cancer—not merely statistically linked to a higher risk of cancer.

Nobody manufactures dioxins on purpose. Dioxins are the unintended by-product of any process involving the burning of chemicals with a high chlorine content.

Pesticides, wood preservatives, and the burning of fossil fuels such as gasoline, and waste incinerator oil are all major contributors of dioxins. Meat, cheese, eggs, and milk products processed in industrialized countries also contain high levels of dioxin, but the primary source of dioxin in our environment is vinyl.

Vinyl is a plastic material used in house siding, windows, PVC pipes, medical packaging and credit cards. Vinyl makes it possible to own beautiful and inexpensive dishes and glasses. Many kitchen appliances, windows, furniture and some food containers are coated with vinyl.

Unfortunately, when vinyl breaks down—as it inevitably does over time or when it is heated or burned—it directly releases dioxin into the environment. When you cover food with a plastic wrap and turn on the microwave, dioxin can literally drip onto your food from the sheets of protective plastic. Your old computers and scanners are probably no longer welcome at your local landfill because they contribute a deadly stream of dioxin into the environment as they break down over time.

Globally, dioxin pollutants persist without restriction in many countries. The dioxin-producing pesticide DDT is still used in South America. Regrettably, dioxin is also a major factor contributing to infertility in men who spray dioxin/DDT to control the spread of malaria by mosquitoes. Dioxin from the sides of our houses, our furniture and appliances subsequently filters into our water and soil contaminating the food chain. Dioxin we absorb from foods enters our bodies by eating contaminated fats and meat by-products. Our livers are able to detoxify this poison by tucking it away in our body's fat.

This powerful hormone-disrupting chemical has become associated with testosterone deficiency. Testosterone deficiencies caused by dioxin in unborn babies can interfere with normal sexual development in males and affect fertility in adulthood.

The problem of infertility has spread to most of the Western world. A fertility rate of 2.1 births per woman is needed to maintain population levels. Instead, the U.S. rate hovers around 2.0 births per woman and in Europe has dropped to 1.42. Even in less developed countries where the impact on the population of a high birthrate is modified by high infant mortality rates and a short lifespan, the birthrate has dropped from 6.2 to 3.0 in the past thirty years. As a result of these trends, over the past four years the United Nations has reduced its projections for the world's total population in 2050 from 9.8 billion people to 8.9 billion. Experts estimate that another billion will be cut from the estimates within a few years.

Pollution from environmental estrogens has become a worldwide problem producing low sperm counts, miscarriages, and reproductive disorders. Babies exposed to dioxins before birth are more likely to have a lower IQ, learning disabilities, a short attention span, and damaged immune and nervous systems. Contamination from dioxin leads to a higher risk of asthma, allergies, diabetes, endometriosis and miscarriages.

Testosterone deficiency is becoming a pandemic, a worldwide epidemic. Future generations may be affected with decreased testosterone production after being exposed to dioxin as children. The failure of world leaders to take this threat seriously now endangers our planet's population. Our delicately balanced hormonal system that has evolved unchanged over eons is brittle and in danger of being damaged beyond hope of repair.

The facts are alarming, but little is being done about it. It's time to stop and listen to our hormones. Let's do something about them while we still have a chance.

## Let's Stop Poisoning Ourselves

How can we protect ourselves against pesticide exposure? One way would be to stay indoors or wear gas masks during dust storm activity when chemicals waft our way on the jet stream from Asia. Or we could only eat plants and avoid all animal fats. We could stop smoking, drinking and having fun. None of these would help much because poisons have permeated other aspects of our lifestyles!

Another group of hormone-like chemicals, a new batch of toxins, is threatening your testosterone levels. These newly discovered chlorine-based molecules are called "phthalates" and are derived from a relative of the dioxin molecule.

Phthalates are routinely used in soaps, shampoos, and nail polish and in medical products like tubing and plastics to keep them soft and flexible. Tests for phthalates on human urine samples from across our country show levels that exceed safe or acceptable levels. The levels were highest for two phthalate solvents used in American cosmetics, hair dyes, fingernail polish, and soft plastic containers. Undoubtedly, all plastic dishes, containers and plastic grocery bags contain phthalates. Phthalates are everywhere in our environment.

How do phthalates affect testosterone levels? They quickly block the androgen receptor. You will recall that when testosterone converts to DHT (dihydrotestosterone) at puberty, it exert a masculinizing effects on boys. DHT triggers the onset of puberty, penis development, sexual drive and other bodily changes by stimulating the androgen receptor. DHT increases muscle strength and causes the deepening of the voice, the growth of hair and enlargement of sexual organs, as boys become adolescents.

Studies indicate that phthalates can interfere with sex hormones and impair reproductive health by directly blocking the action of DHT on the androgen receptor. Researchers at the Harvard School of Public Health in Boston found phthalates in both semen and urine samples of at least seventy-five percent of volunteers attending a clinic for couples experiencing difficulty conceiving a child. Could there be a relationship?

Mature sperm counts rise in order to make reproduction possible. Phthalates interfere with this process by decreasing sperm counts and sperm maturation. Authors of a study from the journal *Epidemiology* in May of 2003 believe that dioxin exposure and the presence of phthalates could explain why semen quality in men is declining worldwide.

Phthalate and dioxin exposure has devastating effects on both young men and women. By acting as a potent estrogen, dioxin feminizes males, creating problems in sexual function and in the ultimate size of the sexual organs. To offset these negative effects, early testosterone monitoring and future supplementation as needed is essential if we are to restore fertility and normal sexual function in any affected males.

Environmental estrogens and androgens may be major contributors to the pandemic of breast, uterine and prostate cancers around the world. Estrogen-like compounds are not the only problem. Excess male hormones that can duplicate the action of testosterone seep into the rivers and streams in runoff from pulp and paper mills. These testosterone-like compounds affect fish and frogs in the wastes from these mills by masculinizing female fish. Fake hormones are all around us!

An excess of DHT from too much testosterone in the water around these old paper mills has been implicated in the changes seen in these fish. Sex ratios in fish swimming in pulp and paper wastes change dramatically, with more males than females. Herbicides, which are usually estrogen-like in rainwater, have been found to feminize male frogs. Testes with ovarian tissue have been found in wildlife and fish throughout the Great Lakes. Excess androgens may be masculinizing females in our society, while estrogens are feminizing males. This is a form of "equalization" of the sexes that is intolerable.

Active forms of all hormones are being detected in sewage wastes dumped into the oceans, eaten by fish and subsequently consumed by the public. When these affected fish are used as feed in salmon "farms," they increase the levels of pollutants in the tissues of this fish. Farmed salmon have been found to contain three times the amount of dioxin and thirty times the amount of PCBs of wild salmon. Excess dioxin can randomly alter the entire testosterone pathway of our bodies. In androgen target tissues such as the brain, dioxins cause permanent damage leading to conditions such as attention deficit hyperactivity disorder or ADHD.

While we can't totally avoid these toxins, we can minimize their potential effect by eliminating certain foods containing animal fats, including farmed fish. In most cases this means increasing carbohydrates, easily achieved by following a plant-based diet. But not everyone likes the idea of becoming a vegetarian. Many Americans are looking to low carbohydrate and high animal protein diets to help them lose weight. Chef-prepared meats and fish are considered a delicacy among our citizens. It takes real commitment to modify your diet and your lifestyle.

Even with a totally plant-based diet, it would still be almost impossible to avoid the plentiful plastics and cosmetics in our world. But eating more foods lower in the food chain definitely reduces our exposure to these toxic chemicals.

There are other things we can do, too. Using the indigestible fat Olestra™, for example, can remove up to seventy percent of the dioxin in the fat of our bodies. Cooking can also destroy fifty percent of the dioxin in foods. Watch out for raw meats and raw fish in sushi bars.

Foods placed in the microwave in plastic containers release phthalates that mimic estrogen directly into our foods. There is no such thing as a "safe," microwaveable plastic wrap, although the plastic industry is now promoting this feature. The best solution is to use only ceramic containers in the microwave oven. For similar reasons, plastic dishes and glasses should not be used for hot foods or foods with a high acid content. The acid can leach toxins directly from the plastic itself.

The use of cosmetics such as hair dyes and fingernail polish is a choice, not a necessity. You can take a big step in protecting yourself from harmful chemicals in our environment by decreasing your exposure to them.However, healthy and safe cosmetic products including lipstick, face cream and makeup removers are available if you make the effort to find them.

Organic food, including meats from animals organically raised without pesticides or hormones, are now widely available in American supermarkets. Fresh fruits and vegetables grown without pesticides are another way to enjoy good food that is free from harmful poisons.

Vitamins A, C and E are antioxidant vitamins. When used in conjunction with the beneficial bioflavinoids from fresh fruits, seeds, nuts and vegetables they can remove bioactive compounds, which cause DNA mutations and tissue damage. Locally grown fruits and vegetables are still the best reservoir of these beneficial anti-oxidants and phytonutrients. Antioxidants and other plant-based phytochemicals are helpful in stopping some of the harmful effects of dioxin in the diet.

I believe that the health of our children is worth the small extra cost of organic products or hormone therapy. Our future fertility and the lives of our descendants are in our hands. We need to do more to let our government representatives know that we want air, water and food that are free from toxins to protect our children and our fertility.

## Meat and the Development of Man

Killing animals for food is morally wrong for Jews, Buddhists, and Hindus. A growing number of people around the world feel for religious and other reasons that the flesh of animals should not be consumed as food. And for millions of others on the planet, meat eating is not an economical choice. Nonetheless, meat is a major part of the diet for one out of three people in the world today and has been a staple in the human diet for centuries.

Our need to survive influenced our biology. Primitive peoples hunted animals to supplement their diet of nuts and berries that they could forage. Women, who excel in verbal ability, in order to communicate with their children, probably developed language. Or, perhaps spoken communication was developed among men in order to improve their hunting strategies. Basic gender differences were based on the hunter-gatherer lifestyle, with men trained for the hunt and women for cooking and serving food.

On the plains and grasslands of the African savannah, primitive man developed the skills needed to hunt animals. Mankind would not have evolved to this point were it not for the cooperation of these early humans in their quest for meat.

High-quality protein obtained at the dawn of mankind made a definite contribution to the growth and refinement of the brain. In the early days of hunting and gathering for food, meat was a quick and easy supply of nutritious protein. The high protein load from meat apparently helped man's brain to grow, and hunting probably helped early humans to advance socially and physically.

Man continues to evolve today, still using animals for food, but the continued development of the brain no longer requires the proteins of animal flesh. The reality is that we do not have to eat meat for survival.

Another fact we need to consider is that in the early days of human history animals were not grain-fed but rather subsisted on range grasses, which are high in the healthy omega-3 fatty acids. This is definitely not the case today. Cattle, sheep, and pigs do relatively little grazing of grass-like plants, feeding instead on formulated mixtures of feed enhanced by additives often containing hormones and sometimes chicken manure or ground-up intestines from sheep and cows to enhance the protein levels of the feed. Livestock are kept in horrendous conditions and are often sick. Antibiotics are used routinely, often mixed in every meal the animals eat.

As a result of this practice, bacteria that are resistant to antibiotics have evolved, threatening the health of animals and people. The first case of "mad cow disease" in the US occurred at the end of 2003 in an infected cow in Washington State. Ironically, these animals that are fed body parts of other creatures are strict vegetarians who would eat only grass if allowed to graze at will.

Meat continues to play an important role in the diets of many people in "enlightened" countries and for those who can afford it, meat is often the primary source of food.

Meat is the major source of iron in the diet of carnivorous Americans, but this is not healthful. You may recall hearing that the free "heme" (iron), obtained from eating red meat, has been implicated in the creation of free radicals and damage to the heart muscle. High iron levels have also been blamed for an increased risk of heart attacks.

A study focusing on the differences between fatal and nonfatal cases of myocardial infarction (heart attack) indicated that the presence of heme iron was more pronounced in fatal cases, suggesting that a high dietary heme iron increase the fatality rate from heart attacks.

The huge waste of food involved in producing meat is another reason why meat does not make sense in today's world. About sixteen pounds of grain are required to grow one pound of beef. As little as one pound of grain can make a loaf of bread. Meat is prepared as food much less efficiently than a loaf of bread. Cornell researchers have calculated that meat from the most efficient factory farm returns 34.5 percent of the fossil energy it takes to provide the meat as food energy. The least efficient plant food, by contrast, delivers 328 percent as much energy as it consumes from fossil energy sources.

Another reason for avoiding meat is the tremendous amount of waste produced by animals harvested for food. A cow delivers 120 pounds of wet manure to the environment every day. Grazing livestock produce 250 to 500 liters of methane gas per animal per day. Methane has sixty times as much power as carbon dioxide in contributing to the "greenhouse effect," although it has less impact on our weather because it only remains in the atmosphere for ten years, compared to one hundred years for carbon dioxide.

Other sources of pollution that we would not have without our huge meat industry include the absorption of liquid manure into our groundwater, and the effects of supplying additional electricity and gasoline for preparing, refrigerating, and transporting meat products.

Almost every day new research into the effects of lifestyle and diet on the health of the individual explodes old myths. Undeniable facts emerge from this research about the contribution eating animal flesh makes to environmental pollution. "The beef industry has contributed to more deaths than all the wars of the century, all natural disasters and all automobile accidents combined. If real meat is your idea of 'real food for real people,' you'd better live real close to a real good hospital," says Neal Barnard, MD, President, Physicians' Committee for Responsible Medicine, used with permission from Johns Robbins' book, *The Food Revolution.*

Let's take a look at how meat eating affects immunity, a system so complex that we can't possibly explain it in a few pages. Healthy tissue does not become infected with viruses or bacteria unless our built-in resistance fails us due to high stress, poor diet, hormonal imbalance, deficiency in vitamins and minerals, low levels of solar energy, or some other factor.

Once we are sick, our immune system springs into action, fighting the invaders. The immune system will always recognize these foreign agents, called antigens and can remember the experience by producing antibodies to destroy the invaders the next time they enter the body.

Since toxins in meat can weaken our immune systems, doesn't it make sense that people who limit their diet to fruits, vegetables and grains, will have healthier immune systems than will meat eaters?

Edible mushrooms such as Shiitake, Coriolus and Reishi have been used in Asia for centuries to improve the function of the immune system. A new class of medicinal food products is manufacture by Mycological

Research Laboratories. In the UK clinical studies using these mushrooms as medicine are being conducted in patients with hepatitis, herpes and tuberculosis. Consuming food with fewer bacteria means fewer toxic products causing less disease. A few definitive studies have been published showing that vegetarians have more robust immune systems. Their exposure to dangerous bacteria such as *E. Coli* and salmonella, plentiful in spoiled or contaminated meats, can be close to zero.

We have abundant scientific evidence that meat is not essential for normal physiologic functioning. Since meat can be readily polluted with environmental estrogens, it is not a great leap of logic to assume that at some level contaminated meat may be noxious to humans.

Some say that meat once played a major role in the evolutionary development of intelligence, but if that is true, it does not follow that meat is essential in our diet today. Perhaps we have evolved past the point of needing to rely on meat. At the very least we should consider the fact that meat and other estrogen-laced foods can be hazardous to our health.

## Proteins, Fat and Energy in Meat

To qualify as obese, you must weigh twenty percent or more than your ideal weight. More than sixty percent of the American population is obese, and the rate of obesity is increasing so rapidly that if we keep it up every man, woman and child in the United States will be obese within the next decade!

The main reason Americans are getting fat is that we eat too much food and get too little exercise. In other words, we consume more calories than we burn. Too many of us live to eat instead of eating to live. One of the most fattening foods in the American diet is meat. We've always looked to meat as a primary source of energy. Remember that energy comes to us in food as calories, and if calories are not burned they become fat.

Many Americans are aware that meat contains a high percentage of fat in the form of cholesterol. They also know this is bad for them, but the taste hooks them. Meat is advertised as inexpensive, healthy, and nutritious, essential for energy and strength. The reality is that meat is very expensive, contaminated with bacteria, ecologically destructive and not at all healthy. In the end, meat just makes you fatter and is a major contributor to disease!

Meat in the process of breaking down delivers low fiber, rotting flesh laden with fat. In order to be used for fuel, meat and the fat it contains must first be converted into protein fragments known as amino acid molecules. During the digestive process, animal proteins are metabolized and reconfigured as amino acid portions to be used for human protein.

Meat requires high stomach acid concentrations and high digestive enzyme levels to break it down into these amino acid components. The process uses up quite a bit of energy, requiring an increase in the intestinal blood supply. Eating meat actually uses up energy in the short run. This is why most people feel tired after a large meat meal.

Dietary fat, on the other hand, is broken down to provide extra glucose to be stored in the muscles as glycogen or returned to the fat cells as fat. Although in the long run, the reserves of fat and muscle-stored sugars or glycogen might increase stamina, meat is definitely not a high-energy food, nor is it a good source of high quality protein for delivering quick energy.

In commercially processed meat today, bacterial putrefaction, parasitic infestation and contamination with fecal and urine are standard findings in animal carcasses from the slaughterhouses. In addition, synthetic hormones, pesticides and other chemicals have infiltrated this food source. At least one scientist, Deborah Cadbury, *The Estrogen Effect*, believes that meat with its high content of pesticide residue could be responsible for loss of sexuality early in life.

How can animals raised for food become a destroyer of sexuality? Animal fat, the basis of so many chronic diseases, contains the highest amount of dioxins, which act like estrogen. These toxic products, concentrated in animal fats, contaminate much of the meat, eggs, fish, poultry and dairy products eaten in industrialized countries. Estrogen mimics ultimately result in a hormonal imbalance, particularly in heavy meat eaters.

Meat can hardly be considered essential for life when two thirds of the people in the world are vegetarian. In minimal subsistence societies such as primitive villages in Africa and in Asia, the rain forests of South America or the slums of major cities in the US, people are starving and do not really care whether the meat they manage to scavenge is toxic. They simply want their bellies to feel full, and they think that meat is the only source of a complete food.

Americans can afford any diet they chose, but they like meat because of its taste. The smell of meat cooking over an open fire or on the barbecue stirs the primordial instincts and taste buds, stimulating our digestive juices. But meat today is not as good as it was in the days of our grandparents. Animals are no longer tended lovingly as barnyard pets or raised in small herds. Farms have become high-tech factories using hormones, antibiotics and special additives for the animals' feed instead of letting cows and sheep graze on the range or chickens scratch the soil for insects.

As a result, some of our supermarket meat is now high in deadly *E. Coli* bacteria and deficient in the essential fatty acids, the omega-3 fatty acids, created in the past by animals grazing on grass. The fat content of meat has risen dramatically in meat from commercial farms. Bison raised on the prairies, for example, contains 2.4 grams of fat per one hundred grams of cooked lean meat compared with today's beef, which contains 9.3 grams of saturated fat. In other words, beef from the supermarket contains about four times the amount of fat as bison raised on the plains.

Animal rights advocates express disdain for the way animals are treated before being sacrificed for human consumption. This perspective is slowly receiving acceptance in mainstream America. An example of the outrage some people feel can be found in the book, *Eternal Treblinka: Our Treatment of Animals and the Holocaust,* by Charles Patterson. The author compares our daily slaughter of millions of animals to the atrocities of Nazi Germany. In the foreword to the book, Lucy Rose Kaplan, a daughter of holocaust survivors, states, "I came to understand that the oppression of non humans on this Earth eclipses the ordeal survived by my parents." That may seem an exaggerated statement of passion, but it shows that people can be deeply upset about the amount of suffering involved in producing meat products for consumption in our society.

Research into diet and its effect on the health of the individual is correcting ancient tradition with undeniable facts. We know without a doubt that eating animal flesh contributes to pollution both within our bodies and in the environment. Compounds from meat and meat products are not essential for fabricating the hormones used by the brain and the body. Cholesterol, for example, is produced by the liver and does not need to be provided from the animal fat of meat, eggs or dairy foods.

The role food plays in disease is known only in part at this time. A new theory has emerged suggesting that the high cholesterol levels we observe in older people may be due to a deficiency of the enzymes needed to produce the hormones that are synthesized directly from cholesterol. The body, as it ages, tries to produce more cholesterol in order to increase the amounts of these hormones. Restoration of hormonal deficiencies could restore cholesterol levels back to healthy low normal levels.

Harmful metabolites of meat protein such as sulfates, phosphates, and nitrates are hard for the kidneys to filter out of the system. John Robbins, who advocates a plant-based diet for many reasons, states in his book, *The Food Revolution,* that a high meat protein diet in old age contributes to early kidney failure, osteoporosis and premature aging. Americans already have the world's highest incidence of cardiovascular diseases, due in large part to our meat-based diet.

If we factor in the cost of polluting our air, water and soil, the actual cost of meat is about ten times higher than the retail price consumers pay for meat at the supermarket.

Meat subsidies from the government keep the prices down. Direct US government payments to farmers totaled $12.2 billion in 1998, $22.7 billion in 1999, and an estimated $17.2 billion for 2000. Prior to its sale in the supermarket, the government subsidizes the meat industry so that a $35 per pound piece of meat ends up costing the consumer an average of $3.21 per pound for USDA choice cuts of beef. Because meat becomes contaminated with high numbers of bacteria, it must be refrigerated constantly to delay spoilage. If one considers shipping, trucking and the processing of meat, the actual cost of production is even greater.

Not all meat is laced with hormone additives. It is possible to find range-fed, cage-free meat, organically raised without hormones and considered safer to eat. In the Jewish tradition, meat is rendered kosher—safe to eat—by killing the animal in a merciful fashion and then draining all its blood. This theoretically removes all the traces of hormones released at death and disease-causing bacteria from the meat. Salting the meat repeatedly also helps to draw out the last traces of blood, the medium in which organisms multiply to transmit disease. You may not be excited about asking for kosher meat, but you'll have to admit that it cuts down on the risk of blood-borne disease.

The bacterial count of meat increases geometrically from the moment of death of the animal whether it is cooked, refrigerated or frozen. By the time meat is consumed by the public as hamburger, steak or chicken breast, the dead flesh has become loaded with harmful bacteria and parasites, among them salmonella, *E. coli*, trichinosis and tapeworms. Robbins asserts that meat has become the number one cause of food related deaths and illnesses, including heart disease related to high cholesterol levels.

The adulteration of beef from feeding entrails of other animals to the cows has created an environment for mad cow disease, which decimated livestock in England and France. In the wake of the mad cow scare, beef consumption has plummeted in Europe to half its former level.

In the US we keep eating meat at a level that is almost beyond belief. Meat comprises over *fifty percent* of the American diet, and advertising by fast food restaurants encourages higher consumption. The idea that there might be a market for vegetarian fare is making slow progress in the restaurant business. When Burger King became the first fast food restaurant to offer a plant-based burger on its menu in 2002, the event was world news.

In spite of a growing number of vegetarians in our midst—at least twelve million in the US at latest count—meat was purchased for food at the highest level ever in 2003. According to the US Department of Agriculture, Americans ate an average of 219 pounds of red meat, pork, and poultry that year, a staggering increase of 32 percent since 1960 when the average US citizen consumed 166 pounds of meat, including 64.5 pounds of beef per year.

Beef consumption in the US rose steadily in the sixties, seventies and early eighties, rising to an all time high in 1987 of 82.4 pounds per person. As a result of the tremendous amount of publicity and discussion following the 1987 publication of *Diet for a New America,* it dropped by twenty percent in the following five years and then began increasing again.

In North America we produce enough grain products to feed the entire world. The fact that almost one half of all the corn and one third of all the grain grown is used to feed and fatten animals is catastrophic. An estimated 130,000 cows and calves are slaughtered each day, according to the US Department of Agriculture. Not counting fish and other aquatic creatures, ten billion birds, animals, and other creatures are slaughtered for food every year in the U.S.

Some experts like John Robbins and Peter Burwash, who founded an environmental group known as "EarthSave" believe that our dependence on flesh-based diets creates most of pollution on our planet. "Moving away from an animal based diet to a plant-based diet will decrease world pollution and decrease all chronic diseases," said EarthSave's scientific director, Dr. Michael Klapper in 1996.

## Cutting our Toxic Load

Every day we lose large chunks of earth trampled and loosened by overgrazing cattle, sheep, and pigs and blown or washed out to the sea. This amounts to a net loss of about a thousand acres of topsoil per year. Iowa has lost half of its fertile topsoil over the past century and is continuing to lose topsoil at an alarming rate.

When our natural resource base deteriorates as a result of topsoil depletion and pollution of our groundwater, we pass on a weakened capacity for future generations to prosper and enjoy good health. Consider the decline of ancient civilizations in Mesopotamia, the Mediterranean region, Pre-Colombian southwest U.S. and Central America. Historians believe that these cultures disappeared into vapor because of their failure to make a successful transition from subsistence farming to an agricultural economy robust enough to support large populations.

To help preserve our farmland, we could alter our diet and become healthier by eating more of a plant-based organic diet. Vegetarianism involves a highly rewarding lifestyle that fosters respect for oneself and other animals. Not eating the flesh of dead animals gives us a longer lifespan, decreases chronic disease and improves our ability to control our weight. Vegetarian or not, we would all be better off if we stopped eating so much meat. At the very least we should avoid animal fats because of the very real possibility that they are laden with deadly bacteria and too much dioxin.

Toxic chemicals such as dioxin affect our farm-raised animals as well as our wildlife. Fortunately, toxic residues are not readily incorporated into many fruits, vegetables, cereal grains or other plant materials if they are present in the soil or sprayed on the growing plant. Many pesticide residues can be washed off or peeled off in the outer leaves of plants or the skin of fruit. Toxic substances in meat are embedded into the cells of the meat tissue and cannot be removed.

We should never eat the brains of any animal and should avoid all organ meats because these are the body parts most likely to be contaminated with toxins from the environment as well as brain proteins called "prions," which can reproduce themselves and can cause mad cow disease.

Of course we can't avoid all exposure to environmental toxins in the food chain and in our water and air, but by modifying our food choices we can reduce the toxic load on our bodies by almost fifty percent.

## Recommendations for Healthy Living

I am going to share with you seven simple recommendations that will make it easier for you to follow a vegetarian or Asian/Mediterranean type diet. We would all be healthier by substituting meat with soy, consuming eggs only from free-range chickens (if at all), insisting on low-fat dairy products from organically fed cows and focusing on soy, tofu, seeds and nuts. Here are my recommendations—

**Avoid animal fats.** Most types of meat, but especially organ meat, as well as eggs, milk, cheese and margarine are high in saturated animal fats. Most of these foods are also contaminated with toxic amounts of environmental xenoestrogens. If you must eat meat, use organic chicken without the skin and avoid farmed fish. Remove the skin and cook all fresh fish thoroughly (baking, poaching and broiling is best). Better yet, eat soybean products such as tofu, vegeburgers, and tempeh instead. John Robbins' books on alternative diets will give you more details on this subject.

**Eat more fresh fruits, vegetables and seed oils.** These colorful foods are your best source for vitamins and other nutrients essential for good health. Fruits and vegetables do not contain fat or processed sugar. Choose healthier fats such as flaxseed, safflower, sunflower seed, peanut, walnut, avocado, pumpkin seed, sesame, and grapeseed oils. Most seeds and nuts are also healthy options for high quality proteins and make delicious additions to salads, snacks and baked goods. Lentils, soybeans and fat free refried beans are great protein sources.

**Do not use plastic containers and plastic wraps for storing food.** The toxins in plastic can leach into the food you are trying to protect. Be safe and replace plastic with wax paper or glass jars. Use ceramic dishes only for serving or heating food. Never microwave food in plastic containers.

**Ask your doctor to test your hormone levels.** If your levels test low in serum or salivary testing, request a prescription of the deficient hormone. Remind the doctor to test free hormone levels as well as total and protein-bound levels.

**Stay away from saturated fats and trans fats.** Avoid all fried foods, refined sugars and corn syrup or diet foods, as they contain chemicals associated with an increased risk of cancer. Commercial products such as trans fatty-acid-free Smart Balance® buttery spread sold in supermarkets and health food stores across the country are great sources of healthy unsaturated fats. To avoid contamination from mercury, avoid or cut back on eating fish from the Great Lakes and all farmed salmon. Nordic Naturals (Watsonville, California) is one company that removes all the mercury as well as the "fishy" taste from their fish oil capsules. For those deep-fried snacks that you love, make sure they were made with Olestra, an indigestible fat substitute, which may help to eliminate dioxin.

## Elevate your mood by eating more foods that encourage production of serotonin in your brain.

Bananas, tomatoes, plums, avocados, pineapples, eggplant, walnuts and dates and figs are high in compounds known as serotonin precursors. These compounds do not directly produce serotonin but make it easier for your brain to manufacture and release this natural mood-elevating hormone into your bloodstream.

## Eat more natural foods rich in healthful minerals.

Increase your intake of minerals such as selenium, zinc, calcium, magnesium, iron and copper by eating more fresh fruit, vegetables, seeds and nuts. Incorporate one antioxidant supplement (picnogenol, quercitin, ginger, garlic) into your daily diet to reduce the toxicity from dioxins, PCBs, and phthalates and other toxic compounds. You'll also want to eat more bioflavinoids, bioactive antioxidants as found in Juice Plus®, Vitamins K, A, C, E, D, ubiquitone, and folic acid.

Lycopenes are antioxidants found in watermelon, grapes, tomatoes and some shellfish. Lycopenes are only released by cooking the food. They seem to help to treat dioxin-induced infertility in men. Lycopenes are one class of the 650 carotenoids found in high concentrations in the testicles of normal males and in low levels in infertile males. Physicians are studying the use of lycopenes as a nutrient useful in preventing prostate cancer.

Hope is alive that one day we can clean up our environment and produce a safe food supply for the American people without the presence of toxins destructive to our endocrine system such as PCBs, PVCs, TCDDs, and dioxin. Until that time, if you want good health you should modify your food choices and focus on a plant-based diet with an intelligent selection of supplements of bioflavinoids, antioxidants and vegetable oils free from trans-fatty acids. Again, if you must eat fried foods, try those made with Olestra.

Each person is a powerful force for change. We should make a noble effort to save our planet for our children. If someone becomes a vegetarian, awareness of this lifestyle choice can help to stop the senseless slaughter of animals, and one small change can help to decrease the ongoing pollution of our world.

## Can We Still Save the Planet?

In view of the fact that our food is contaminated, our water polluted, our fish filled with mercury, PCBs and dioxins and our animals loaded with toxic waste, some people feel that there is nothing safe to eat. This is not true.

The safest and healthiest choice for a well-balanced diet is one with an abundance of fruits and vegetables. Compared to the situation in some other countries, our food is generally very safe. Fruits and vegetables are much "cleaner" than flesh foods and far less likely to cause disease.

Nevertheless, we should maintain strict monitoring of fruits exported to our supermarket from countries that continue to use banned pesticides such as DDT and a group of closely related pesticides known as organophosphates that affect the functioning of the nervous system. Bananas and many other kinds of fresh fruit in the supermarket are examples of fresh produce that come to us from Central and South America after being sprayed with pesticides that have been banned for use in the US. These contaminants can be washed off or peeled away with the skin. Mother Nature wraps bananas in a tough and effective barrier against toxic chemicals.

Beef and meat from turkeys and chickens that are organically fed and raised free from hormones are safer to eat than those injected with hormones and other growth-enhancing substances. Of course, hormones are not inherently bad. We carry them in our bodies and have developed an intricate hormone-regulated system over millions of years. Problems occur from hormonal imbalance caused by exposure to environmental toxins and the natural loss of certain hormones with aging.

The FDA approves the use of animal hormones through their Department of veterinary medicine. The FDA states that agricultural hormones leave only small residual concentrations in the meat. The European Economic Community does not agree and has banned the use of hormones in meat and dairy production. I hope that FDA regulators will consider the long-term effects the hormones might have when they spill into the environment and enter our food chain. A substantial portion of the hormones pass unchanged through the cattle into their feces and end up in the environment. Hormonal drugs do not become neutral over time but retain their effects in the excrement of animals.

Instead of hunting for meat, modern man raises animals in large commercial farms. We devote more land in North America to raising cattle, pigs, chickens, sheep, and other farm animals than to acreage inhabited by people. We also lavish half of our total water supply in the US on animals we raise as food and use twenty-five hundred gallons of water to produce a pound of beef. Only twenty-five gallons of water are needed to grow one pound of wheat.

Every year American farmers send thirty million head of cattle to feedlots where the animals get "beefed up" on high protein chow. The feedlot diet consists of corn and other grains with soy fillers added for protein. Sometimes body parts of sheep or chickens are ground up as protein boosters and fed to cattle, which never consume animal products in their natural state. This practice has led to problems with meat safety, including the risk of mad cow disease.

Then there is the use of steroids. To enhance the production of more lean muscle, livestock producers now treat more than 90 percent of all feedlot cattle with steroid hormones.

Cows typically receive steroids from a controlled-release device implanted in their ears. These hormones offer a bonanza to the breeders. It costs farmers only about one to three dollars per cow to treat their livestock with hormones and boost the animal's growth by as much as twenty percent. For each pound it gains, an animal on steroids consumes fifteen percent less feed than does an untreated animal. This works out to a cost saving of about forty dollars per head. The farmer gets more beef for less money.

Much of the food we eat is tainted with pesticides. Toxins from these pesticides along with active hormones are added to the feed of cattle and chickens. These chemicals are stored in the animal's fat, especially in milk, butter, cheese and eggs, a major part of most American diets.

Toxic dioxin-like pesticides mimic and disrupt normal hormone action in both people and animals. Yet the weakest of these steroid growth promoters found in animal tissue is one hundred to one thousand times stronger in biological activity than the most potent industrial pollutants. By disrupting our hormonal balance, hormone-like agents have the potential for greater harm than almost any other substance we can ingest.

What about global warming? Greenhouse gases generated by our power plants are destroying the earth's protective layer of ozone. The amount of electricity required to refrigerate dead animal flesh to stop it from spoiling is a major factor in electrical energy shortages. Trucks, airplanes and trains used to transport frozen meats, result in heavier use of fuel and by-products that are major contributors to the greenhouse effect. Global warming could melt the glaciers at the poles, raise ocean levels and flood coastal cities. The resulting weather changes would lead to drought and an acute water shortage or another Ice Age.

Can one person make a difference in stemming the tide of toxic pollution and destruction of our planet? Of course! All improvement begins with one person, one idea and one purpose. Albert Einstein expressed it like this: "Nothing will benefit human health and increase the chances for survival of life on earth as much as the evolution to a vegetarian diet."

Evidence abounds on every hand that the foods we eat are not only making us fat but are also exposing us to a high risk of debilitating illness and inability to have babies. It's time to start paying attention to the evidence and make life-style changes that will put us in harmony with the natural forces that make life as a human so rewarding.

We need to listen to the warning signs. It is not too late.

# 5

## Please share this chapter with your physician

# A Hormone Checkup

## Self-Esteem, Aggression and Testosterone

Bobby is bullying younger children at school. Barry is biting the baby-sitter. Tom is yelling at everyone because he is convinced that they're all scheming to drive him crazy. As Mary goes through her "time of the month" she is sure that everyone else has an attitude problem.

Are these examples of emotional problems or too much—or too little—hormone?

The answer depends on which sex hormones are at play at what point in an individual's life. During puberty boys are expected to become more aggressive due to increases in testosterone. Girls going through puberty also may show disrespectful behavior triggered by outpourings of estrogen.

Aggressiveness is commonly defined as a generalized disposition to engage in physically combative or competitive interactions with male peers. Is this what's happening with Bobby or Tom, or are they merely developing their ego and self-confidence? The picture is considerably more complex than it may appear at first glance.

Sometimes aggression is associated with irritability or anger. Does that mean testosterone is the culprit? Not at all. Sharp increases in testosterone levels can produce aggressive behavior that may include competitiveness related to job performance and physical and verbal aggression. These activities have been labeled "testosterone behaviors," but that does not necessarily mean they are bad.

Competition and desire for dominance are usually associated with aggression, and in this way aggressive behavior can be seen in a favorable light as an inspiration for motivation, high self-esteem and strong leadership qualities. In men, a competitive drive for financial success is related to testosterone dominance. Studies show that younger men are more competitive than older men in a variety of areas, but they are also more physically and verbally aggressive than women. These behaviors are often related to the higher testosterone levels commonly seen in these young men. So high testosterone does drive certain types of behavior.

The highest testosterone levels are seen in prosecuting attorneys, actors, doctors and business executives. You probably know of aggressive women who have succeeded in these occupations, but their success is generally thought of as demonstrating "masculine characteristics."

In general, men are driven to succeed by testosterone. They want to prove their manhood and believe this requires playing a dominant role in the family, workplace, and society. In their desire to surpass others, some men will turn to drugs to give them that "edge." Drugs, which increase testosterone as a rule, affect the self-regulating system creating serious problems down the road.

Higher levels of testosterone have often been blamed for physically aggressive behavior in men. In one study using four times the normal dose of testosterone, self-reported ratings of aggressive feelings did not increase.

Contrary to common wisdom, this study was one of several which seemed to point the finger at the sudden drop in testosterone, rather than elevated testosterone levels, that result in aggressive behavior in both males and females, as was generally assumed.

This paradox in the interaction of "male" and "female" hormones relies on the actual effect of free testosterone on the brain, which creates more estrogen. An enzyme called aromatase encourages the rapid conversion of brain testosterone into estrogen. This might explain how testosterone action on estrogen receptors can cause moodiness and feelings of violence.

Aggression has several components, which we can classify as either physical or sexual. "Physical" aggression is expressed as socially acceptable conduct. "Sexual" aggression, on the other hand, is often not acceptable in social settings. It may make itself known as increased sexual activity in healthy young men. Physical aggression seems to correlate most closely with high estradiol levels while sexual aggression is associated more closely with high dihydrotestosterone or DHT levels. Whether it is physical or sexual, aggression engages the brain in a complex interaction of hormones because both DHT and estradiol originate from the conversion of free testosterone.

Whether it makes itself known by a lack of desire or the inability to perform sexually, hormonal dysfunction that results in aggression can interfere with life's basic social and physical needs. Yet, the human body is amazing in its efficient self-regulating systems. Hope is therefore available for people with less than their fair share of hormones.

Accurate testing and appropriate therapies can restore normal function in the majority of men—and women—with hormone deficiencies. All you have to do to do is to take the time to stop where you are and listen to your hormones. Paying attention to them is the first step in restoring the harmony.

## The Big T

Testosterone leads the parade of hormones in importance, especially for men but comes in dead last in terms of understanding by medical and non-medical persons alike. I call testosterone "The Big T" because powerful hormone has such a huge impact on our bodies.

In the first chapter of this book we looked at several of the distinguishing functions of testosterone in the male, including penis and beard growth and the enabling of the penis to become erect for sexual intercourse. Because of its power to create manliness, testosterone is the undisputed king of the hormones. The Big T has total sovereignty in men.

Like other hormones we have discussed in this book, testosterone is a steroid hormone produced by our body to perform vital tasks in regulating, stimulating, and controlling our body and our brain. Similar to other fatty compounds, testosterone consists of molecules of hydrogen and carbon bound so tightly together that they shed water and dissolve only in oil or alcohol. This fact allows testosterone to enter the brain.

All steroids, including DHEA, androstenedione, androstenediol, and DHT, are variations of the same basic configuration. They are called endogenous hormones, meaning the body produces them naturally. Other steroids, manufactured by chemical manipulation to mimic the structure and effects of naturally occurring steroids, are called exogenous steroids because they originate outside the body.

The word "testosterone" has found its way into everyday vocabulary because of its association with male virility and raw muscular power. Testosterone has been around for ages, but in the 1960s it was discovered by athletes as a way to gain an edge, by becoming bigger, stronger, faster and better than their opponents. The athletic use of testosterone rapidly deteriorated to abuse, eventually leading to prohibitions by the Food and Drug Administration in 1969 when it was reclassified as a Class III substance.

As important as the Big T may be, when testosterone falls below acceptable levels, a man's sexual performance and physical and emotional security suffer. Unrecognized and untreated, testosterone deficiencies cause untold physical and emotional problems for millions of men and women. The misuse of this powerful hormone can have devastating effects on men—and on women as well.

How can you find out if you have a problem with any of your endogenous hormones and treat it appropriately? Read on.

## Diagnosing Testosterone Deficiency

Mark and Phil share office space in their family practice center, and one afternoon they pause to chat a bit about testosterone testing.

"My patient wants me to check his testosterone," Mark says, "so I'm just going to run a test to see what his total T level is. That should be enough tell me if there's a serious deficiency, shouldn't it?"

"Not necessarily," Phil replies. "I've been reading up on this, and what I'm finding is that a blood test for total testosterone doesn't give a complete picture. The amount of testosterone that is actually available to tissues and organs is more important, even though it's only about one or two percent of the total testosterone. We've been looking at the wrong part of the testosterone supply, seems to me."

"Yeah, but is the extra testing worth the expense? Can't we just extrapolate?" Mark tucks his stethoscope into his coat pocket and disappears into an exam room as he mumbles, "We've always measured total T."

Phil is on the right track, but too many doctors stop where Mark did, assuming that testing total testosterone test is sufficient.

Both Mark and Phil should be using newer sensitive tests that have been developed to measure "free" (or circulating) hormone levels of testosterone and other hormones in saliva or blood. Physicians who specialize in endocrinology get a comprehensive hormone profile and want to know a patient's levels of bioavailable testosterone (BT) and dihydrotestosterone (DHT) in addition to their total testosterone levels. They will also test for the pituitary hormones—prolactin and luteinizing hormone, as well as the sex hormone binding protein known as SHBG.

However, primary care doctors are too busy to do all these hormone tests. You may be getting the idea by now that knowing your blood levels of free testosterone as well as other hormones is a good step to take in planning for your future health. I couldn't agree more.

Free testosterone increases sexual drive and permits firm long-lasting erections in males. In females, free testosterone helps lubricate their sex organs and contributes to orgasmic ability. Research indicates that the frequency of ejaculation and sexual drive are all related to how much free testosterone is circulating in the body. Free testosterone provides a much more accurate prediction of a man or woman's hormonal deficiency than total testosterone.

Even if total testosterone levels could measure sexual activity, there is a huge variability in levels of this hormone among the sexes. At this point, there is no single value indicating a "normal" blood level of testosterone for the different age groups. In addition, testosterone levels in an individual vary from hour to hour. Because the highest testosterone levels occur in the morning, sometimes taking an average of three morning specimens proves more accurate. The generally acceptable range of total testosterone values falls between 270 and 1,200 nanograms per deciliter (ng/dl). A nanogram (ng) is one billionth of a gram, and a deciliter is one hundredth of a liter. A liter is equal to about one quart.

An even more precise assessment of testosterone activity is to measure bioavailable testosterone, a fancy word for testosterone that is available to interact with the androgen receptor. In simple terms, bioavailable testosterone includes the free testosterone component of human blood. About one third of the total testosterone is bioavailable. About two percent of testosterone in men and one percent in women is free testosterone.

We have learned that measuring free or bioavailable testosterone gives us a much better estimate of how masculine (androgen) hormones are functioning in the body than does measurement of total testosterone. Certain labs have now determined age-specific normal ranges of bioavailable testosterone and have been able to document the fact that it declines with aging. (See Appendix A.) When bioavailable testosterone levels drop too low, symptoms such as loss of sexual drive, lack of orgasms, and erectile dysfunction result.

Nonetheless low testosterone levels cannot always be easily identified by a physical examination, even with a clinical profile showing the amount of testosterone in its various forms. Only a complete picture of the hormone interrelationship: bioavailable testosterone, DHT, SHBG and estradiol can provide a proper diagnosis, but some medical detective work is still required. How can you help your doctor in this regard?

To assist your doctor in determining a possible testosterone deficiency, men should provide a detailed medical and sexual history. Major illnesses, all prescription and non-prescription drugs currently being used, past hormonal and drug or steroid use, family or other relationship problems, sexual difficulties and major life events or changes—as well as information about the health of immediate family members will help the doctor pinpoint the basis for the problem. The doctor can use these bits and pieces as clues to make an accurate diagnosis.

You can't refer to a simple chart on the wall to check to see if there is a testosterone deficiency. Hormone levels vary widely from person to person. Age, sex, sexual orientation and race each play a role in the diagnosis of hormone deficiencies. Asian men and women, for example, develop lower testosterone levels as they age, and African Americans have higher testosterone levels at any age than do white Europeans. Homosexuals seem to notice a testosterone deficiency at a much earlier age than heterosexuals.

On average, male testosterone levels drop by about 110 nanograms per deciliter for each decade of life. By age fifty, men's levels may be 550 points lower than at birth. Ideally hormone levels should be checked at around age thirty-five to determine a baseline for future evaluation. Differences in age, race, activity, sexual appetite, prior use of hormones and drug or alcohol use can all affect hormone test results.

As complicated as detailed laboratory testing may be, without an accurate hormone determination, precise hormone replacement therapy is impossible. One reason is that too much hormone in the dose can change its action completely, causing a totally opposite effect to what was intended. One more common problem is the huge variability of testosterone numbers from one man to another and throughout his lifetime.

If you have a sexual dysfunction such as a loss of libido or sexual desire, your personal physician might also want to test the two common by-products of testosterone conversion, estradiol (E2) and dihydrotestosterone (DHT) that are commonly associated with these problems.

In my clinic we routinely test major hormone levels in my male patients at the initial visit and for those on replacement therapy to be sure they are absorbing adequate testosterone and not getting too much or too little. We monitor testosterone for about one to three months until levels stabilize. Then we fine-tune estrogen, testosterone, DHT and DHEA levels, measuring as often as every three to six months, using a reputable endocrine laboratory for all testing. I recommend testing for all men over the age of thirty-five.

All men notice less intense sexual arousal as they get older, but a man who suddenly loses his erections and starts getting "hot flashes" definitely has a hormonal problem. It could be due to low testosterone or some other hormone. The same can be said for a young man who is unable to grow a beard and a mustache or cannot develop a muscular physique after working out for years with weights. Specific penile reflexes will also provide a clue to testosterone deficiency or hypogonadism.

I am seeing younger and younger men with testosterone deficiency (hypogonadism), some of whom I refer to hormone specialists. Endocrinologists, our primary hormone specialists, usually follow guidelines from the American Academy of Clinical Endocrinologists (AACE) for the treatment of men with low testosterone. While these guidelines give clear information about hormone replacement for any man with a testosterone deficiency, most family practice doctors do not follow them and do not even know that they exist.

Guidelines recommend but do not insist on the types of testing a doctor should order when total testosterone is in the normal range but symptoms of hormonal deficiency are still present. Like Mark, the physician we overheard earlier in this chapter, many physicians are unaware of these new findings, and keep on measuring total testosterone, telling their patients they are "normal" when results are within the normal range even though they may have symptoms of possible deficiency. Consequently, millions of men are not being properly diagnosed—or treated.

The complete AACE guidelines for testosterone prescribing, published in 1998, are too complex for most non-medical people, but if you've carefully read the definitions and explanations, you can probably understand much of the information.You can find them at www.aace.com/clin/guidelines/sexdysguid.pdf.

Translated into plain English, the guidelines state that all men with symptoms of a testosterone deficiency should be treated with hormone replacement therapy. These guidelines are written for doctors but are usually followed only by endocrinologists who treat hypogonadism. If you are having trouble finding an endocrinologist, you can find a list by state in the URLs in the appendix of this book. Also the Endocrine Society 2001 andropause consensus meeting provides recommendations for the diagnosis of hypogonadism. These are available at www.endo-society.com.

The guidelines suggest further testing for patients with symptoms of low testosterone whose test results indicate normal levels. These patients should be retested for free testosterone and sex hormone-binding globulin levels.

A single low testosterone measurement is not enough to establish a diagnosis of hypogonadism. Levels of follicle-stimulating hormone, luteinizing hormone, and prolactin should also be measured—and maybe semen analysis, pituitary imaging studies, genetic studies, bone densitometry, testicular biopsy, and specialized hormonal dynamic testing should be included.

Any medical laboratory can perform most of these tests, but certain endocrine labs specialize in these types of evaluation and are better able to provide consistently accurate and reproducible results. These labs are listed in the appendix for your reference.

The guidelines do not attempt to explain why physicians are seeing more cases of testosterone deficiency in civilized countries. Though numerous environmental factors have been mentioned, more research is needed in order to understand how these factors might be creating the epidemic of testosterone deficiency.

If your doctor is unable to help you and you would like a consultation, I have made myself available through our online service at my website at www.WellnessMD.com or you can obtain a secure email consultation with me at www.Kryger.medem.com.

## The Origin of Testosterone and Estrogen

The human body manufactures testosterone from cholesterol, so we call all such related compounds steroids. Steroid molecules form a four-ring structure that supports additional side rings, and these rings give the molecule its special characteristics. Cholesterol turns out to be the primary substance from which our bodies form testosterone and estrogen. You don't have to go on a high-fat diet to make enough cholesterol to manufacture the hor-

TESTOSTERONE

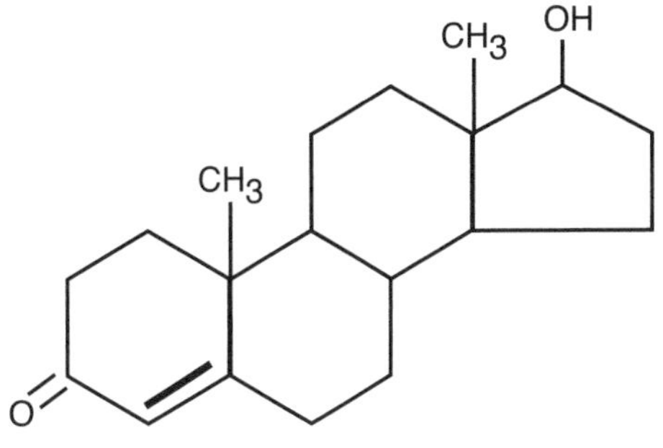

$CH_3$ OH

$CH_3$

O

Testosterone

mones your body needs because only a small amount is required to make all of the hormones that govern your body.

The word "steroid" points to the origin of these substances, coming from "sterol" in the word, "cholesterol." The first step in fabricating all the hormones is the conversion of cholesterol to pregnenolone. Pregnenolone itself is not a true hormone, but is the immediate precursor for the synthesis of all of the steroid hormones. Sometimes pregnenolone is called the "grandmother of all hormones" because it is essential for the production of all sex hormones. Pregnenolone is found in many places in our bodies, including the adrenal glands, liver, skin, testicles, ovaries, and even the brain and the retina at the back of our eyes.

The pollutant dioxin interferes in the development of pregnenolone from cholesterol. Unfortunately, cholesterol added to our body from a high animal fat diet contains components such as oxidized low-density cholesterol (LDL), which can plug up our blood vessels. Newly incorporated cholesterol does not always convert to essential hormones because some of the enzymes needed to make the conversion possible are destroyed by dioxin. Unaware of the futility of the task, the liver keeps making more and more cholesterol.

The amount of cholesterol in our bodies increases with aging even if we don't consume more cholesterol in our food. This could be because the pathways that convert cholesterol to the various steroid hormones become

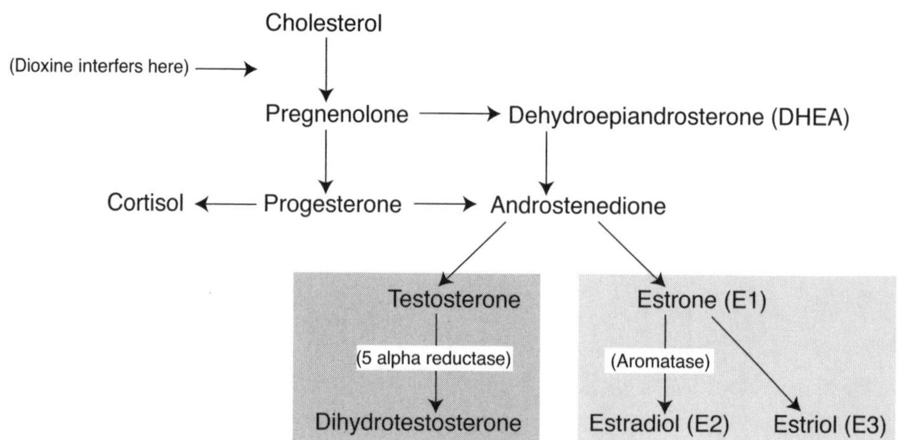


SYNTHESIS OF HORMONES

impaired as we age. Life-long exposure to dioxin could interfere with the development of the entire hormone sequence from cholesterol. Recognizing the decline in hormone levels, the body signals its need for more hormones and, as a result, there may be a corresponding increase in cholesterol production.

"Hormone restorative therapy," is a term coined by Sergey Dzugan and Arnold Smith, two physicians who undertook to correct hormonal deficiencies in aging persons in a six-year study on the factors affecting cholesterol levels. By receiving broadly based hormone replacement therapy, the sixty-three patients in the program were not only able to correct their hormone deficiency but also to restore their cholesterol levels to normal. This relatively new theory has not been proven.

We need more research about toxic exposure. Perhaps we could then better understand why the accumulation of environmental toxins over time could increase our cholesterol counts and decrease the levels of other hormones such as DHEA and DHT.

## Do You Know Your Hormone Levels?

"A single measurement of testosterone is not sufficient to diagnose hypogonadism," according to Dr. Adrian Dobbs, a respected Johns Hopkins endrocrinologist. Your doctor can order a blood test that shows your blood levels of the different hormones. For some men the optimal testosterone level is below average; for others it is higher. In addition to your total testosterone, your doctor should have your circulating or free testosterone level measured because sexual desire is more closely associated with this form.

At a level of free testosterone that is just right for you, you should enjoy enhanced erotic urges, experience the desire for frequent sexual activity and feel more sleep-related erections. The effects of total testosterone on spontaneous erections are not totally clear.

Hypogonadism (low levels of total testosterone) must be detected and treated early with adequate doses of testosterone replacement in order to restore normal sexual function. We know that morning or night-time erections should occur daily in a man with normal penile function. The diagnosis of hypogonadism requires an early morning blood test to check the testosterone level before starting any hormone therapy in men under forty. For the most accurate results in younger men, samples can be collected between 6 and 8 a.m. on three different days.

You may experience some physical or psychological symptoms associated with low testosterone even if your testosterone levels are within a normal range. Be sure to discuss these symptoms with your doctor. In some cases determining your levels of free testosterone, the sex hormone binding globulin (SHBG), and dihydrotestosterone (DHT) will provide more useful information than will measurements of total testosterone alone. These values plus estradiol and prolactin will assist your own doctor in making a diagnosis of hypogonadism.

Tom, a 34-year-old married man with two children, wrote to me about his low sexual libido was beginning to affect his marriage.

"I get lots of exercise," he wrote. "I watch what I eat, am not depressed, get a good amount of sleep, and have a satisfying job. I seem to have not much interest in sex and have not had sex yet this year. I also feel old and tired. My lack of sexual enthusiasm is hurting my relationship with my wife. I have heard that there may be new ways to regain a more active sexuality and I would like to try."

Tom's story seems compatible with low levels of free testosterone, the major enabling ingredient for sexual enthusiasm. In addition, Tom may be deficient in another hormone, oxytocin, which we have discussed as critical for a man to climax with a strong erection and produce a maximum volume of ejaculate.

Orgasm is therefore a neurohormonal response. That is, it requires both hormones and neurotransmitters to come about. Dopamine and norepinephrine, two essential neurotransmitters, are fundamental for nerves to communicate properly. These compounds peak with orgasm, at which point endorphins flooding the brain create feelings of pleasure and contentment. A drowsy or sedated feeling often follows. This post-orgasmic relaxation time is known as the refractory period and lasts from one to twelve hours in men but is much shorter for women. You may recall that prolactin, released in the brain, regulates this refractory period.

The time required after an orgasm for a man to develop another erection increases with age. Young men can ejaculate as many as four times in a night but as they age, this thrilling ability drops to only once each day. As we mentioned earlier, women can experience orgasm repeatedly, the frequency of multiple orgasms depending on their level of oxytocin.

Once the trapped blood leaves the penis after ejaculation, the sexual act is completed. The penis subsequently becomes "flaccid" or soft. A satisfactory erection involves a sequence of activities as previously outlined, each driven by different hormones and their interactions. Ignorance of the actual stages involved in the sexual act can occasionally lead to embarrassment.

Email from a twenty-two-year-old illustrates this confusion about what is normal or abnormal in terms of erectile function.

"Hey Doc," Michael wrote in cool email prose. "how ya been....?"

Michael and his girlfriend had spent a weekend of sexual pleasure—"a ton of sex"—but on the second day when he went for "Round Six," he found he'd lost his steam. "I couldn't keep an erection," he said, "but the next morning I was fine and we went at it a bunch of times and then the same thing happened later that evening. I just wanted to make sure this was normal, and that guys can wear out so to speak. I wanted to know if there was anything I can do to help shorten the recuperation time."

Michael, only twenty-two years old, didn't stop to think that after six rounds of sex with multiple organisms he might need time to recuperate. Even during youth, the recovery time lasts more than an hour. Erections cannot simply be called into service any time a man wants to have sex.

## Saliva Hormone Testing—Is It Accurate?

It might seem strange that both sexes, which are so different in so many ways, need the same sex hormones to function normally. As you know by now, a firm erection depends on multiple steps occurring in a specific sequence. When anything goes wrong with this sequence, most men realize they have a problem.

Whether you are a man or a woman, you might be wondering, "How do I know if I am at risk of a hormone deficiency? Is there any way to know which hormones or chemicals are most at risk in my body?"

Special laboratory tests are available for testing the level of these substances in your body. How can your doctor determine exactly how much of each hormone you need? Fortunately, there is an inexpensive option.

Hormone levels can be determined with analysis of your saliva. Saliva test kits are available to anyone without prescription except in the states of New York and California. In states where individuals may obtain saliva tests without a prescription, many individuals do not realize that hormonal levels can be accurately measured in a teaspoon-sized sample of saliva collected in the early morning.

Saliva test kits can be ordered over the Internet and are less costly than blood or serum tests for the same hormones. These evaluations can prove lifesaving for individuals who cannot afford traditional blood tests. In all states blood serum tests are more commonly used for diagnosis, but their higher cost makes them unpopular with patients.

Salivary hormone testing is uncomplicated and economical. Saliva testing allows anyone to take hormone testing into his or her own hands. Only a few medical laboratories in the United States do not require a doctor's prescription for hormone testing using blood samples. Hormone testing labs, which perform salivary hormone testing, are listed in the appendix.

Measurement of free testosterone level in saliva has been found to be more accurate than total testosterone measured in blood both in the diagnosis and treatment of diseases characterized by androgen deficiency. In any case, measuring salivary testosterone can be a practical method of assessing levels of circulating or bioactive testosterone.

Saliva can now be used for testing LH and FSH, the regulating hormones that reflect pituitary function. Benefits of saliva testing include the absence of any risk of disease, pain or cross infection. Minimal time and effort are required at one-fifth the cost. Best of all, the tests can be conducted in the comfort of your home without spending time in a doctor's waiting room.

Not all physicians accept saliva testing for screening and diagnosing hormone deficiencies because it is only eighty-five to ninety percent accurate. However, saliva testing provides a convenient way for a patient to track the effectiveness of testosterone therapy once a person has been diagnosed with a testosterone deficiency.

Appropriate therapy can make all the difference in the world for a man whose life lacks the inner zest that makes a sexual relationship fulfilling. Jonathan is someone who epitomizes this conclusion. Healthy at fifty years of age, Jonathan made an appointment with his doctor. After a physical, his doctor told him he was in perfect health, but Jonathan knew better. He made an appointment to see me instead.

"I have been experiencing low libido in the last few years as well as low energy," he told me. "I seldom experience morning or spontaneous erections. I have only a mild interest in sex, which is very alarming considering my past healthy sex drive." He had mentioned these concerns to his previous doctor.

Jonathan had explored possible causes, and it seemed to him that hypogonadism was the logical answer. His father told him that he had experienced a loss of sex drive at the same age, and he was aware that there could be a genetic component in his experience. Jonathan was motivated to find serious answers to his questions.

We ran a complete battery of tests and found significant deficiencies in Jonathan's bioavailable testosterone levels. It was relatively easy, in this case, to prescribe testosterone replacement therapy and put Jonathan back on the road to full recovery.

Three months later he telephoned me at the office. "If I keep improving at this rate," he told me, "I don't know what my wife is going to do. She says she wants a honeymoon before our twenty-fifth wedding anniversary this summer. She says I'm a new man."

I've already mentioned that in young men values from serum or blood hormone testing are time sensitive. Testosterone or DHEA should be measured between 6 and 8 a.m. for significant results. Melatonin tests must be measured between 11 p.m. and 1 a.m. for testing to be accurate. Cortisol levels should be measured during four specific times during the day to determine the pattern of secretion. If you think this is complicated, you are right. But there is an easier approach to using blood testing for hormones.

A simple early morning saliva test can screen for sex hormone deficiencies. Saliva is secreted by the salivary glands in the mouth. Although levels vary with the time of sampling, levels of free or circulating hormone should easily be detected in saliva. Research shows that results of tests from saliva match those collected from blood samples. Other research indicates that testing saliva for testosterone actually provides a better measure of bioavailable testosterone than blood tests. Most major insurance companies will pay for this form of testing.

Multiple hormone tests are sometimes needed for a correct diagnosis, but not all medical laboratories are equipped to perform melatonin, DHEA or testosterone testing using saliva. Refer to the appendix for a list of laboratories that provide accurate hormone testing.

The ideal testosterone treatment plan involves an adjustable form of testosterone delivery that raises hormone levels in small increments to restore optimum sexual function. Your doctor who is prescribing testosterone may be concerned about the risk of prostate cancer. More information about the prostate gland to help you and your doctor realize the benefits of testosterone replacement therapy in preventing prostate cancer follows in the next section.

## The Prostate: An Important Sex Gland

A few pages ago I announced that the prostate is man's second most important sexual gland after the penis. This is true because the prostate gland helps deliver semen to the penis, and without semen the sperm has no reproductive function. Important they may be, but prostate glands get very little respect from their owners. Some men dread the prostate examination so much that they avoid going to the doctor even when they have painful urination or cannot urinate standing up. They'll sit down to pee rather than finding out that a prostate problem exists.

Synthetic testosterones have been used for decades without increasing the risk of prostate cancer, although the long-term effects of their use need further study. Some evidence indicates that low testosterone may, in itself, present a risk factor for prostate cancer.

A long-term study in Finland involving of thousands of men over twenty-four years showed no increase in the occurrence of prostate cancer following high levels of SHBG, testosterone, progesterone or androstenedione.

Doctors are still reluctant to prescribe testosterone products to their older male patients for fear of triggering prostate cancer. "Better safe than sorry" is a good motto for the doctor and his male patients in their older years. Nonetheless, regular examinations can be life saving.

As troublesome as the risk of prostate cancer may be, a far more worrisome risk involves testosterone replacement therapy and age-related-prostate enlargement. Male sex hormones (androgens) such as testosterone and DHT provide the primary signal for the start of cell division in a normal prostate. If unchecked, this effect could result in non-cancerous enlargement of the prostate gland, known medically as BPH for benign prostate hyperplasia.

This condition occurs in most men as they age but does not result in cancer. The entire story is not in, but evidence indicates that testosterone may block some age-related changes that promote increased growth of the prostate. Dihydrotestosterone (DHT) and estrogen may be more important factors in causing prostate cancer than testosterone.

The conversion of free testosterone to high levels of DHT is now blamed as the primary cause for the enlargement of the prostate gland. The process of converting free testosterone to DHT within the prostate causes cells to grow and multiply in the gland. Hormonal changes probably precede the enlargement of the prostate gland to a certain degree, and high levels of DHT have been blamed for the condition.

The prostate specific antigen (PSA) is a protein normally produced by prostate cells but manufactured in excess by cells in prostate cancers. The PSA test, approved in 1986, measures levels of prostate-specific antigen and has been credited with detecting prostate cancer in its early stages eighty percent of the time. This test can also detect an increase in volume of the prostate as occurs in benign (non cancerous) prostate enlargement.

The test is not foolproof. A research team evaluated 6,691 volunteers at the Washington University School of Medicine in St. Louis and found that men under sixty with prostate cancer had a "healthy" PSA reading eighty-two percent of the time.

A limited number of studies in 1997 by Adrian Dobs, an endocrinologist with Johns Hopkins, found only mild increases in the prostate-specific antigen (PSA) after administering testosterone injections weekly for up to two years. Normal functioning of the prostate appears to depend on the balance between testosterone and estrogens or between DHT and testosterone. These ratios are crucial for endocrinologists as well as for the FDA in evaluating the safety and effectiveness of hormone therapy.

While the PSA test misses many cases of prostate cancer, it is effective enough to justify its widespread use in detecting early cases of prostate cancer. Because of the possible effect of testosterone on the development of prostate cancer, the physician should always perform the PSA test and a digital rectal exam before prescribing any hormone treatments for men. The size of the prostate, as determined by the physical exam or ultrasound visualization, is usually proportional to the prostate specific antigen.

Men from families with a history of prostate cancer are more susceptible to this type of cancer if their circulating testosterone falls below the minimum range for their age. A more serious consequence is one of the most deadly outcomes of extremely low free testosterone—a heart attack.

Prostate cancer is still not easy to detect early and it cannot be detected merely with a digital rectal exam and testing for PSA. If a physician is suspicious of a hidden prostate cancer due to a positive family history and a low ratio of testosterone to estrogen, a diagnostic ultrasound should be added to the screening examination.

Although physicians are trained to diagnose and treat sexual diseases and disorders, many do not feel comfortable dealing with these problems. One reason is simply that men do not like to talk to their doctors—or anyone else—about their sexual problems because they are embarrassed about their masculinity being at stake.

This policy of silence creates problems for the doctor, the patient and the spouse. When health issues are not addressed until it is too late, sexual dysfunction can become permanent. Prostate infections, for example, may progress without detection and lead to infertility and impotence.

Sex is important to married couples as a form of communication and an expression of love. The lack of an orgasm, for either person, or the presence of infertility can ruin a marriage.

Men need to stop playing the silence game and start paying attention to their sexual organs, especially the prostate gland. Women also have a critical role to play in the listening game. They need to encourage their men to obtain medical help for sexual problems—and to be alert to possible problems with their own sex life. It's time for all of us to listen to our bodies and pay attention to what they are saying to us.

George writes to thank me for sending him information about prostate cancer. "It looks like I should probably do the prostate biopsy," he says, "since my father had prostate cancer which was discovered when he was in his late seventies. He had radiation and now is fine at eighty-seven, although he might still be fine if he had done nothing."

George has obviously been thinking of all the options. He continues, "It may turn out not to have been such a good thing that I've been using the testosterone. On the other hand, if I do have cancer I might never have found it otherwise."

George brings up an important point. A reliable blood test for cancer does not exist. Multiple hormones are involved in the growth of the prostate and its enlargement. The problem is not simply one of too much or too little of this hormone or that. An imbalance of hormones in either direction can lead to unwanted prostate growth and resulting symptoms. In addition, men with a benign or non-malignant enlargement of the gland are statistically more likely to develop prostate cancer at a later time.

Family history plays an important role in this very common cancer of elderly men. The risk multiplies in men with low testosterone levels. A world-renowned urologist, Wayne Meikle at University of Utah, has done considerable work in this area and finds that transdermal testosterone does not seem to lead to enlarged prostate glands or prostate cancers.

A balance of all of our hormones appears essential to maintain normal function and structure of the sexual organs including the prostate. The presence of more estrogen than testosterone has been linked to both prostate cancer and breast cancer.

The finger points more and more to the role of estrogen in the form of estradiol rather than to testosterone as a cancer promoter in the prostate as well as in breast tissue.

Estrogen primarily affects the body of the prostate, while DHT's effects arise predominantly in the tissue lining the prostate. Cancer most commonly occurs in the body of the prostate gland. This leads to the theory that concentrations of DHT in these two parts of the prostate may play different and opposing roles in prostate growth. If this turns out to be true, testosterone may actually be protective for the male prostate.

Testosterone replacement might someday be considered more important in preventing cancer of the prostate rather than causing it, as many doctors mistakenly believe. What we know now is that testosterone is not the culprit it has been thought to be in prostate cancer and that testosterone may play a role in protecting men from the negative effects of estrogen excess.

## The Real Culprit in Prostate Cancer

Doctors are still afraid of testosterone because studies indicate that there is a small chance that testosterone will accelerate the growth of cancer cells in the prostate even if the man is not aware of any problem. "Hidden cancers" of the prostate are more common in men over the age of fifty, so few doctors are willing to take a chance of causing harm to these patients. This is remarkable because the odds of serious side effects from cancer treatment are far worse than the risk of cancer from testosterone therapy, but patients with cancer are routinely treated with chemotherapy and toxic drugs.

A more important practical issue, however, is that low testosterone may predispose men to developing prostate cancer. This observation has been confirmed with research. Doctors also need to consider research indicating that testosterone may help to shrink enlarged prostates and does not cause prostate cancer.

Controversial research suggesting that low, rather than high testosterone may cause prostate cancer was reported over a decade ago by two highly respected urologists, Wayne Meikle mentioned earlier and Robert Prehn, at the Cancer Institute. Regardless of these findings and others, the safety of testosterone is not fully accepted thus far. According to Dr. Prehn, testosterone may protect the prostate by blocking some of the age-related changes, which promote its increased growth. Dr. Meikle, a well-known researcher in transdermal testosterone, has found that low testosterone is a risk factor for prostate cancer in men with a positive family history for the disease.

The entire story is not in. However, considerable evidence exists to point to the fact that DHT (dihydrotestosterone) and E2 (estradiol) may be more important than testosterone in causing prostate cancer. Testosterone is not the villain in promoting prostate cancer that the FDA has made it out to be. In their zeal to put a stop to the abuse of testosterone, the FDA may have put this hormone out of reach of people who really need it.

The myth that increased prostate cancer results from testosterone restrains the prescribing habits of other physicians. As we have noted, there is no positive link between the use of testosterone and prostate cancer, but even a hint that such could be a case is enough to dampen the use of testosterone as a clinical treatment for hypogonadism (low testosterone levels).

# 6

# Testosterone's Role in Sex, Aging, and Health

## Aging and Testosterone

**A** tombstone reads—

Remember, Man, as you walk by,
as you are now, so once was I;
As I am now, so you must be.
Prepare for death and follow me.

Chilling thought! The only way you and I can avoid aging is to die before we get old. Or so it seems. However some people enjoy a vigorous, fulfilling life well into their eighties, nineties and beyond. As you might suspect, hormones are big players in the drama of aging, and the good news is that you can manage your hormones for a pleasure-filled life in your "elder" years.

All hormones diminish through the andropause, the male equivalent of the menopause, which usually affects men fifty-five to eighty years of age.

Testosterone is a major indicator of the aging process. As a male you enjoy your highest levels of testosterone during adolescence and at about twenty-one to twenty-four years of age. From that point on, testosterone declines. At about age forty, your total testosterone level begins to decline at rate of about one percent per year. By the age of seventy your testosterone levels will be less than half what they were when you were young.

Lower testosterone levels affect your sex life by weakening your ability to achieve and hold a hard erection during intercourse. In addition to a weak erection, a testosterone deficiency erodes your ability to increase lean body mass. Simply put, you don't have enough testosterone to enjoy life to its fullest, become muscular, or "do anything till you die."

A dramatic drop in testosterone is usually followed by weight gain, and the more fat a man accumulates, the less testosterone he has. This is because the aromatase enzyme in the body's fat cells transforms most of the body's testosterone into estradiol, the most active form of estrogen. Higher estradiol levels stimulate the sex-hormone binding globulin (SHBG) to bind up the small amount of testosterone remaining. SHBG thus acts like a switch that turns on testosterone availability.

Less available testosterone also leads to the loss of your sex drive, and higher estradiol levels generated by body fat increase the risk of prostate cancer. Lifelong exposure to pesticides and environmental estrogens may also contribute to an oversupply of estrogen in its various forms.

Estradiol is not all bad. A certain level of estradiol is apparently required for men to have a normal amount of sexual aggressiveness. We don't know as much about this as we should because most studies of estradiol's effect on male behavior have examined men with very low testosterone levels. More studies are needed on the role of testosterone and estradiol in the regulation of behavior in healthy, normal men who do not have a hormone deficiency.

Some men become alarmed when they feel they are losing their sexual energy and take steps to do something about it. One of my patients, Bob, was such a person.

Bob told me that in his twenties and thirties he'd had plenty of sexual energy and led an active sex life. By age forty-five when we tested his total testosterone level, it was 321, down from 471 the previous year. He was upset because he felt he needed testosterone levels higher than the normal range of 300 to 1200.

Since Bob's testosterone level has already fallen to 321 at age forty-five, in another ten years it could fall below the lowest normal measurement of 300. This is the level of an estimated twenty percent of men aged sixty to eighty years with low sexual energy.

The amount of testosterone working in Bob's body depends on how much is bound up and therefore inactivated by the SHBG protein. Functional problems in Bob's pituitary or his testicles may be the cause for his drop in total testosterone. Whatever is to blame for his disappointing sexual drive in his mid forties, Bob can almost certainly enjoy an improved quality of life with supplemental testosterone bringing his levels into the middle of the normal range.

## Slowing the Aging Process with Testosterone

Like Bob, many men are thrilled by the results of testosterone replacement therapy in slowing down some of the deterioration associated with aging. The physical benefits of testosterone replacement are well documented, but we need more studies on how supplementary testosterone affects moods and sex drive.

A 67-year-old man I'll call Jim reported to me after a year and a half on AndroGel that he loved the benefits of his testosterone therapy. Results have been gradual, but now he's hearing all sorts of affirmation. "People I haven't seen in a while have said, 'Man, have you been lifting weights or what?' Friends tell me I'm less stressed and more patient. I don't seem to lose my temper as much as I used to. I seem to be in a better mood more often and have more self-confidence."

As far as sex is concerned, Jim says he experiences more frequent morning erections, a fuller penis even in the flaccid state, and erections that seem to be harder and last longer. Sounds pretty good, but there's more.

"Something happened the other night that was pretty good," he said. "I was having sex with my wife, and we had been at it for about ten or fifteen minutes. She had not climaxed yet. I couldn't hold back any longer, but my erection did not go away. I stayed just as hard as before. I kept going and she came shortly thereafter, but I was able to continue just as before for another ten minutes or so and was able to climax again! I can't remember ever doing that before. How do you explain that?"

Jim was a happy man with great sexual performance.

Testosterone replacement therapy improved not only his sexual drive and his moods but also shortened his recovery time after sexual intercourse. Testosterone replacement therapy eliminates symptoms of androgen deficiency, and, over time appropriate testosterone therapy helps avoid heart disease and mental deterioration. As with any long-term treatment, there are always risks to consider, but Jim wouldn't hesitate to recommend the therapy that renewed his sexual pleasure at the age of sixty-seven.

Impotence is just around the corner when a man begins to lose interest in sex and doesn't wake up with an early morning erection. When these signs occur in relatively young men, chemical castration from estrogen in a polluted environment (see page 138) might be the villain. Castration—chemical or otherwise—dramatically reduces the frequency of sexual desire, masturbation and ejaculation for many men. Loss of early morning erections warns us that we should listen to our hormones.

Be sure to listen to your doctor explain the pros and cons of testosterone therapy and make your decision based on your doctor's recommendation to you. Appropriate hormone replacement not only provides a rebalancing of hormones, but also is a much safer, more effective option than receiving hormone injections twice or three times a month.

## The Penis and Castration

Long before the benefit of modern scientific research, primitive humans ascribed great importance to the penis. Male erection was perceived as a reflection of raw masculine power, and the phallus—the erect penis—was revered as a symbol of strength and virility. For thousands of years, rituals of pagan worship and tribal bonding in diverse cultures revolved around the sex act. Various representations of the form of the erect penis were used as altars. Obelisks are artistically modified upright phallic symbols once fashioned as altars to the gods.

According to stories passed on from the past, ancient warriors consumed the genital organs, hearts, and brains of lions, tigers, and other animals in an attempt to transfer the vigor of the animal to themselves. They believed that the sex organs of animals contained the animal's physical power.

In Oriental markets today you can find tiger penises and rhino horns offered for sale as aphrodisiacs. This is unfortunate because the sale of such items accelerates the extinction of these species. Koreans collect deer antlers, which are formed by the action of testosterone on the young buck, and consider them to be powerful aphrodisiacs. In Africa men of some primitive tribes adorn and accentuate their penis rather than covering it as we do in today's society. For many in our civilized society, pictures of human genitals provide visual stimulation leading to sexual arousal. A large penis is still considered a sign of increased masculinity and sexual dominance.

The removal of the testicles in certain animals and humans has been practiced for centuries. Before the pyramids were built, ancient people knew that castration made animals more submissive as beasts of burden or pets.

Male servants of the Chinese emperors were castrated, creating the first "eunuchs." They were considered safe to care for the Chinese empress since their sexual drive was greatly reduced. In Egypt the king's slaves were castrated to keep them docile.

The characteristics of castrated men depend on the age at which their testicles were removed. Merely a century ago, young choirboys in Italy were castrated before puberty to keep their sweet soprano voices intact. Boys castrated before puberty develop a tall, slender, feminine body type with very high voices and tiny sexual organs. As they age, they not only look much younger than their non-castrated counterparts but also tend to outlive them by a few years.

Men castrated after puberty continue to develop normally but are usually infertile, have no sexual drive and never develop enlargement or cancer of the prostate. Because the development of both the prostate and the penis depend on the action of testosterone and DHT (dihydrotestosterone), castration late in life inevitably results in lower testosterone levels and the loss of sexual arousal.

Decreased testosterone production later in life may also be caused by the loss of one or both of the testicles or any form of chemical castration. Castration today is limited to treatment for metastatic (spreading) prostate cancer or for the removal of retained, diseased or cancerous testicles. Chemical castration is also occasionally used as punishment for violent sex offenders and child molesters.

Dogs and cats are routinely castrated (spayed) to stop them from wandering or becoming aggressive, to stop territorial spraying behavior, and to reduce the multiplication of puppies and kittens. Horses are castrated to create geldings, which are preferred for riding.

Far more disconcerting than these forms of castration is the inundation of chemicals that effectively neutralize testosterone and result in chemical castration without the knowledge of the affected person. How can this happen?

Environmental estrogens proliferate as a by-product of our industrialized society. These unwanted chemicals create excess estrogen in the body, which can block the effect of testosterone on the penis.

The dramatic reduction of androgens in the body from the onslaught of artificial hormone-like substances in the environment is known technically as "chemical castration." This can result in a loss of libido by affected men, including much less frequent masturbation about six weeks after exposure. Fortunately, this form of castration can usually be successfully treated either by removing men from the source of the polluting chemicals or from treatment with testosterone supplements.

An interesting case illustrating this involved men recruited from Haiti for agricultural work. They accepted the work assignment and stayed in housing units provided by their employer, carefully spraying their bedding and clothing with chemicals to kill lice. They escaped infection by lice, but soon were dismayed to see their breasts bulging and other "feminine" traits. They had experienced chemical castration—loss of male sexuality—from the excess of environmental estrogen in the delousing sprays, resulting in the development of female characteristics.

If you are man with sexual problems, don't hesitate to talk to your physician about what you are suffering. You don't have to just chalk it all up to "getting older." One of the specifics I most want to convey in this book is that there are things that can be done to restore male virility and optimum health and function.

## Penis Size—Does It Really Make a Difference?

You would think from the load of annoying email messages coming your way that everyone in the whole world is dying for a longer, fuller, larger penis either as a personal possession or as the primary feature of a sexual partner. Really now—how important is penis size in experiencing a satisfying sexual relationship?

According to Richard Kaye, a professor of English at Hunter College, everybody is obsessed with penis size and other physical attributes. From his piece entitled, "The Masculine Mystique," Kaye makes the following comments (used here with permission):

> At the moment, an ever-wider array of new images of the male physique permeates the culture, subjecting the body of the American male to more scrutiny than ever before as. Television shows like "Ally McBeal" and "The View" depict fictional and real-life women giddily discussing male performance and penis size. Magazines devoted to male fitness and health break circulation records, and advertisers become bolder and bolder in purveying hardened *übermenschen* (supermen of sexuality).
>
> Adolescent boys—the newest focus for worried psychologists and social workers, according to *The New York Times Magazine*—fret over the relative scrawniness of their physiques, worrying about the shape of their "abs" and penis size much as young women long for ample

breasts and slim waistlines. It's a democracy. Everyone has an equal right to be anxiety-ridden about his or her physique.

It sometimes seems that all men are obsessed with the size of their penis. Men with no medical deficiency in that department have somehow equated the size of their sex organ with their masculinity. The bigger their penis, the better.

Men in search of a larger sex organ rush to questionable medical sources on the Internet for penis pumps, penis extenders, and penile surgery to increase their penis size. I'm sure that at least a thousand companies or individuals are offering a miracle product guaranteed to increase penis size by a greater dimension than seems humanly possible, and hundreds of thousands of men are buying penis enlargements products on the web.

Two researchers reviewing the Kinsey studies on sexuality found that heterosexual men are more likely to be preoccupied to the point of obsession by the size of their penis than are homosexual men.

By the time you read this, the longing for large penises along with the craze for huge breasts may have faded away as a blip in society's evolution. Or maybe not. But since we're here, let's take a look at penis size and see if there is any relationship between sexual bliss and an oversized male sex organ.

The actual length and girth of the penis depends on the action of DHT and other androgens in the body of a developing youth. Testosterone itself creates very few of the secondary sexual characteristics such as increased hair and beard growth and deepening of the voice. DHT, a metabolite of testosterone, is the hormone that is responsible for normal development of the penis and urethra. Without DHT, malformations of the penis can develop. Besides an abnormally small penis, the urethra may not fuse with the penis, a condition called hypospadias that has become more common than in the past, apparently due to the action of environmental estrogens on the developing male fetus.

The penis grows in size during various phases of fetal, childhood, and adolescent development. When erect, the normal penis is five and one-half inches long. Both dihydrotestosterone and testosterone are androgens that are responsible for the normal growth and development of male sex organs and the maintenance of secondary sex characteristics. These effects include growth and maturation of the prostate, penis and scrotum; the development of male hair distribution such as beard, pubic, chest and armpit hair; vocal cord thickening, and alterations in body musculature and fat distribution. Aside from androgens, other hormones including the growth hormone and thyroid hormone have some effect on the growth of the human penis and its eventual size.

Hypogonadism—literally, "less than normal genitals"—is a condition of extremely low levels of testosterone and is a disease that can occur in men of all ages. Depending on the age at which it strikes, hypogonadism can have life-altering effects including abnormal penis formation, an unusually small penis and undescended testicles in younger boys and sexual dysfunction in older men.

A penis less than four inches long when erect is considered to be abnormally small and is known in medical terminology as a micropenis. Therapy may be available to correct the situation in a boy whose penis has not fully developed by puberty. A man with a micropenis may feel emotionally devastated even if it is fully functional.

You may remember Todd, back in Chapter Two, who had marital and other problems because of his small penis.

At age thirty-six Todd was diagnosed with hypogonadism after suffering four years with fatigue, loss of libido, headaches, hot flashes, night sweats, severe loss of penis size, depression, and lack of concentration. "I carry all my excess weight in my abdomen and chest. I have severe loss of muscle tone and mass," he said.

Todd's penis was always undersized. An illness as an adult caused his testicles to swell and become sensitive. He took antibiotics, and the swelling and discharge went away, along with his libido and other symptoms described above. Listen to his story.

"I fathered three children in my twenties," he said, "but my wife made comments about how my penis was undersized compared to that of her first husband. We divorced, and I have since remarried. My current wife and I have had a very hard time dealing with my condition. She becomes very distressed when we have intercourse because of my inability to get and maintain an erection. When I do achieve one she complains that she can't 'feel' me. Because of my condition our sex life is non-existent and has been extremely unsatisfactory."

Could Todd have low testosterone though he is obviously not infertile since he has fathered children? If low testosterone during adolescence resulted in failure of his penis to develop fully, how could his fertility have remained intact?

For one thing, fertility does *not* depend on penis size. Sperm production depends on the action of estrogen and testosterone, while the penis develops as a result of the action of DHT (dihydrotestosterone). Boys suffering with low DHT levels at puberty may not develop a full-sized penis and may endure sexual dysfunction later in life. Even so, these men can still father children.

What's the real story? Is it possible for a man's penis to grow after puberty? For men whose penis completed its full growth during puberty and for adult men diagnosed with hypogonadism, penis growth after maturity can be a reality.

One method of achieving penis growth for these men is by applying testosterone directly to the skin. The added testosterone triggers production of growth factors (example insulin-like growth factor-1 or IGF-1), and free testosterone converts to DHT. The effects on the penis are not merely from local tissue expansion. Researchers at University of California at San Francisco have found that applying testosterone directly to the genitals of boys before puberty can result in penis growth.

A study of Israeli boys with abnormally small penises—less than 4.5 inches long when erect—used a high strength topical testosterone cream applied twice daily for several months. Serum DHT and free testosterone levels were measured over several months, and the average penis grew sixty percent longer and fifty-three percent larger in diameter. Imagine the outcome if this could happen in an adult!

Frank, a patient of mine who was using a ten percent testosterone cream, shared some remarkable observations with me. "I'm still making steady progress with the testosterone topical cream that you had made for me," Frank wrote. "My strength has come up at least ten pounds on every lift, and my libido continues to rise. Will it continue to get better for me sexually and physically? I have fantasies now! Also, my penis is getting thicker! Six inches around! I'm very proud of my muscular accomplishments to this point. You've changed my life! Well I've been using your testosterone cream for almost three years now and have gained an inch in penis length and one and one half inches in thickness. Now my wife really has a conversation piece."

Frank sounds like a satisfied guy, but we have to wonder how much of his perceived penis enhancement is real and how much is from increased confidence. Maybe he should recheck his measurements. Six inches around—could that be correct? Can the penis grow in adulthood?

Yes, it is possible. Testosterone encourages gradual penile growth after it has been converted to DHT. It does this by activating androgen receptors in the corporal bodies on either side of the shaft of the penis.

For a male to develop a normal-sized penis and a normal sex drive, androgens like testosterone and DHT are essential. This is why administration of androgens to boys soon after puberty results in rapid growth during adolescence and a normal penis in adulthood.

Until recently, medical researchers believed that the penis stopped growing during adolescence because of testosterone's final action on androgen receptors in the penis. Now we believe that these receptors decrease after puberty but do not totally disappear. Accordingly, it is possible to increase the size a man's penis at any age.

Reports of studies supporting this concept were welcomed by scam artists looking for text to include in millions of email messages.

The age of a man plus his DHT level is the key factors role in determining whether his penis can increase in size after puberty.

A study involving boys with a growth hormone deficiency found that treatment before puberty with the human growth hormone improved the growth of their genitals. Following this study the question arose about whether the penile growth was influenced by testosterone, DHT, or both. Researchers at UCSF Children's Medical Center concluded that androgen receptors remain sensitive to testosterone stimulation through adulthood.

As we have mentioned earlier, local application of testosterone can stimulate the growth of the penis. Most doctors do not know this fact and go along with the consensus that penis size cannot be altered except by surgery. This myth ultimately leads many men with small penises to feel that they were cheated by nature without realizing that potential treatments are available to help them overcome their problem.

Larry wrote to me from Michigan reporting that he had been on AndroGel for hormone replacement therapy for nearly two years and was enthusiastic about the program.

"The libido has gotten better, the memory got better, and I actually wanted to get off the couch and do stuff," he told me. "Also," he added, "I noticed in increase in the size of my Johnson. Prior to AndroGel it would sometimes retract into me so far you could barely see it. Now, while it's not huge, it doesn't disappear like it did. As for the testicles, I think they got a little smaller, but not by much, which I'm glad to report."

Besides making big gains in physical performance, Larry was doing well on the social front and was getting into the dating scene again. "I haven't had a chance to test everything in 'battlefield conditions,'" he said, "but I think I'll be OK when the big event happens, which I'm hoping will be soon. Starting to see someone on a serious basis. Another thing is the irritability is gone. I'm a lot nicer than I used to be. I used to get nasty with people, especially on the phone."

Finally, Larry likes his doctor a lot better these days. "I was just checked out by the Doc," he said. "He seems to be getting better (or is it me getting better?) I interact with him better. I asked and he gave me the Viagra sample pack—I want it just in case. Got my T levels from April. My results were not astronomically high, but I don't think I'd want them real high. What I'd like to do is get the free T up a little higher. Isn't zinc the way to boost that? I take a multi-vitamin, but haven't taken zinc in a while."

As we have mentioned earlier, the penis usually stops growing sometime after puberty. Larry's experience indicates that an apparent increase in the flaccid or non-erect size of the penis can be caused by an increased amount of blood in the penis. New research indicates, however, that penis growth is still possible with topical hormone application in adults with hypogonadism. Some men using topical testosterone have reported dramatic changes.

My patient Brian told me that though he had a normal-size penis, he decided to use testosterone cream. Several weeks after he began rubbing it on his scrotum and penis he noticed a dramatic increase in the fullness and sensitivity of his penis, and his testicles also grew.

"My libido increased markedly as well," he told me, "so the entire experience was very gratifying. Furthermore, my arthritis improved, I put on muscle like crazy, and my whole sense of wellness improved. Then gynecomastia (enlarged breasts) appeared, and I stopped completely. Maybe I was taking too much, although I was simply following the prescription except in the genital application of the cream. I can't remember what the dosage was on the applicator. I would love to get those same positive effects without the breast problem."

Brian's over-zealous use of testosterone made him feel much better, but it created an excess that was converted to estrogen. Too much estrogen in the system is one of the most common problems faced by bodybuilders and others self-medicating with too much testosterone. Excess estrogen can cause other problems in men as well, including sexual dysfunction, breast enlargement, aggression and moodiness.

Too much testosterone, and we produce estrogen. Too much estrogen is feminizing. DHT has more to do with penis size than testosterone does. The study of our sexual hormones is both intriguing and incredibly complex. You may be thinking that we'd all get along better in life if our sex organs came with printed instructions—an owner's manual.

This book is an attempt to make some of the physical aspects of enjoying the pleasures of sex a little clearer. Whether you're just curious or are struggling to achieve a higher level of satisfaction with your bodies and your sex life, why not learn everything you can to enjoy the sexual experience to the fullest?

## Myths about Testosterone

Some "old wives' tales" and legends passed on from the days of old live on in spite of the scrutiny of modern science. Testosterone replacement, for example, is surrounded by mythology that would do justice to the Dark Ages. Though testosterone has been proven to be a safe and beneficial hormone, many doctors and their patients insist that using testosterone leads to increased aggression, prostate cancer, heart disease and hair loss. All of these are "testosterone myths."

One of the most insidious of all testosterone myths is the assumption that the loss of ability to perform sexually is part of the normal aging process. When testosterone and estrone levels start to decline, men and women are naturally distressed over losing their sexual spark of vitality. But when older men complain to their doctors about their loss of sex drive, they are often told not to worry about it because, they are told, "it's normal."

Of course aging causes our sexual prowess to diminish along with all of our human systems, but they should not fail prematurely. Dr. André Guay, a professor of endocrinology at Harvard Medical School, says that even a ninety-year-old man should be able to get an erection at least twice a week.

It is *not* normal to stop having sex after age fifty-five, nor is it normal to lose interest in sex during your older years. If your doctor tells you that your testosterone is normal, but you are having trouble with erections or orgasms, this is *not* "normal." Men who are over forty should not assume their sexual life is over. It is a myth, and a dangerous one, to believe that losing energy, muscle mass, and getting fat, are normal—and that it's all-downhill from then on. Too many developments in sexual medicine are occurring to justify a pessimistic view of the future.

Not many years ago, men were referred to urologists for impotence therapy unless it was assumed that the problem was due to psychological causes. Therapy was almost primitive, and the possibility of a testosterone deficiency was rarely considered. It was not until 1985, when the FDA first approved testosterone patches, that doctors seriously considered testosterone deficiency as a treatable problem.

That wasn't the end of confusion. For decades doctors considered total testosterone levels as the only effective screening tool to diagnose a deficiency, and most doctors today still go along with this outdated belief. Current research into the numerous functions of testosterone teaches us that bioavailable testosterone (see page 118), not total testosterone, determines the actual amount of testosterone accessible for morning erections and sexual arousal.

Testosterone deficiency is often a multi-faceted problem associated with other hormonal inadequacies. For example, levels of oxytocin, progesterone, DHT and thyroid hormones show a parallel age-related decline along with testosterone. The sad reality is that the myth that testosterone deficiency is merely a natural aging phenomenon stops many men from enjoying a vital sex life during their older years.

Mark suffered from testosterone, DHT, and thyroid deficiency. After a month using testosterone cream and taking a thyroid replacement medication, he was feeling a lot better. "Mental clarity—still fuzzy," he said, "Appetite not great." But Mark was no longer suffering from hot flashes and sweats, felt more strength and was confident performing routine tasks "without loathing it," as he said. His libido and erections were noticeably improved.

Hormones work in concert. Like many men with a testosterone deficiency, hormones originating in Mark's thyroid were also involved. Your doctor should recommend a complete hormone profile as a comprehensive diagnostic tool when dealing with any sexual deficiencies you may be experiencing.

Doctors have assumed that there must be something wrong with the brain of a man who complained about his sexual drive. If it wasn't psychological, perhaps tumors in the brain were sending out an excess of prolactin. You may remember that prolactin blocks the action of testosterone to increase the length of time after sexual intercourse when a man is unable to achieve another erection. Blaming lack of libido on too much prolactin made sense.

I always recommend checking prolactin levels for men with untreated erectile failure and sexual dysfunction. Prolactin, which is regulated by dopamine and certain growth factors, increases during stress or depression. Stressful feelings respond well to a low dose of transdermal testosterone in aging men because the additional testosterone can lower excess levels of stress-aggravating prolactin as well as the "stress hormone," cortisol.

An accurate measurement of both free and total testosterone is the first step in helping a man with erectile dysfunction, and should be done prior to prescribing an "erection enhancer" like Viagra. Traditionally, the next step is to prescribe injectable testosterone and have the patient visit the doctor for monthly injections.

Although injections are the least expensive form of testosterone replacement, problems are associated with this method of delivery. For example, long-term use of injectable testosterone is believed to cause increased thickness of the blood (polycythemia), liver dysfunction, fluid retention, and elevated cholesterol levels. Other side effects may include personality disorders and prostate enlargement with an increased risk of cancer.

Nevertheless, low-dose testosterone has been given by injection to men from sixty-five to eighty-five years of age for up to six years without any increase in the size of the prostate or the development of cancerous tissue, showing that for many men this mode of therapy can still be very effective and safe.

In my practice I prefer the transdermal or skin delivery system because I believe there are greater benefits and fewer side effects.

A recent wide-ranging study exploded another myth—that the long-term use of testosterone is dangerous. In continuing clinical trials over six years there was no significant increase in levels of hemoglobin, hematocrit, or the presence of sleep apnea among men using transdermal testosterone. Prostate size and PSA did not increase, but body weight and abdominal fat decreased significantly while muscle strength increased—without dieting. Sounds encouraging, doesn't it?

Testosterone was used to treat chest pain in men for decades, and a clinical study in 1988 shows that testosterone plays a key role in protecting men against heart disease. Dr. Conrad Swartz studied hundreds of men who had heart attacks. He found that men with abnormally low levels of free or bioactive testosterone had a greater risk of hardening of the arteries (arteriosclerosis), and that increasing their testosterone levels lowered total disease in the blood vessels of the heart.

Swartz was way ahead of his time. Today heart disease is still the number one killer of Americans, but for the first time in history doctors are managing cholesterol levels with diet and cholesterol-lowering medications. At the same time, improved dietary habits, supplementation with the new testosterone forms and more exercise have combined to result in a decline in the incidence of heart disease.

Testosterone replacement therapy helps keep supporting ligaments and tendons strong and speeds their repair. After an injury on the racetrack, a horse will be treated with testosterone, and the same hormone has the capability of healing humans as well. Supplemental testosterone replacement therapy has helped men heal not only their Nevertheless, in spite of overwhelming evidence of the benefits of testosterone replacement after a heart attack or joint injury, many doctors still resist prescribing testosterone.heart muscle but also the rest of their body.

Nevertheless, in spite of overwhelming evidence of the benefits of testosterone replacement after a heart attack or joint injury, many doctors still resist prescribing testosterone.

Why? Most doctors believe the patient could have a greater risk of prostate cancer after taking supplemental testosterone because the prostate gland depends on the androgens testosterone and DHT to develop and maintain its various structures and functions. The concept behind the myth is that more testosterone leads to higher androgen levels, and that this stimulates the prostate gland and raises the risk of prostate cancer. This is simply not true.

A study by a group of Johns Hopkins urologists looked back fifteen years at men who developed prostate cancer to see if their hormones could give a clue to their development of this disease. They compared levels of free and total testosterone, sex hormone binding globulin (SHBG) and luteinizing hormone in these men with the levels of men who did not have prostate cancer. Researchers found no measurable differences in these hormone levels among men who were destined to develop prostate cancer and those without the disease. The study proved that no predictions of prostate cancer could be made on the basis of testosterone therapy.

A much larger Finnish survey published in 1999 collected blood from over one thousand men between the years 1968 and 1972 plus a follow-up period of twenty-four years. A total of 166 prostate cancer cases occurred among men who were cancer free at the beginning of the survey. No evidence was found linking levels of serum testosterone, SHBG, or androstenedione with prostate cancer in the entire study population or in subgroups based on age or weight. The study failed to find a cause-effect relationship between concentration of the male hormone and prostate cancer.

Why does prostate cancer develop mostly in older men? If you think about it, adding more testosterone to the system of men with low levels of the hormone due to aging should not cause prostate cancer. If it could, wouldn't young men whose bodies are loaded with an abundance of testosterone have the highest rate of prostate cancer?

Today the finger of blame for prostate cancer points to estrogen, not testosterone replacement therapy. Testosterone levels decline as men age, and lower production of testosterone does not block the age-related tendency to produce more estrogen. Studies, including one at Tufts University, show that prostate cancer can be induced in laboratory rats by injecting them with low doses of estrogen. Life-long exposure to environmental estrogen (see page 85) could be responsible for excess estrogen in the bodies of older men.

"Use testosterone supplements and go bald" is one of the oldest and hardest reports to dispel. With or without testosterone, the incidence of baldness in men ranges from about twenty-three percent to eighty-seven percent, and baldness may develop any time after puberty. Castration after the onset of puberty halts the progression of human balding, indicating that hormones must play a significant role in this condition. Even so, I've never heard of anyone advocating castration as a way to avert baldness—certainly not me!

Testosterone injections do *not* result in the loss of hair in adult males treated to correct a testosterone deficiency, and there is no noticeable change in the scalp hair of normal men who receive testosterone. Perhaps low testosterone is a greater risk factor for increased balding than high or increased testosterone. Male pattern baldness, with balding limited to the top of the head, also seems to be related more closely to hormone deficiencies than to excess testosterone.

TESTOSTERONE to DIHYROTESTOSTERONE

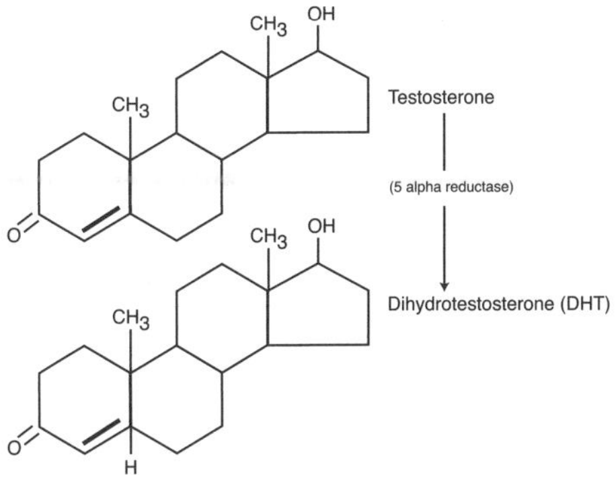

Testosterone

(5 alpha reductase)

Dihydrotestosterone (DHT)

The common pattern of hair loss is apparently the result of increased sensitivity of the hair follicles in those who are genetically predetermined to become bald. The active hormone in the balding scalp appears to be not testosterone but DHT, which is produced from testosterone through the activity of the 5-alpha-reductase enzyme (5-AR).

Detailed studies have confirmed that high 5-AR levels are present in the frontal hairline area of balding men and that males with 5-AR deficiencies do not go bald. Levels of the 5-alpha reductase enzyme are as much as four times higher in balding areas than they are in the back of the scalp. This is why hair transplanted from the back and sides of the head into the bald areas continues growing.

The last myth is that all testosterone deficiencies are due to the uncontrollable effects of aging. One out of ten men over forty years of age has hypogonadism, or below normal testosterone levels, but medical records show that it is rarely the diagnosis. The interpretation of testosterone levels is so complex that the condition is often overlooked.

Plenty of men and women in their eighties have high normal testosterone levels—people who are still enjoying sex and looking ten to twenty years younger than their contemporaries. The shocking reality is that both sexes are running out of testosterone—sometimes for reasons well within their control!

## Hormone Replacement: Injections or Gels

Injections into the muscle has been the standard method of delivering testosterone for years because injectable testosterone products are effective, practical and relatively inexpensive. A major drawback to injecting testosterone is that levels of the hormone rise rapidly immediately after the injection and then drop almost as rapidly. The wildly fluctuating levels of testosterone following the injections can result in mood disorders and withdrawal symptoms.

Another way to deliver testosterone is through patches and alcohol-based gels applied directly to the skin, a method known as transdermal delivery. These preparations are medically as effective as testosterone injections but are far more expensive. Testosterone patches and alcohol-based gels can also be irritating to the skin, although newer testosterone creams have been formulated to eliminate this problem.

A new product, a high potency testosterone cream, which I have developed, is discussed in Appendix A.

# 7

# Gender, Sexual Preference, and Heredity

## Becoming a Boy—or a Girl

After the magic moment of your conception there was a time when you may have been seconds away from arriving with a different gender than the one you have now. For the first seven weeks of your life in the womb, your rapidly growing body was female in form even if you were a male. That's right. The default sex of the embryo is female.

This is true with all mammals. Male and female embryos are identical in their early stages of development. Eight to ten weeks after conception, bulges appear near the kidney of the forming embryo and become the glands known as the gonads. If the gonads receive a signal from the male-determining gene, they develop into testes. Otherwise they become ovaries.

Another way of looking at life before birth is to think of it as a unisex blueprint with two sets of reproductive ducts extending from the gonads to the embryo's urinary tract. Ducts destined for female sex organs are called the Mullerian ducts, and their male counterparts are the Wolffian ducts.

For the fetus that will be born as a baby girl, the Mullerian ducts normally develop into female parts. In males a hormone called the Mullerian inhibiting substance from the male embryo's testicles causes the potentially female parts to wither away. Stimulated by testosterone, the Wolffian male ducts are transformed into testicles.

An interesting feature of this hormone makes the male gender possible. A gene on the Y chromosome unique to males sends signals to the Mullerian-inhibiting substance, which is activated by a powerful gene known as the SRY gene, named for the sex-determining region of the Y chromosome. This action causes male sex organs to develop. Once in a while, part of this sex-determining gene is transferred to the X chromosome. This results in the birth of an XX sterile male with testicles and a penis.

During the eons of evolution, fetuses developed from the female form in order to create a more convenient and efficient model or prototype for the human race. All boy babies develop from a modified girl prototype. Yes, it's true, men. We would all be born female except for the influence of the Y chromosome.

In the process of becoming male, maternal testosterone performs its last role in the unborn baby before the brain begins to develop. At this point the androgen dihydrotestosterone (DHT) takes over, creating the testicles from the embryo's ovaries, which then descend from the abdomen into the scrotal sac. The presence of DHT also allows the fetal equivalent of the clitoris to enlarge and fuse with the urethra to form a penis. At this point, during the eighth week, the fetus is sufficiently masculinized to be born as a fully equipped XY male. Notice that it is DHT and not testosterone that ultimately creates the male sex organs.

The brain, however, is not fully masculinized until more testosterone is present, and the developing male baby's testicles do not start producing adult quantities of testosterone until they descend from the abdomen. In some cases testicles do not descend until after birth, or only one testicle descends while the other is trapped in the abdomen. Undescended testicles must be surgically removed because they often become malignant.

In any case, during the first seven weeks after conception, the external and internal sex organs can become either male or female. By the eighth week the physical process of transformation from female to male is completed due to the action of Mullerian inhibiting substance, but the brain itself has not yet changed from female to male.

Physical capabilities of the male are not enough to be fully male. Our brains must learn to be drawn to the opposite sex, to long for a satisfying relationship with a female. Otherwise reproduction will not occur. Enter testosterone. Only with testosterone can we men modify our original female brain into a male brain equipped with all of the hormonal responses that are necessary for the male to fill a procreative role in the human race.

The level of testosterone in a baby is the same as that of a fully-grown man. After the brain finishes its initial development, between one and four years of age, testosterone levels decline quickly, and boys and girls have about the same testosterone levels from kindergarten until puberty. No wonder boys and girls at these age levels get along so well.

In males, testosterone continues to affect the developing right side of the brain, making it highly compartmentalized. Men are "wired" from the beginning to concentrate on one thing at a time. You can observe this by watching a baby boy learning to walk. Distract him and he falls down.

Females, on the other hand, have more nerves connecting the two halves of the brain so that it is easier for them to carry out parallel tasks while the two halves of their brains are operating at the same time. Men come with the ability to contain their emotions better than women because of the compartmentalization and logic of their right brains and the potential lack of full communication between the two halves of their brains.

Only with testosterone can the male fetus differentiate itself from the female model. Gender differentiation is totally regulated by chromosomes, which control the release of specific hormones. Sexual preference—the choice of a same-sex or opposite-sex partner—is a totally different issue that may be affected by additional factors.

On the evolutionary time scale female babies are much better adapted for survival than are males. Females have two complete X-chromosomes; males have only one. Because the X chromosomes have about two thousand genes, compared to only about twenty-six for a Y chromosome, a girl baby is born with an abundance of genes compared to boys. Girls are able to repair damaged genes because they have a bunch of "spare parts." This genetic fact helps explain the resilience of women. Boys simply do not possess this ability.

Approximately 120 boys are born for every one hundred girls, but about fifteen boys die in early life. Although baby boys are heavier than girls, their brains are lighter and are not as fully developed at birth. Boys are thus more vulnerable to trauma of every kind and seem more prone to certain mental diseases such as attention deficit disorder as well as autism and schizophrenia.

Chromosomes and our hormonal development are the two factors that determine whether we are male or female. In most cases these factors are in harmony, but sometimes nature plays a trick, and babies are born with mixed genitals—part male, part female.

These children are called hermaphrodites. The word comes from the story in Greek mythology of the male god, Hermes, and Aphrodite, the goddess of love, who became parents of a child, Hermaphrodite. The baby was molded in the womb by the gods to be both male and female and grew into maturity with a male penis, female breasts, and the shape and form of a woman.

This condition is not as rare as you might think. In the US there are thousands of diagnosed hermaphrodites, persons with the medical condition known as ambiguous genitalia. *Middlesex,* a novel by Jeffrey Eugenides, tells about growing up as a hermaphrodite. Dr. Richard Raskins, now Renee Richards, the US tennis star, is an example of blurred gender and its possible consequences.

Medical statistics indicate that for every fifteen thousand babies born, one will have ambiguous or mixed sexual characteristics.

Blurred gender leaves confused parents wondering just how to raise their child. Dolls or trucks? Dresses or overalls? Joan or John? Studies have shown that raising children according to their external genitalia regardless of their sex as determined by genetic analysis will result in fewer problems. Apparently our sexual organs determine our sex regardless of our chromosomal pattern.

A child easily adapts to whatever expectations are put upon it. A female child with male genitals, raised as a boy, will think she is a boy until proven otherwise and vice versa.

To understand how our chromosomes can go wrong, we need to go back and look at what happens after the egg is fertilized. The developing fetus carries one X chromosome from the mother and either the X or Y chromosome from the father. An XY combination is usually male, and an XX is female. That's how it is supposed to happen, but accidents happen.

Sometimes an extra X chromosome is incorporated into the developing embryo producing an XXY pattern. This is called Klinefelter Syndrome, and the resulting males have small testicles but cannot produce sperm. Females with one X chromosome (XO) have a genetic condition called Turner's Syndrome and do not develop ovaries.

Rarely, a genetic mistake involving a crossover or mutation of the SRY gene will produce a genetic XX male or an XY female equipped with appropriate external sex organs but the lacking the ability to produce sperm or eggs for fertilization. In some cases, a portion of the SRY gene from the Y chromosome attaches to an X chromosome, causing females to develop male sex organs—and internal female organs. In a similar fashion, XY males with an incomplete SRY mutation can become feminized, looking like a girl at birth.

We have learned a lot about genes in the past twenty or so years, and today we understand far more than ever about how important they are. But they can still fool us.

## The Biology of Homosexuality

We shudder at the idea that sexual preference is fixed from birth, but the concept that a boy or girl consciously chooses to be homosexual or gay at puberty or any other age is a biological impossibility. Indeed, recent studies of bisexual men, homosexual men, and homosexual women tell us that people with alternative sexual orientations not only have different hormonal levels from heterosexuals but also possess different physical characteristics.

According to Dennis McFadden at the Institute for Neuroscience in Texas, evidence has accumulated that "the bodies and brains of homosexual males and females differ subtly in structure and function from those of their heterosexual counterparts." Specifically, homosexual men have larger suprachiasmatic nuclei (SCN) in their hypothalamus and thicker connections between the two halves of the brain than do heterosexual males.

I've saved the discussion of how the dihydrotestosterone (DHT) in the brain may be involved in determining sexual preference for the last chapter of this book, starting on page 238. For an explanation of how the release of melatonin and oxytocin regulates the biologic clock, see page 14.

At puberty, when sex hormones are at their peak, boys become physically stronger, and their brains become more masculine. Boys demonstrate a far greater desire for excitement and risk-taking than do girls of the same age. They also begin to develop a romantic interest in girls.

It may be at this point—at puberty—that the developing brain determines sexual preference, long after physical gender has been established. Perhaps a subtle process takes over as the child's brain matures and makes a neurological and emotional commitment to either a female or a male sexual orientation.

Dynamic differences in the brains of boys and girls appear at puberty as a result of hormonal action. This happens because each half of the brain is wired differently. From puberty onward, the right or more emotional half of the brain tends to dominate in women, and the left or more logical half tends to dominate in men.

This is not to say that women cannot do well in theoretical physics or calculus or that men cannot be brilliantly creative. You probably know a strong-muscled man who writes tender love songs and a pretty woman who can take an engine apart. Our abilities are determined not by the dominance of one half of the brain over the other, but by the way the two sides of the brain work together. Each of us draws from both our right and left brain to form the characteristics that make us unique.

Nevertheless, in general, visual and spatial ability predominate in the left brain of males as more of their brain becomes devoted to vision-related stimulation. This is why men are more likely than women to possess an instinct for finding their way around a strange city or navigating an airplane in stormy weather—and why more men than women turn to pornography for sexual stimulation.

Beginning at puberty boys start to prefer geometry and mathematics and enjoy building mechanical skills. Girls, who are already ahead of boys in verbal and organizational skills, maintain this lead and generally do not follow boys to greater interest in problem-solving or mechanical understanding. In maturing girls estrogen increases the neural connections that mainly affect the right half of their brain so that hearing and speech capabilities develop better. Women's brains also have more interconnections between the two halves, creating a thicker connecting bridge that enables them to process data moving rapidly between both sides of the brain. Men might "see" how things are going better than women can, but women "listen" and "hear" better.

This effect happens not because boys are smarter than girls—or the other way around—but because of the way circulating hormones such as estrogen, progesterone and testosterone are working on the developing brain.

Girls mature earlier than boys because of the role of estrogen in their bodies. Pubic hair and full breasts are signs that estrogen is working. Some girls develop mature breasts as early as eight or nine years of age and reach full sexual maturity as much as five years ahead of boys because of their sensitivity to high levels of estrogens in the environment.

When girls grow to the weight of about 110 pounds, their fat cells contain enough of an enzyme called aromatase to work with testosterone and bring on their menstrual cycle. At that point girls are physically and hormonally ready to mate. Estrogen increases in girls and women until it reaches a peak during their first pregnancy, usually between the ages of eighteen and twenty-two, but sometimes not until they are thirty or forty years of age. For boys, the "male" hormone testosterone takes a more predictable course, increasing until the male is about age twenty-one when it peaks and then starts its slow decline.

We are still exploring testosterone's complexities and are just now beginning to fully understand how this hormone works. We know that testosterone has a powerful effect on the brain and on the sexual drive of both sexes. We now consider testosterone to be bisexual, both a male and a female hormone, because it can convert to the female hormone estrogen in the form of estradiol (E2) as well as to the male hormone DHT (dihydrotestosterone).

Now it gets complicated.

DHT regulates sex drive and muscle growth in both sexes. A burst of this hormone at the time of puberty nurtures the growth of sexual organs in boys and girls. We are beginning to see indications that DHT may affect brain development and sexual orientation—a breathtaking perspective. If it turns out to be true, perhaps we could change sexual preference by manipulating hormones. As boys and girls reach puberty, their sex hormones can create turmoil and change behavior, possibly influencing sexual preference.

Our skin and hair as well as our sex organs contain a concentrated enzyme known as 5 alpha reductase (5-AR). This enzyme is the chemical catalyst that makes the conversion of testosterone to DHT possible (see page 149). In adolescent boys, DHT brings masculinity forward by causing penis growth, deepening of the voice, and increasing a sense of dominance and sexually aggressive behavior.

In young girls, DHT increases breast and clitoris development and stimulates interest in boys. Scientists now know that some girls have a gene that boosts their body's ability to convert testosterone to DHT and that these girls reach puberty earlier than those whose bodies metabolize testosterone more slowly. Girls who go through puberty early develop breasts by the time they are nine or ten years old and in later life have a higher risk of breast cancer.

The opposite effects occur in boys and girls when estrogen instead of testosterone increases at puberty. In girls, estrogen-initiated changes cause breast buds to form and the body to take on a female shape and create a desire within the girl's brain to find a mate and reproduce. In boys, estrogen increases territorial aggressive behavior in the brain, stimulates the production of mature sperm production and increases the size of the testicles. You read that correctly. It is estrogen, not testosterone that makes the testicles grow.

Another interesting observation is that males who develop a female orientation as well as women who would rather be males seem to possess an overactive 5-AR enzyme, the substance that triggers the conversion of testosterone to DHT. For people with additional activity by this enzyme DHT levels automatically increase as they age. Men with high DHT levels are sexually aggressive or, occasionally, bisexual or homosexual in orientation. Women who produce relatively more DHT than testosterone are also more sexually aggressive and more likely to be sexually ambiguous than are women with more normal levels of the 5-AR enzyme and the DHT hormone.

Your body needs both testosterone and DHT. Ongoing studies suggest that men whose bodies produce more DHT than testosterone may be prone toward a same-sex sexual preference. The results are not definitive yet, but evidence seems to underscore the concept that gender preference is probably not confirmed at birth but is set by the hormones functioning in the brain during or after puberty.

Men who are genetically programmed to metabolize DHT efficiently from free testosterone reach maturity far earlier than their peers. They often become super-masculine with more muscle mass, larger penises, hairier bodies, thicker beards, a shorter stature, and a stronger, more aggressive sex drive. If they carry the gene for male pattern baldness, these high DHT men become bald earlier than average.

Is this complicated enough? It gets deeper.

The hormones DHT, estradiol, and testosterone create a biological paradox. Although chemically identical in all human beings, these hormones trigger totally different responses in men compared to women. Each hormone can have a totally different effect on people depending on whether they identify as male, female, or bisexual in their sexual preference.

## Straight or Gay: Biology or Choice?

Sexual orientation is the sustained erotic attraction to members of one's own sex, the opposite sex, or both. For centuries we have been intrigued by the fact that some men choose to make love to other men, and some women prefer a physical relationship with other women. The majority of men and women want a sexual relationship with a person of the opposite sex, although a few seem able to have a satisfactory sexual life with either men or women. These three varieties of orientation are called, "gay," "straight" and "bi"—for homosexuality, heterosexuality, and bisexuality.

The study of sexual orientation is probably as old as the science of psychology, but we are still wrestling with fundamental issues. Our lack of understanding persists in spite of astounding progress in the neurosciences over the past quarter century.

Genetic and hormonal influences are so closely intertwined that it is pointless to attempt to distinguish between them as we delve deeper into issues of gender identity. However, I am impressed by mounting evidence from studies of behavioral genetics that sexual preference may be less a matter of choice and more a matter of biology.

It seems to me that sexual preference is a mindset determined by the influence of various hormones in the developing brain. It may be that homosexuality in both sexes is due to the way that the fetus is exposed to hormones in the womb, leading to homosexual behavior in men and women whose genes would support a sexually "straight" lifestyle.

Homosexuality affects about three to five percent of the population in the United States, Britain and France. A nationwide survey of five thousand Australian adult twins between nineteen and fifty-two years of age revealed that for every one hundred men, fifteen of them reported they had engaged in homosexual behavior at least once, twelve said they had been sexually attracted to someone of the same sex, and six said they were not completely heterosexual. The corresponding figures for women were about half the rate of men: For every one hundred women, eight said they have engaged in homosexual behavior, eleven had been sexually attracted to someone of the same sex, and four said they were not exclusively heterosexual.

From data collected in another survey of three thousand adults, a researcher at UCLA studied sexual orientation and its relationship to illness, distress, and mental health services used by the adults. Results indicated that gay and bisexual men are more likely to experience depression, panic attacks, and psychological distress than are heterosexual men. The study also found that lesbian and bisexual women are diagnosed with generalized anxiety disorder at a higher percentage than are straight women. This is explained in part by the fact that parents, especially fathers, tend to mistreat their gay or bisexual children, blaming them for their "abnormal" gender activity. Often this abuse is both physical and sexual.

The question immediately arises: Do homosexuals have hormone levels that are different from those of the rest of the population?

When hormones in homosexuals were first studied in the 1970s, free testosterone in plasma was found to be significantly lower in male homosexuals than in heterosexuals of the same age. This finding sparked the theory that homosexuality was somehow associated with low levels of male hormone. However, it should be noted that the research was not conclusive because the sample size was small and only older men were studied.

In the mid 1990s larger studies using new, more accurate tests showed that the hormone levels of homosexual men seem to fall somewhere between those of heterosexual men and heterosexual women. Newer experimental evidence suggests that homosexual males and females may have been exposed to elevated levels of androgens while in the uterus.

The theory that sexual preference is related to hormone levels was not accepted when it was presented to the scientific community in the 1990s. Recent studies, however, have provided more compelling evidence to support the thinking that the amount of circulating testosterone and its by-products, DHT and estradiol, play a significant role in body type, sexual drive—and sexual orientation.

For example, studies show that women with higher testosterone levels are more likely to develop a tendency toward homosexual activity or sexual ambiguity. From twenty to forty-two percent of daughters of women exposed to diethylstilbestrol (DES), the first synthetic estrogen had a life-long bisexual orientation. When prescribed for pregnant women, DES created estrogen levels hundreds to thousands of times more potent than natural estrogen levels.

You may find it ironic that higher than normal levels of estrogen, the "female hormone," seem to exert a masculinizing effect on the developing brain. The explanation is that when exposed to DES, a synthetic estrogen, the developing female brain became more female than was possible naturally, and so the body responded by developing masculine characteristics.

A study of males undergoing sex change surgery to take on a female identity was conducted at John Hopkins. The men were given estrogen prior to the procedure, and they developed physical characteristics of the opposite sex, such as softer skin, less hair growth, and breast development. Not only did their bodies change, but their sexual preference also intensified.

The ability to shift preferences from one sex to another under the influence of sex hormones verifies the concept that the human brain is incredibly supple. Just as sexual arousal is the result of testosterone stimulation, sexual preference in both sexes may well be determined by the predominance of one hormone—DHT—and its effect on the developing brain.

Researchers today tell us that the same "sexy trio" of hormones—testosterone, estradiol, and DHT—that affect reproduction also affect sexual orientation. Gay and bisexual men report an earlier age of puberty, defined as the age of first pubic hair, than do heterosexual men. In women, puberty, marked as the beginning of menstrual cycles, occurs at about the same age in all women regardless of their sexual preference.

No one has discovered the gene or hormone responsible for sexual preference, or what triggers the differences, but I believe there is strong evidence that high hormone levels can definitely modify sexual orientation in women and can probably do so in men.

You won't find all of this in the medical literature because established medicine does not support a hormonal basis for sexual preference. I want to make it clear that I do not believe that levels of the hormones testosterone, dihydrotestosterone, oxytocin or cortisol can predict sexual preference. While the evidence is coming in, however, let's listen to the hormones of animals studied by researchers for clues to help us understand the phenomenon of same-sex orientation.

Pregnant rats subjected to stress at certain times during their pregnancy are more likely to give birth to male rats that behave in the submissive sexual manner of females or female rats that mounted males and other females in typical male sexual behavior.

Are these homosexual characteristics or are the rats simply responding to stress? Higher levels of cortisol during pregnancy could affect the developing fetus, and we know that high levels of cortisol can cause depression and other mood disorders. We also know from other studies that both lesbians and gay men are at higher risk for stress-sensitive psychiatric disorders than are straight persons.

An interesting study in Germany involved interviews of a large group of male homosexuals born in 1944 and 1945 in the middle of World War II. A German scientist named Dorner wondered if the stress of living in a crowded wartime environment caused an increase in the number of homosexuals born. To test this hypothesis, he designed an experiment using rats. He found that if he gave the stressed male rats testosterone, he could avert stress-induced feminization. These studies supported the fact that hormones play a role in sexual preference—at least for rats.

A word of caution is relevant here. Animal studies can provide useful theories, but since human sexual orientation is probably unique, conclusions about human sexuality based on animal research are automatically suspect until they can be verified in studies of humans.

In my own clinical practice I have observed that homosexual and bisexual men seem to notice a drop in their free testosterone levels at a much younger age than do heterosexual men. We regularly screen for sexual preference in order to see if the studies are verifiable in real life. Non-heterosexual men I have observed in my practice are also sensitive to the effects of low circulating testosterone and to the premature loss of their sexual drive.

It could be that homosexual males and females require higher testosterone levels to feel "sexually normal." Or, perhaps their sexual orientation was induced by higher levels of testosterone, but they became accustomed to testosterone levels at the high end of the normal range. In any case, my experience is that gay men seek treatment for testosterone deficiency earlier than straight men do. They start to feel their hormone levels slipping as early as their late twenties and early thirties rather than in their forties and fifties as do straight men.

## Handedness, Hormones and Sexual Identity

When hands and fingers are developing in the fetus, testosterone affects the growth of bones by causing fusion of the growth plates after bone growth has been stimulated by growth hormone. The amount of testosterone present seems to have an effect on the final length of the fingers. During the transformation of the rapidly growing fetus into a male, the normal growth of fingers make the second—or index—finger shorter than the fourth finger and the middle finger the longest. Take a look at your own hands.

You would expect the growth stimulating effects of testosterone to be applied equally to all fingers. Shouldn't the left hand be an exact mirror image of the right? It isn't always. The middle finger is always the longest, but the fourth finger isn't always longer than the index finger. We know that testosterone causes the fingers of the fetus to grow, but why do some fingers grow longer than others?

Dr. John Manning, professor of Biological Psychology at the University of Central Lancashire, has a theory about this. He states that testosterone is likely to affect finger length via androgen receptors in the connective tissue and bone. He believes that the fourth (ring) finger is stimulated to grow in the fetus by testosterone and the index finger is more affected by estrogen. More about this can be read in his book, *Digit Ratio: A Pointer to Fertility, Behavior and Health,* published in 2002.

Humans also show hand preference. A number of studies have shown that left-handedness is more predominant in homosexuals than in heterosexuals. This could be significant when we consider the fact that the right half of the brain controls the actions of the left hand and vice versa.

Early in the development of a male's brain, testosterone slows the growth of the brain's left hemisphere while it accelerates growth of the right. Although the evidence linking testosterone and handedness is largely indirect and sometimes contradictory, the association of sexual orientation with brain changes during development is supported by considerable research.

We have been able to observe that ordinarily females have a slight difference in finger length between the second and fourth fingers on the left hand compared to the right hand. This occurs in all heterosexual females. Check your finger lengths by putting your hand on a piece of paper and tracing around the tips. Make sure you label the index or first finger for proper orientation.

By comparison, for heterosexual men, the index finger is always shorter than the fourth finger on both hands. In other words, the hands of typical straight males are mirror images of each other while straight women have a slight difference in the lengths of their index and fourth fingers of their right hand compared to the fingers of their left hand.

It gets interesting when we examine the finger lengths of homosexual men because they are not mirror images from the left hand to the right hand as they are with straight persons. Instead, there is a variation in finger length between the left and the right hand, and this variation is the opposite to that of women. Also, in both homosexual men and women, the left hand predominates, and the index finger is often longer than the fourth finger. What does all this have to do with sex and listening to your hormones? What makes this happen? And does it occur on a predictable basis?

If increased testosterone enhances the right half of the brains of homosexual men, could this also affect their finger lengths and result in a variation in length in the opposite direction than for heterosexual men? Patterns of finger length might be a response to the effects of testosterone, with excessive amounts causing hypermasculinization of both the right brain and the left hand. The index finger on the left hand would grow in response to the effects of testosterone.

If varied patterns in finger lengths and influences on handedness by testosterone gives a clue for recognizing the sexual preference of other humans, could this phenomenon be associated with another male body part? Yes—the penis! Scientific investigations in large groups of young military men have shown that the length of the index finger is closely associated with penis size.

These are interesting views, but hormonal effects still do not explain sexual orientation completely since there is little evidence that the size or shape of the genitals of homosexual men and women differ from those of heterosexual men and women. If higher hormonal levels before birth are underlying factors in sexual orientation, then it seems logical to assume that dimensions of sexual organs would also be affected by these biologic factors.

The vast number of cases in the Kinsey report gave researchers the opportunity to examine statistical data on the relation between sexual orientation and genital size. Kinsey suggested that homosexual men had larger penises than heterosexual men, and the researchers were able to confirm this using the power of statistics.

Moving along, it is logical to assume that if higher than normal testosterone affects the developing penis, it might also affect the brain. Actually, the penis develops in the male embryo when the fetus is eight weeks old, much earlier than brain structures that are important for sexual identity and sexual orientation.

What about gay men? By now you may begin to notice that dihydrotestosterone is a very powerful hormone in the human body. The size of a man's penis depends on DHT. The influence of testosterone through its conversion to DHT may play a role in anatomical differences between gay or straight males, and gay or straight females.

Hormone levels may play a role not only in determining sexual preference and handedness but also in the development of the auditory portion of the brain that controls our hearing.

A researcher at the University of Texas, Dennis McFadden, demonstrated that the auditory system including the inner ear or cochlea differs between men and women. He discovered that the ear could produce an echo-like response to audio stimulation. By sending clicks and measuring the time of return (much like sonar) McFadden found the women hear better than men and that the hearing ability of gay persons is more acute than it is in straight persons.

This fits the general assumption that feminine gay men tend to be more talkative, more sensitive and more emotional than straight men. Women with a homosexual orientation have a similar leaning towards speaking and feeling. This raises the question: Are "better listeners" those with improved hearing ability or those with more perception? It could be that men or women with more feminine brains seem to hear better because of the increased interconnections between the two brain halves.

The brain is rich in aromatase, an enzyme that converts high testosterone levels to estradiol, creating changes that drive the brain more toward the female model. Extra testosterone present in the brain could result in a return to the so-called "female brain" in a male body, a phenomenon that seems to occur in homosexuals. Perhaps the additional testosterone feminizes a boy's brain, affecting specific areas of the hypothalamus and leading to attraction to the male sex.

Studies with transsexuals have confirmed some of these observations, but more research is needed concerning the phenomenon of a female-type brain in homosexual men. Theoretically, the two halves of the brain connect more readily for these men, resulting in the traits of more acute hearing and better-developed speech capabilities that are commonly seen in homosexual males. The only fact that has been proven is that the hormone testosterone somehow plays an essential role in sexuality and probably in probably sexual orientation or preference.

One day studies may show conclusively that our hormones drive our sexual identity. In the meantime, new research supports the concept that either variations in hormonal levels or some other biological mechanisms influence our sexual orientation before birth.

I am intrigued by the fact testosterone, the hormone that masculinized a female prototype and transformed it into a male fetus, is released from the mother's ovaries. In some situations an excess amount of testosterone may alter the sexual preference of the unborn baby. This finding is in contrast to earlier theories, which suggested that lower than normal testosterone was the factor causing sexual identity disorders.

So which is it, too much or too little testosterone? The answer is not clearly established. Specific brain structures in addition to hereditary factors seem to play a role in sexual ambiguity.

We have enough evidence to suggest that testosterone plays a key role in determining sexual orientation. I am certain that controversy about sexual preference will continue for years. Meanwhile, the complete deciphering of the genetic code may give us significant information to determine the degree to which homosexuality can be inherited.

## Heredity and Homosexuality

Many studies support the theory that sexual preference has a genetic component, but not much light has been shed on exactly how heredity fits in. We do know that homosexual men are statistically more likely to have older brothers than are straight men. Gay males are also more likely to have other gay family members than are straight males, and identical male twins are often gay as well. When human gene markers in some gay males were studied, it was found that they shared a gene on the X chromosome linked to failure to reproduce.

Females have two X chromosomes and plenty of backup genes to protect their brains from conditions such as autism or schizophrenia, which are more common in males. Since many of these "extra" genes are redundant, nature shuts off one of the two X chromosomes in every cell in females.

Neurophysiologist Arthur P. Arnold of the University of California at Los Angeles explains that brains respond differently, depending on which X gene of a pair is inactivated. Sometimes the X gene donated by the father is neutralized; in other cases it's the X from the mother. The parent from whom a woman gets her functioning genes determines how vigorously her genes perform. This parental effect is known as genomic imprinting of the chromosome.

It doesn't matter much which sex genes you have or which parent provided them, except for the fact that it is the Y chromosome that determines male gender and promotes the growth of extra dopamine neurons. These nerve cells are involved in reward and motivation, and the release of more dopamine enhances the pleasure of addiction and novelty seeking behavior. Dopamine neurons also affect motor skills in people with Attention Deficit Disorder (ADD), which strikes twice as many males as females.

Perhaps genes instruct the brain to develop a different sexual orientation when extra testosterone increases feelings of pleasure triggered by sex with someone of the same sex. At present there is no evidence to substantiate this theory, but Daryl J. Bem, professor of Psychology at Cornell University has written about same sex attraction in his paper, "Exotic Becomes Erotic" (www.dbem.ws), which proposes that feelings of being different produce heightened physical arousal.

At this point we have no idea of the purpose that nature intended for homosexuality or bisexuality to fulfill. What we do know is that although our faces may differ in the color of our skin and that we may have different ideas about sexual orientation, we are all humans.

Over two decades of research has been based on the assumption that homosexuality can be traced to heredity, prenatal brain differentiation, or the effects of regulating hormones from the pituitary gland. From a scientific standpoint the studies are not conclusive. For example, the methods of determining hormone levels have often been inaccurate, the number of subjects studied was too small, or the study was conducted without controls.

Scientists are uncertain about the process of sexual differentiation in human brains and do not agree among themselves regarding the role of hormones in human behavior. As a result, their studies are sometimes based on unwarranted assumptions growing out of popular beliefs and produce results that are fundamentally flawed.

An American and a Canadian researcher, Hershberger and Bogaert, used a large sample size and paid attention to detail in a study examining the timing of fluctuations of hormone levels in the pregnant female and their role in determining sexual orientation. They found that homosexuality is closely related to changes in genital anatomy including an increased penis size due to higher levels of DHT in the developing gay adolescent. Is this beginning to sound familiar?

Considered along with findings of auditory differences between homosexual and heterosexual women, this study indicates that physical distinctions do exist between these groups. The fact that handedness and finger lengths seem to play a role as physical manifestations of gender nonconformity makes it more likely that these differences are due to abnormally high testosterone levels or genetic factors—or both.

Perhaps it works like this. Some mothers in high-stress situations might transfer a genetic tendency for homosexuality via their extra X chromosome. When this marker pairs with increased testosterone exposure at specific times in the developing male or female brain, the portions of the hypothalamus that regulate sexual orientation could be affected. These same parts of the brain also regulate hormone cycles influencing oxytocin and vasopressin, which, in turn, affect bonding, sexual arousal, aggression and the formation of DHT.

As research advances in this area and specific characteristics are examined, physicians may find that sexuality, gender identity, and fertility are all intertwined as part of the symphony of human evolution.

Plenty of questions beg to be answered. Some may wonder why we expect a biological basis for sexual orientation or why biologists go to great lengths to explain homosexuality but not heterosexuality.

Personal beliefs and cultural prejudices inevitably color the interpretation of biological research. Nevertheless there are clues that hormone levels play a major role in gender identity. The answers will come when we do more research and listen more closely to our hormones. Now look at your hands again. Notice any difference between the length of your right and left fingers? Do you see what your hormones can tell you?

# 8

# The Testosterone Conspiracy

## A History of Testosterone Development

Testosterone was discovered rather late in the annals of medical marvels of the nineteenth century. Slightly more than a century ago, in 1889, Charles Edouard Brown-Séquard, the founder of the branch of medicine we know as endocrinology, concocted a "rejuvenating therapy" for body and mind with the use of extracts from testicles. He reported increased vigor and mental capacity after injecting himself with fluid he drew from the genital glands of different animals.

Arnold Berthold, a French physiologist, had conducted the earliest testosterone animal experiments forty years prior. In his experiment he took four roosters, removed the testicles of two of them and transplanted them into the abdominal cavity of the other two. The two castrated roosters, capons, grew fat and lazy, and their combs turned a pink color and stopped growing. The pair with extra testicles continued to behave normally. They crowed, they fought for territory, they chased hens, and their bright red combs continued to grow.

The red comb of the roosters acts as a secondary male sexual organ. The color and size of the comb indicate degrees of superiority in the roost. The potency of early testosterone products developed in the late 1800s was originally tested in roosters. The redder the combs grew, the higher the potency of the testosterone preparation. This simple test inspired continuing research that proved that testosterone is the primary male sex hormone in all animal species, including man.

The active ingredient in the testicles of bulls was discovered and analyzed in 1927 by McGee. This component was able to promote the growth of secondary sexual organs such as the underarm hair. In those days the only way scientists could tell if a substance caused sexual growth or activity was to inject it into castrated roosters (capons) and observe the comb.

Two years later DHEA, dehydroepiandrosterone, extracted from men's urine was found to demonstrate a similar activity. Following these discoveries, scientists were able to isolate a pure substance responsible for sexual growth, in 1931 and it was named androsterone for its properties as the definitive male androgen (Greek is "andro" for "man" and "sterone" for "hormone"). Today an androsterone derivative, androstenedione, is promoted as a sure way to increase a man's testosterone. Andro, using the popular name, is still sold without a prescription.

A German scientist, Adolf Friedrich Johann Butenandt, won the Nobel Prize in Medicine in 1935 for his work in isolating the first testosterone molecule. Within four years another scientist, Leopold Ruzicka discovered that testosterone had a beneficial effect in diabetes and could also improve the blood supply to the legs and the heart. Physicians of that day jumped on this research.

By 1945 testosterone was being used as a treatment for pain in the heart (angina). Digitalis, the only heart drug available fifty years ago, was not very helpful for this problem. Six years later it was discovered that testosterone could increase lean muscle mass by promoting protein synthesis. Athletes started using testosterone to increase their muscular development and gain an advantage in their sport. By the 1960s, testosterone use was popular in this group.

Athletes used testosterone to improve muscular strength and to decrease recovery time after intense physical activity. By the 1970s the positive effect of testosterone on bone density in both men and women was validated, and testosterone achieved status as a "miracle drug." An American, Earl Sutherland Jr., was awarded the 1971 Nobel Prize in physiology for the discovery of a form of bioenergy known as cyclic AMP, which regulated hormones. Cyclic AMP is involved in energy production and testosterone metabolism.

A decade later, Swedish and British physicians discovered prostaglandins in the prostate glands of sheep and concluded that they played a role in testosterone regulation through feedback to the pituitary gland. Today prostaglandins are used for many different conditions from asthma to ulcers. When certain prostaglandins are injected directly into the penis they produce an erection in impotent men. Two old drugs Caverjet® (Upjohn), injectable prostaglandin E or Muse® (Vivus), a pill inserted into the urethra, the opening of the penis are still used to create erections for impotent men. Testosterone ultimately regulates prostaglandin secretion.

## Players in the Marketing of Testosterone and Other Hormones

Stakes are high with billions of dollars at play in the development, marketing and distribution of potent hormones and erection enhancing products. The players with the most leverage in the hormone war are the Federal Drug Administration (FDA), the Drug Enforcement Agency (DEA), and the privately owned pharmaceutical houses that manufacture these products. Other players include the patients suffering from hormonal imbalances at the other end of the distribution chain and their physicians are caught in the middle, holding the prescription pad.

Sports and bedroom athletes are always looking for ways to enhance their strength or their manhood. This group also plays a role in the supply and distribution of bodybuilding and sex-enhancement products. These people go outside established channels if they cannot obtain the drugs they want from the medical community. In the fashion they support an underground industry consisting of an informal network of unscrupulous drug dealers who distribute illegal drugs that often contain phony or inactive ingredients.

This creates an interesting set of conflicting goals.

The purpose of the Food and Drug Administration is to protect the health and safety of the American public. The Drug Enforcement Agency was established to enforce US laws dealing with illegal drugs or controlled substances. The FDA and the DEA work in tandem. Once the FDA determines that a hormone such as testosterone poses a threat to public safety, the agency declares that it is a controlled substance, and then the DEA will apply all the regulations related to the use and abuse of a controlled product.

Enter the drug companies with profit as their primary motivation. The biggest pharmaceutical houses at the moment this paragraph is being written are Astra-Zeneca, Bristol-Myers Squibb, Eli Lilly, GlaxoSmithKline and Pfizer. Mergers and acquisitions change the playing field continually, but these companies manufacture and sell more than $40 billion of the $317 billion prescription and over-the-counter medications, sold around the world—roughly half of them in the US.

All pharmaceutical firms with operations in the US come under the protective arm of both the FDA and the DEA, but some companies are able to manipulate the system to their financial advantage. Stories are plentiful about drugs that failed to be approved by the FDA, following intense lobbying by a competing drug company or group of companies defending their financial interests by keeping out drugs they do not want marketed.

No wonder the drug manufacturers have so much influence on laws affecting their industry. Today there are more lobbyists on Capitol Hill, representing the pharmaceutical industry, than there are Senators or Congressmen. A common cause for these companies is to do battle with generic drugs, which sell for far less than brand name medications. Out of the eighty million dollars spent each year on lobbying efforts by drug manufacturers in Washington DC, ninety-seven percent comes from companies defending the position of their brand-name drugs in the marketplace. Firms that provide lower cost generic products spend practically nothing on lobbying.

The physician who writes the prescription for a specific pharmaceutical product and justifies its use in the treatment of a patient ends up being held hostage to the big business and big government maneuvering the availability of medications. Decisions about hormone replacement therapy are based on information provided by pharmaceutical houses and evaluated by government agencies.

The lowliest player in the game is the patient. Although they outnumber all other players, patients do not have as much to say about their treatment as the numbers indicate. They rely on their physicians to tell them the best course of treatment to follow when they report problems, and if the doctor matches the complaint with the best medication, the patient probably feels better and moves toward recovery. If not, he returns for another prescription or with a new symptom.

The doctor, at the next level up in the hierarchy of drug control, may not know exactly how to treat the symptoms the patient presents or may simply be ignoring new data supporting a certain form of treatment. Either way, men with severe symptoms of hormonal imbalance remain untreated. Of the estimated six million men who are affected with hypogonadism, or extremely low testosterone levels, only about a million—one out of six—will be treated for their testosterone deficiency. Then there is the group that takes treatment into their own hands.

Another group of patients are those bent on building muscle size and strength so that they can compete or win in sports. These people won't wait until the doctor tells them they do or do not need hormone-related products. They will order them on the Internet, obtain them from illicit sources on the web, or resort to other means to obtain the benefits they think they can obtain from an anabolic (bodybuilding) steroid shot or pill

## How Your Government Looks Out for Your Best Interests—or Says it Does

The FDA walks a narrow plank in looking out for our best interests. Since no substance known to mankind is totally free from every possible risk or side effect, the agency cannot keep all drugs that might cause harm out of the marketplace. In the words of the FDA itself, "There is always some risk of an adverse reaction." A lot of risk, you might conclude when you consider the fact that an estimated 125,000 people die in this country every year from drugs the FDA determined to be "safe and effective."

How does the FDA decide on the level of acceptable risk? The FDA explains this as follows, stating "when the benefits outweigh the risks…the Food and Drug Administration considers a drug safe enough for approval." According to the FDA, it's a matter of calculating the risks and comparing them with the benefits in making the appropriate decision. This is not totally an objective process because opinion and judgment are involved in identifying and measuring benefits versus risks.

Since natural hormones cannot be patented or "owned" by a commercial interest, the FDA does not investigate, approve, or regulate them. You can buy sixty tablets of melatonin, for example, without a prescription for less than ten dollars. Advertisers call melatonin a "life extender" and assure you that this naturally-occurring substance will protect you from harmful free radicals in your system, stimulate the beneficial activity of the body's growth hormone, help you sleep better, and give you many other life-extending benefits.

Many companies sell dozens of anti-aging hormonal products without a prescription, including "nutrients that accelerate your own natural production of hormones" and not only "slow down but actually reverse the aging process," according to unsubstantiated claims. Hundreds of Internet pharmacies also package and advertise "natural" hormones and prescription drugs without FDA approval. Why does the FDA leave these groups alone?

The FDA does not monitor "natural" hormones and becomes involved only when they bring about injury, medical problems, or death. The problem with using unregulated "natural" hormones is that many of them are low grade or bogus concoctions with little or no positive effect and usually contain no hormones.

It can take years from the preliminary testing of a drug until it is available by prescription or direct sale to the public. The FDA usually takes anywhere up to a decade. The process of drug approval begins when the drug sponsor presents the results of scientific studies to the FDA to show that the product is safe and effective. These studies include animal testing for toxicity by the company requesting approval.

The next step requires testing of the product in humans, usually volunteers, to see if there are any adverse effects. This is followed by clinical studies on persons with medical problems the drug is designed to treat to determine how effective it is compared to a placebo (a neutral substance) in achieving the desired result. The application process costs millions of dollars per drug and hundreds of patients are usually required.

The actual process is far more complicated than that, but this gives you a general idea of what is involved in drug approval. Although the FDA claims to have reduced approval time dramatically in recent years and now offers fast track approval requiring as little as six months for drugs treating certain serious diseases, on average it takes between five to ten years from the time a new prescription drug is developed until it becomes available to the general public. The costs are astronomical—about eight hundred million dollars per drug—and only one of twenty-five drugs that are developed by pharmaceutical firms makes it to the marketplace.

Obviously, only large, well-funded organizations can afford to pay the huge fees required to belong to the exclusive club of manufacturers of brand name drugs. Though the United States government officially endorses free competition in the marketplace, when it comes to medicine, a free market does not exist.

Instead, the high price of drug approval creates a protected and privileged market for pharmaceutical giants who can afford to pay top dollar to get their drugs legalized in this country as quickly as possible. The new pharmaceutical company Auxillium, which released the new testosterone gel, Testim®, spent about forty million dollars for clinical trials to bring the drug to market at a breathtaking speed of only twenty-two months. Most of its staff had previously worked for a competitor.

When a market is artificially protected, innovation is stifled and the consumer ends up paying a grossly inflated price for the final product. Testim costs about $185 per month, for example, and the price for Andro-

Gel, a comparable product, is $175. High prices bolster the myth that the more you pay, the better the product.

As a result, drugs such as Viagra are approved for treating sexual dysfunction while competing "me-too" drugs may face almost insurmountable barriers from entering the marketplace. Too much caution by our government means that the FDA and a few powerful pharmaceutical companies effectively direct the medical treatment of sexually related conditions.

An example is the drug Cialis® from Lilly. Dubbed as "the weekend pill," this drug is similar to Viagra but longer acting and safer, according to results of head-to-head clinical trials. Nevertheless, after extensive lobbying by Pfizer, the manufacturer of Viagra, the FDA put Cialis on hold for several years, requiring Lilly to conduct further testing. Meanwhile in Europe, where the FDA has no authority, Cialis was readily available for years and late in 2003, it finally found its way to the US market. The cost of Cialis rose to ten dollars per capsule. As a result the price of Viagra has dropped from ten dollars to one dollar for each little blue pill.

The FDA has categorized testosterone as a Class III medication, putting it into a class along with narcotics, sleeping pills and tranquilizers. Testosterone is controlled much more tightly than estrogen, which is a far more dangerous hormone (see page 84). The FDA's concern about the potential abuse of testosterone has led to heavy regulation of the prescribing of testosterone by physicians, fostering an illegal market for testosterone-related products.

Bodybuilders responded to these regulations by buying their own anabolic steroids. They call these products their "juice" or "roids" and purchase them over the Internet or from Mexico and Europe without a prescription or medical supervision. Even worse, many of these steroids sold on the black market are counterfeit.

Uncontrolled trade in illegal steroids has led the government to insist on preventing the widespread illegal access to injectable testosterone. The abuse of anabolic steroids does not cancel the fact that when a qualified physician manages testosterone therapy, it can be used therapeutically with positive value and minimal side effects. In their zeal to close the underground pipeline for injectable steroids, it seems that the Food and Drug Administration has taken an extreme position on testosterone that does not make sense from a medical perspective.

Nevertheless, several forms of testosterone are available today as medical therapy. As of the writing of this book, five major pharmaceutical houses are involved in testosterone distribution around the world. Organon, a Dutch company, is the largest. Schering-Plough, a German company, produces most of the injectable steroids that are sold in the US and Europe. Solvay, a Belgium company, owns Unimed, the manufacturer of AndroGel®, the first topical testosterone gel. Watson Pharmaceuticals, located in Salt Lake City, manufactures the Androderm® patch, known in Europe as the Andropatch®. These companies have been in the testosterone business for more than two decades.

Other testosterone medicines approved by the FDA and rarely used include Testopel®, testosterone pellets—common in the UK. In the United States TestoDerm® or Androderm®, plastic T patches and AndroGel or Testim® topical transdermal gels are the standard. Synthetic injectable testosterones such as testosterone enanthate, cypionate, and propionate were created as bodybuilding or anabolic steroids, derived from testosterone. These injectable hormones are available under a wide variety of names including Sustanon®, Virilon® and Androlan®.

Oral bodybuilding hormones such as methyl testosterone and oxandrolone can be very toxic to the liver. For this reason their use in this country has been abandoned by most men, although the drug oxandrolone (brand name Anavar®) is used in treating HIV/AIDS, while methyl testosterone is still used in some European hormone preparations for women.

An oral testosterone preparation, Andriol®, developed in Canada, will soon be available in the United States as a lozenge which can be placed in the cheek pouch, like chewing tobacco. Apparently Andriol circulates exclusively within the lymphatic system avoiding the liver-related problems that have been observed with the use of oral anabolic steroids. The disadvantage is that Andriol is short acting.

Early in 2004 four new companies were jockeying for a piece of the testosterone pie. Proctor and Gamble, partnered with Watson, is testing a testosterone patch for women. Release was expected within a year. King Pharmaceuticals and Novagen each have two testosterone products in the pipeline. Cellegy, a South San Francisco company, and BioSante from Illinois, are competing with two new transdermal testosterones: Tostrex® and Bio-T® gel. These companies are working to develop new topical testosterone gels for both men and women.

Each of these drug companies has negotiated a license to market testosterone. Operating somewhat like a testosterone franchise from the FDA, the Food and Drug Administration, these licenses permit manufacturers to market their product legally. A franchise is a privilege granted under franchise law to a corporation or an individual in exchange for business rights that most corporations and persons would not otherwise have. The FDA gives itself permission to issue franchises as it sees fit.

The problem is that virtually no one, including FDA insiders, understands the decision making process at the FDA. Dangerous drugs like Accutane® (Roche), which was prescribed to treat acne but caused severe psychiatric problems leading to suicide, stay on the market. Other medications with a proven track record such as DHT gels, successfully used by European men, were kept off the American market. As I was preparing this book for printing, Solvay was petitioning the FDA for approval of their new DHT gel, Andactrim®, in the US.

Because the FDA and the Drug Enforcement Agency (DEA) consider the abuse of testosterone to be a serious problem, the DEA closely monitors the prescribing of testosterone, and attempts to interfere with the vast illegal market for steroids, which are derivatives of testosterone. Meanwhile, the FDA acknowledged the importance of testosterone in men's health by approving two new transdermal gel preparations in less than two years.

These preparations have become increasingly valuable in treating "low testosterone syndrome," a phrase used to describe the negative effects of not having enough testosterone circulating in the body. The most common problems for men with low testosterone include a lower sex drive, less muscle mass, memory difficulties, increased risk of heart attacks, and more fragile bones with lower mineral density.

The good news is that men with dangerously low levels of testosterone can be treated successfully with replacement doses of testosterone and enjoy better muscle and bone strength, improved moods, and less body fat in addition to increased sexual drive.

Ironically, testosterone is often used to restore life to men suffering with AIDS, but is not readily available for normal men when they become testosterone deficient. The aging American public has no idea about the benefits of balanced hormone replacement, particularly in terms of improved vitality. Even though estrogenic hormones are given to women to help protect them from age-related changes, testosterone is not made readily available to men who need it.

The FDA approved testosterone for the treatment of impotence in men in the 1970s, but many physicians were reluctant to use it, largely because they were not trained in the management of impotence with testosterone. Paradoxically, other, more potentially harmful products are sold over the counter (OTC).

The FDA considers testosterone a highly dangerous and abused drug and looks askance at the idea of making it available to anyone without a prescription. Even as it takes a hard line on testosterone, other potent hormones such as androstenedione and DHEA are readily available over the counter, and athletes can buy testosterone products without a prescription or from unscrupulous doctors on the Internet, creating a type of international pharmacy black market.

Athletes seem to care about only one thing, winning. To do that, they believe they must be faster and stronger. Prohormone precursors such as androstenedione, DHEA, pregnanediol, nor-testosterone, Tribulus, pregnenolone and nor-androstene, sold OTC, are regularly promoted in muscle magazines and the popular press as effective stimulants and alternatives for testosterone activation. Most of them don't work or create another set of problems by increasing estrogen levels.

Occasionally so-called precursor compounds lead to higher estrogen or cholesterol alterations. Erectile dysfunction can develop in young men using these OTC products for a short time because of higher estrogen levels. These men think that hormone precursors will raise their testosterone level without needing a doctor's prescription. Not true. OTC testosterone products are neither reliable nor effective for increasing muscle mass in testosterone-deficient men.

Why would men buy their drugs on the Internet rather than going to see a doctor for a prescription? The reality is that most doctors, even when the patient has clear laboratory evidence of a deficiency, will not prescribe testosterone products because of its association with illegal drug use. Internet businesses have jumped in to fill the gap, selling bogus products to unsuspecting men who may have hypogonadism that is not being diagnosed or appropriately treated.

Harm to the body from unauthorized use of hormone supplements is not severe. For those buying "undiluted" or unadulterated steroids, actual side effects are mild, and serious problems seem to occur only if the injection of steroids is suddenly stopped. A Canadian study showed that most of the side effects of anabolic steroids are reversible, although abrupt withdrawal from steroids can produce problems similar to those in other types of drug withdrawal. This indicates that addiction may play a role in anabolic steroid abuse.

## Testosterone Delivery—Shots, Patches or Gels

Testosterone therapy can be delivered in a variety of ways, including injection, pellet implants, pills, gels, and skin patches.

The problem with injected testosterone is the erratic swings in testosterone levels that result. Testosterone injected into the bloodstream raises the level of the hormone rapidly at first and then diminishes until the next injection. While levels are exceptionally high, the person may experience severe side effects, including headaches, acne, unwanted erections, and liver and sexual problems.

Testosterone patches applied to the skin deliver a steady stream of the hormone without these side effects. In 1985 the FDA approved testosterone treatment in the form of medical patches to treat testosterone deficiencies and to prevent osteoporosis. Clinical trials confirmed that muscle strength, mood, and sexual energy were enhanced in men of all ages after they received supplementary testosterone from skin patches.

After the FDA granted marketing approval for AndroGel in July of 2000, it approved another one percent testosterone gel named Testim in November 2002. Auxillium conducted the largest placebo controlled trial in testosterone history with over 400 men receiving either Testim or a placebo gel. The trial results showed that these products are very safe and Testim was more effective than AndroGel. No negative effects, other than occasional skin reactions, have been reported with the skin patches Androderm or TestoDerm after almost two decades of use. Nevertheless, today only four testosterone products are available for application anywhere on the male body.

The skin patches are safe and effective for most persons, but the same products do not work equally well for everyone. Brian, for example, was pleased with the effects of the scrotal patch but had no benefit from AndroGel®.

Despite numerous studies proving the safety of delivering testosterone via gels applied directly to the skin, the DEA still considers testosterone to be a dangerous drug. This attitude endures from years of dealing with the abuse of injectable bodybuilding steroids.

Clinical trials by Bob Swerdloff and Christina Wang at UCLA demonstrated that AndroGel is safe for increasing muscle mass and reducing osteoporosis in men with HIV/AIDS. Researchers are now looking at dihydrotestosterone gels as a superior treatment for these conditions in older men.

The DEA is the official drug enforcement agency of the FDA and takes its work seriously in cracking down on people misusing testosterone and illegal pharmacy sites on the Internet. Men who self medicate with steroids or are caught selling them are subject to federal punishment, often without testing them to determine their testosterone levels. One look at a muscular man, and the doctor sees another "red flag" for the DEA. Treating the patient with testosterone regardless of hormone levels places the doctor under suspicion for being a drug pusher. The doctor knows that refusing to treat is the only sure defense against being accused of prescribing steroids inappropriately.

Most physicians are oblivious to the benefits of testosterone for aging men and women. Fostered by the media and supported by the FDA, misinformation that runs counter to studies produced by the large pharmaceutical testosterone manufacturers is distributed to the doctors. The cycle of misinformation assures that little testosterone will be prescribed until doctors become better educated in this area of hormonal therapy.

Once a pharmaceutical company is given approval to market a drug, the FDA makes suggestions about how the drug should be marketed and medical indications for the drug. If testosterone is approved for treating low testosterone levels (hypogonadism), for example, as are TestoDerm and AndroGel, or Androderm, then it cannot be used for any other purpose, or the FDA would consider that "off label" use.

The irony is that doctors routinely use several FDA-approved products for off-label use to benefit their patients. I believe that we could call the relationship between the FDA and the large pharmaceutical companies "financial nepotism." This built-in conflict of interest might help protect some drugs from scrutiny when they are used "off label" while others are carefully watched—and restricted.

Mergers and acquisitions are as common in the pharmaceutical business as they are in other industries. Bentley Pharmaceuticals purchased the license to produce Testim, a newly approved low potency testosterone gel, from the start-up company Auxillium. Solvay bought Unimed as a subsidiary to manufacture AndroGel. In 2000, Johnson and Johnson purchased Alza Pharmaceuticals, the maker of TestoDerm TTS®, the first testosterone transdermal plastic patch applied to the scrotum. Although it delivered a physiologic dose of 4 to 6 mg of testosterone per day, the patch was too awkward and uncomfortable for general use. Johnson and Johnson decided to discontinue the scrotal patch in 2001 because it was not delivering adequate profits. This is unfortunate, especially for my young friend Brian.

When I first talked to Brian, he was thirty-four years old and spilled out a list of his sufferings for the past ten years or so, including horrible joint pain, major depression, weight gain for absolutely no reason up to two hundred and fifty pounds with a small frame.

Because of his pain and emotional discomfort, Brian's doctor prescribed Prozac and various strong pain medications. Over the years all of Brian's tests years came back normal, but his testosterone was never checked.

One day Brian was "playing doctor" on the Internet and learned that all of his symptoms led to the idea that his testosterone levels were extremely low. By then his symptoms had worsened to the point that his doctor was recommending that he see a shrink, but Brian knew everything that he was experiencing was not in his mind.

"After my research on the Internet," he told me, "I discussed my findings with my doctor and he finally agreed to test my testosterone, which came back at levels in the hundreds—extremely low for someone my age. My doctor immediately prescribed patches to be worn on my scrotum, and the effects were amazing and immediate. To date, I am off all medications for depression, pain, etc., and in one month lost ten pounds without changing my diet. I ran four miles the other night and wasn't even breathing heavy."

After a month of "feeling human" again, Brian asked the doctor to let him discontinue the patch and just apply the testosterone gel every morning.

"The results were horrible," he told me, "and just as immediate as were the good effects from the patch." In less than a week Brian got all of his problems back and gained three pounds in the process. "We doubled the dosage of the gel, but still I was going downhill and fast." Brian recognized that he was headed for serious trouble so went back on the scrotum patch. I'm feeling great again!" he said, "and I don't plan to come off the patch."

He was puzzled about why there should be such a huge difference in response. Why should he do so well on the scrotum patch, while the gel did nothing for him? "I am frightened to ever come off the patch now because my return to suffering so quickly terrified me," he said. "Can you please give me your insight as to why the scrotum patch is so effective, and what, if any, changes I should or can make in the future?"

Brian wasn't thrilled with the possibility that the scrotum patch would be the only or the best thing that would work for someone like him. After all, he noted, applying and wearing the patch is just plain awkward.

Brian is definitely the exception to the scrotum patch rule, proving that products do not work the same way for all people. Because of unfavorable reactions to testosterone applied directly to the scrotum, today all testosterone products have clear warning labels to avoid scrotal application.

Today pharmaceutical companies promote the newer plastic patches and testosterone gels as safe and effective in men with low levels. These forms of testosterone were first released in 1985 for application to the male scrotum but were seldom prescribed at first because of their high cost and safety concerns. The cost of the patches was almost ten times that of synthetic injections, and the rather large patches (over two inches wide), were uncomfortable and created frequent skin reactions.

Scrotal testosterone patches have now been phased out of promotion and production due to their lack of popularity with both patients and physicians. The new alcohol-based testosterone gels have taken over market share from the testosterone patches.

Low potency testosterone gels are the darlings of the FDA and all the "me-too" drugs submitted by the new companies, which are looking for market share and are practically guaranteed testosterone franchises. Since it release, AndroGel by Unimed, has taken over almost forty percent of the testosterone market from Watson Pharmaceuticals. Solvay, Unimed's parent company, is earning over two hundred million dollars annually from AndroGel sales. Any new competing testosterone products attempting to enter the market will not only cost their parent companies several millions to clear through the FDA but most will be approved.

Of course, in time, other companies will in due course develop new topical versions of the testosterone as well as estrogen, progesterone, and DHT. Some companies will develop generic forms or cheaper equivalents of the current market products, but I do not believe that testosterone will ever be released over the counter.

Testosterone supplementation is indicated for any man or woman who has a testosterone deficiency. You and your personal physician may want to review the indications for testosterone replacement in this book, but be aware that a medically standard screening test for testosterone deficiency is only partially adequate. Only a physician using either a blood serum or saliva test can determine testosterone deficiency. It cannot be diagnosed by responding to a questionnaire or a quiz about hormones.

## Contrived Hormone Shortages Don't Help Anyone

Control by limiting supply is an attractive marketing tool to inflate prices. Despite all the safety studies, clinical trials and large-scale manufacturing, production of testosterone generics and its injectable forms have become difficult for pharmacies and physicians to obtain. Several small suppliers have been unable to obtain any testosterone derivatives at all from their distributors due to restrictive FDA regulations and drug recalls.

Generic drugs are supposed to contain a certain percentage of the same "active ingredient" as those with a brand name. They have been on the market for decades. Generic anabolic steroids were much cheaper than the brand names, but suddenly they are no longer available to physicians or pharmacies.

We face a nationwide shortage of certain injectable testosterone products due to removal from the market by the FDA. Generic testosterone cypionate has been unavailable in San Francisco since 2001 and presumably throughout the United States, although some stocks may still remain in distribution houses. No one is currently manufacturing generic testosterone cypionate or Nandrolone for the U.S. market, and there are no immediate plans to resume production. Why has this happened?

Organon, the major supplier of synthetic testosterone to the modern world, was being investigated by the FDA and had to account for unusually large inventory losses of their anabolic steroids. Most of the losses were probably being diverted to the black market.

Few are aware that multiple middlemen between the manufacturer of injectable medications and the pharmacy give criminals ample opportunity to confiscate and duplicate or dilute injectable hormones by accessing the distribution channels and subverting the delivery of the medications.

If generic drugs are unavailable, physicians must use brand-name versions that cost several times as much—or switch to other more expensive options for testosterone replacement such as patches or gels. Since these products are almost impossible to abuse, we have to consider the possibility that the FDA is attempting indirectly to drive the market for topical applications.

Hypogonadism among HIV-infected patients is marked by decreased muscle mass and functional capacity, fatigue, and reduced quality of life. Synthetic testosterone analogues, such as Oxandrolone and Nandrolone Decanoate, also have been studied in AIDS, the wasting syndrome. Trials of both steroids resulted in significant weight gain at certain doses, but also demonstrated a significant risk of liver damage.

At least one nongeneric testosterone product, Depo-Testosterone® 200mg/ml, has been back-ordered since late 2001. Though the less expensive generics are nowhere to be found, the brand name injectable testosterone enanthate—Delatestryl®—is available, with no supply problems expected. The real problem is the high costs of brand name injectables, which have doubled and tripled since the FDA investigation.

Generic testosterone enanthate has been out of stock in many pharmacies, and more shortages are soon expected. Testosterone enanthate, available only under the brand name Depo-Testosterone was $120 for ten cubic centimeters (about two teaspoons) in 2003 compared to $35 two years earlier. Depo-Testosterone is essentially the same as testosterone cypionate, which is still available as a generic, and can be substituted in most patients. According to two leading HIV physicians, Nandrolone Decanoate, which is very effective for reversing AIDS wasting syndrome, is in drastically short supply.

The additional expense is especially problematic for physicians working under certain managed-care contracts. In San Francisco some leading HIV specialists have been forced into contracts with no AIDS "carve out"—which means they are paid about five dollars a month to cover office visits for a person with AIDS. The additional reimbursement for a testosterone injection barely covered the cost of the medicine for the cheapest generics. Many physicians who specialize in AIDS care are losing money on every patient and being forced to pay for their AIDS practice by taking on other work. They cannot count on a built-in margin to cover the sharply increased cost of non-generic testosterone.

One San Francisco physician I interviewed has had no problems with patients filling their prescriptions at local pharmacies. In the meantime another physician, whose managed-care contract requires that he inject the drug in his office, has been unable to obtain supplies after calling distributors around the country.

The FDA has reasons to be concerned about anabolic steroid abuse through a black market of underground sales of injectable testosterones. This concern has triggered their restrictive position on testosterone.

Because bodybuilders abuse this hormone in any form they can get it, they are willing to pay top dollar for a supply. This has created a huge market for counterfeit testosterone products that are available illegally. Today only two companies provide brand name anabolic steroids—Organon and Upjohn Pharmaceuticals.

Generic anabolic steroids have all been recalled because the FDA wants to regain some control over the availability of testosterone products. Nothing was wrong with the generic products; the FDA was merely investigating the marketing practices of certain companies and wanted to stop illegal availability of testosterone.

Illegal steroids are smuggled into the US from Europe and Central and South America on a daily basis. Holders of testosterone marketing franchises continue to lobby to keep their products in the FDA's Class III category as a controlled drug. Ironically, these same companies, willingly or not, are the major suppliers to Europe of illegal anabolic steroids.

Organon Pharmaceuticals, the number one manufacturer of synthetic testosterone in the world, sells most of its injectable testosterone in Europe and Asia. Organon manufacturing plants could not account for huge inventory losses in 2001, although Organon's salespeople said they had plenty of brand name testosterone to sell.

It does not seem likely that this large conglomerate would want their competition to make any testosterone available. Solvay Pharmaceuticals has been selling testosterone gels in Belgium for about five to ten dollars a month but has set the price of their skin delivery gel, AndroGel, at over $175 a month.

The franchise for testosterone is lucrative and has been granted to only a handful of manufacturers worldwide, assuring an intact monopoly. No new competitor has entered the testosterone market in over two decades. As a result, men are being denied the opportunity to replace their hormones because of attempts to block illegal testosterone use by bodybuilders.

Neither estrogen nor progesterone is regulated so strictly. Progesterone, which converts to testosterone in the body, is readily available over the counter in a low potency cream for women.

The FDA has approved more than thirty-five testosterone preparations from about a dozen different companies, but numbers showing how many are currently on the market are not available.

The FDA guidelines for testosterone replacement with generic testosterone are narrow and rigorous. Though testosterone has been shown safe and effective in protecting against cancer and decreased immune deficiency in HIV-infected patients, inexpensive generics were not available. By limiting distribution to one of the five major testosterone franchises, the FDA could more closely monitor inventories and maintain control.

As a result, many men have been forced to seek their own sources of testosterone. Roger, who was unable to persuade his doctors to check his hormones to see if they were at normal levels and if not to find a solution to his problem, turned to illegal sources of steroids. A year and a half later, a combination of feeling unhealthy and being fearful of getting caught convinced him to eliminate the use of steroids. He suffered severe withdrawal symptoms along with less testosterone production after "cycling off" steroids. I call this condition "Post Anabolic Steroid Abuse Syndrome" (PASAS). True chemical dependence, which is more common than previously recognized, can result from the use of anabolic steroids.

Six months later, Roger felt so rotten that his physician referred him to an endocrinologist, who diagnosed him with hyperthyroidism. "My thyroid was burning up," Roger said, and he had low levels of free testosterone. At this point Roger's total testosterone was at normal levels of 500 nanograms per deciliter, but his free testosterone was only 17 picograms per milliliter compared with a reference range for his age group of 19 to 41. Close to normal, but in Roger's words, "I sure didn't feel normal at all."

Roger worked with his endocrinologist for months. "He kept saying that despite what I felt my testosterone wasn't too low and my problems were more likely due to my malfunctioning thyroid. It's true that soon after I met him became hypothyroid, the opposite of my previous condition."

Roger waited while the endocrinologist adjusted his thyroid medication over the following months, hoping that this would bring back his energy, libido, and muscles. In the end Roger's thyroid levels were normal, but he still felt tired during the afternoons, his libido was poor, his strength continued to decline, and, most importantly, his free testosterone levels dropped further and were hovering around 15 (normal is 19 to 41 picograms per milliliter). To the endocrinologist this was a borderline case of what he called secondary hypogonadism.

Though Roger's condition came about following steroid abuse, the reason he was affected is still unknown. At this point you're probably thinking, "Too bad for Roger, but what's that got to do with me?" Brace yourself. The connection might surprise you.

Roger felt he was suffering from the main problem steroid users had assured him would not happen—incomplete recovery of his testosterone levels. Somehow his pituitary (the control center in the brain that tells testicles to produce testosterone) never turned all the way back on after he stopped the steroids. "To make matters more confused," Roger recalls, "I was only a borderline case. Because of that, my endocrinologist would not suggest testosterone replacement regardless of how I complained of those classic symptoms of low testosterone."

Roger was desperate and tried many new diets and various supplements. "I did find some that helped," he said. "Zinc at fifty to one hundred mg/day really helped my libido. Aerobics five times a week combined with heavy lifting seemed to help as well. Yet with all my efforts, my free levels remained around 15 ng/dl, even with total testosterone rising slightly to the low six hundreds. Now, my doctor was more resistant to any further action because my total testosterone levels were over six hundred—well within the normal range!"

This doctor was so sure that total testosterone was the definitive measurement of testosterone in the adult male that he told Roger that the test results for free testosterone were probably erroneous. Finally, he refused to test Roger's testosterone levels any more and recommended that he just give it "more time."

Like Roger, many testosterone-deficient men are made to feel as if there is a medical conspiracy to deprive them of access to this essential hormone. Testosterone control through regulation is the status quo for the FDA, and the extreme conservative position of the FDA is unlikely to change. As a result most hypogonadal men are made to feel as if they are asking for an illicit drug when they request testosterone supplements or ask about testing for a deficiency they suspect they may have.

"More time?" Roger said. He was getting angry now. "I had already lost all the strength I had gained though years of lifting weights and was wasting further! And to make matters worse, I felt tired and depressed all the time. So there I was with no one to help me, desperate for a solution." Then he found out about my clinic in Monterey, California.

Roger's total testosterone was at a level considered normal for most men, but Roger was only thirty-one years old.

Let's let Roger tell us what happened next.

"I gave Dr. Kryger a call and to my surprise he answered the phone. Already I could tell he was different. Over the phone he spent at least thirty minutes talking about what was going on, and he followed up the discussion saying he wanted to see me in only a few days! It was like a hundred pound weight had been lifted off my shoulders. Here was a medical professional specializing in helping ex-bodybuilders, among the brightest in his field, who wanted to help me at a reasonable price! I was delighted!

"It was a bit of a drive to Monterey from the San Francisco bay area, but it was worth my time. Dr. K was just as friendly and genuinely concerned with me in person as he was over the phone. He knew the concerns and problems of getting off steroids, and addressed every problem thoroughly. He conducted himself in a professional manner but not in a cold or distant manner. He seemed more like a friend who just happened to know a lot about my problem.

"Dr. K prescribed testosterone cream. I had heard of transdermal testosterone creams before, but I was a bit skeptical about them being messy or leaving a sticky residue. I was also scared of potential side effects like sterility, often associated with injection-based testosterone replacement therapy. To my pleasant surprise, the cream is neither sticky nor messy in any way. The white, nearly odorless (slightest scent of tofu) substance is very easy to apply. It rubs in quickly leaving no trace. The doctor also explained to me that testosterone cream might reduce or raise sperm count, but that only time would tell how it would affect my fertility.

"Only a week after having begun the cream, I noticed a huge difference in my energy levels! My depression lifted, and my libido was in full swing! I have been using your testosterone cream for only a short time now, but it is awesome! It's extremely anabolic too; I have made gains in the gym after almost a year of mostly losses!"

Roger's hormone levels were restored to normal with a compounded high potency testosterone cream, which allowed Roger to use a tiny volume of medication.

Let me emphasize here that adding more and more testosterone does not solve every problem of low libido and other symptoms of an inadequate sexual life. If you take in too much testosterone, the excess can rapidly convert to estrogen, causing distressing problems such as sexual dysfunction, breast enlargement, shrinking testicles, aggression and moodiness.

Achieving a proper hormonal balance requires guidance from a doctor trained in hormone regulation along with regular monitoring.

Scott's story describes the problems that result when a person tries to achieve hormonal balance on his own.

Scott's doctor gave him injections of testosterone cypionate, starting with an injection of one hundred milligrams. "I felt nothing," Scott said. "The second injection ten days later was two hundred milligrams, and I felt great, but my nipples enlarged a little and got sensitive, and three days later I felt my usual not-so-hot self."

The doctor's plan was to give Scott two hundred milligrams every ten days and then to check his blood levels thirty-six hours after the third two hundred milligram injection.

The doctor was out of town when Scott had another flare-up of gynecomastia (enlarged breasts). "Every time I've mentioned aromatase inhibitors he says we'll cross that bridge when we come to it," Scott told me. "I've been on that bridge for three months now, and I'm very frustrated."

Scott is convinced that injections are not the best route for him because of the severe letdowns after the initial rush of the dose. The doctor, who uses testosterone injections himself, told Scott that he didn't feel any letdown at all between injections.

"I certainly did," Scott said. "I also felt great when I was using the cream before. Evidently, I'm just one of those cases that's sensitive to the way injections delivers the hormone to my body."

The reality is that injections of testosterone always overshoot their mark. The initial gush of hormone when the shot is given leads to the feminizing problems we've just noted because the excess testosterone converts to the female hormone, estrogen.

Men like Scott are usually given injections to counteract the drop in testosterone with aging. Older men suffering from classic testosterone deficiency are told that it is normal to have lower testosterone with aging. Occasionally they are prescribed testosterone by injection to correct their deficiency. Then the wildly fluctuating levels of testosterone associated with injections too often create a whole new set of problems.

When the FDA finally approved the first low potency one percent testosterone, they were careful not to give the impression that they wanted to restrict men's access to testosterone if there was a proven need. You may recall that the female requirement for testosterone is about one-half to one milligram of one percent per day while two and a half to five grams of gel are recommended for testosterone replacement therapy for most men. This gel product was made for a man but was strong enough to work for a woman in a smaller volume.

Several men who tried AndroGel when it first came out on the market sent me a letter asking for testosterone testing to see if their levels were adequate after they found they needed at least ten grams of AndroGel. Here are some of their comments.

A young man named Gerry from San Francisco had this to say: "AndroGel works really good and has cleared up nearly all of the symptoms I had, including a whole slew of other minor ailments I didn't know were related. What a blessing, but it was bittersweet. You practically have to paint yourself with the stuff due to it being so weakly formulated."

"I was unsuccessful in convincing my primary Doc to go with a compounded gel in a higher strength, but I practically had to beg to get the AndroGel," said Frank, from Illinois. "In fact," Frank continued, "his resistance has cost him my business. He wanted to continue trying other pharmaceuticals on me. I told him to let me try this for a month just to 'get it out of my head.' Actually it was just so I could prove I knew what the hell I was talking about. Point made. I had no idea what a difference a little hormone can make in nearly every facet of my life. My joints are healing up for the first time in many years. I'm making gains on the weights after three years of nothing. I'm getting out and fixing my beautiful boat and getting it running. I get more done in three hours at work than in three days before in the fog."

Randy in Florida says he thinks that AndroGel is still "a little too weak," and that while he was beginning to feel more like his old self, he wasn't quite there yet. "I used to be very aggressive," he said. "Nice, but a hard charger. Now I am getting my low secret snarling attitude back the way I remember, but it's not quite as distinct as before. I'm at 7.5g/d and maybe 10g/d or 12.5g/d would be closer to normal. That's two or three packages at about four hundred dollars a month."

As with most medications, some responses are positive and some are negative. The main problem is that with the gel testosterone concentration is almost always too low.

AndroGel is made for men but contains only enough testosterone in a single gram for a woman's dose. The FDA in its zeal to outlaw testosterone abuse has allowed only limited strength testosterone products like AndroGel on the market.

This is just another way that testosterone-deficient men are made to feel as if they need to beg for a prescription or deal in illegal markets to get their testosterone supplements since transdermal products are so expensive or of such low potency. A man would have to use one 2.5 gram packet of

AndroGel at about $100 a month (without insurance) to receive the equivalent of twenty-five milligrams of testosterone a day. At ten percent absorption, this amount would provide about half the daily normal output of the testicles.

Sam, a frustrated testosterone deficiency patient in California, said he felt he was lucky to have an endocrinologist subscribe AndroGel at the age of fifty-three years. Sam's problem was not loss of sexual interest or function, but severe back problems and sore joints. "I looked at my medical records and found that in 1993 my total T dropped from the five to six hundred range to three hundred. A month ago it was two hundred and seventy. That's when I confronted the internist and said maybe there's a relationship."

With misgivings, Sam's doctor prescribed a few months' worth of AndroGel at fifty milligrams a day. Within two weeks Sam said he was sleeping better and his wrists stopped hurting. "I'm also less cranky and do not think that the world is a black hole any longer," Sam said. "I still wonder why the drop in 1993, and nobody seems to know the long-term impact of this therapy, but I have to tell you I would rather run the risk of prostate problems then return to where I was a month ago, and my endocrinologist says he doesn't expect full impact of therapy to begin until I've been on it at least a month or more."

## Changing Attitudes: Our Greatest Challenge

For all its boasting about how safe and scientific the pharmaceutical industry is, a drug-approval system riddled with incompetence and corruption has been exposed in the media. The system results in the death of over 125,000 Americans every year from drugs the FDA says are safe. The revolving door between the FDA and multi-national drug companies creates a system that excludes smaller firms and virtually ensures that access to drugs is limited in America to those guaranteed to make billions of dollars for large companies.

The recent trend is for companies to develop high profit "life-enhancing" drugs such as Viagra®, at the expense of life-saving drugs that usually return less profit. The FDA supports the pharmaceutical giants who take extraordinary steps to keep out foreign competition, especially if the offshore medication is safer, cheaper, and more effective than its American counterpart.

The net result is that Americans pay the highest prices in the world for pharmaceuticals. At the same time we suffer the highest rate of drug-induced adverse reactions. Deaths from prescription drugs are the fifth or sixth leading cause of dying in the United States. Inflated prices for bad products reflect a system that is corrupt and must be changed if Americans are to live healthier and longer thanks to the benefits of medicine.

Drug manufacturers openly criticize the FDA for the delay and high cost of getting new drugs through the system. Drug companies claimed that from 1977 to 1996, they increased spending on new pharmaceutical compounds fifteen fold, but the FDA approval of new drugs remained relatively flat during that time. Additional problems cited by the drug industry include turnover of FDA personnel, limitations of drug reviewers' technical knowledge and communication problems between the FDA and the drug companies.

All of this points to a bureaucratic quagmire that enables large drug companies to dominate the market, making it far too expensive for smaller companies to compete. Americans endorse a deregulated market, where economic success is predicated on a company developing effective products at a fair price.

Once a profit-generating substance has been approved for marketing to the public, the FDA is so overburdened with investigating new drugs in the application process that unless there are serious complaints or deaths linked to the use of a specific drug, they do not usually follow up.

What should be done?

We must shine the light of full disclosure through public education and communication on the following government issues related to hormone therapy—

1. Extensive lobbying by pharmaceutical houses to block or delay competing drugs from entering the marketplace.

2. A lengthy approval process that lends itself to challenge and manipulation by competing forces.

3. The high cost of obtaining approval for new drugs, resulting in high barriers for competing companies to surmount.

4. Confusion by doctors and law enforcement individuals about the cancer risk of testosterone.

5. Limited or nonexistent supplies of less expensive generic testosterone and other hormone replacement products.

6. Ready supply of fake or low-quality products for sale by unscrupulous dealers.

7. A shortage of low-dosage generic testosterone preparations for sale without a prescription.

8. Widespread ignorance of the facts and total unawareness of the issues involved.

The only way we can meet these problems head on is by educating the public about the risks and benefits of carefully prescribed hormone replacement therapy programs and by putting pressure on our law-making bodies to allow less costly generic drugs to have access to the marketplace.

Doctors need to hear you tell your story and describe your frustration and your sense of being left out of hormone therapy benefits. They need to stop buying every sales pitch from their drug reps and listen more carefully to their patients.

It's time for all doctors to pay closer attention and listen to their patients' hormonal needs.

# 9

# Living Longer with Your Hormones

## Marketing Mania for a Better Life

It's no feat of rocket science to figure out what human beings want. We want to live long and satisfying lives. We want to fight off the demons of old age. We want to be young and sexy forever. We all want to be able to "do it till we die!"

When we discuss aging, we must consider two definitions of lifespan. Average lifespan is the average age at which members of our species die. Improvement in average lifespan can be achieved by assuring a clean food and water supply. Maximal lifespan, or the age achieved by the longest-lived human, is usually what researchers study. Lengthening the maximal lifespan is much more difficult than increasing the average lifespan.

Clever marketers watch trends and look for ways to offer eager buyers what they want. One "famous formula" weight loss program, for example, claims it can help you "drop your dress size" from size eighteen to eight in six weeks. Once you're fashionably thin, you can sign up with another company with a bosom-boosting breast cream that will help you fill a Size D cup bra. Then there's a "love gel" for sale that you can rub on your body so that your husband will be yours forever.

All of these inducements are supported by half-truths veiled with empty promises. But they do sell! For businesses with an ear tuned to the cash register, testimonials and promises are often enough to turn a healthy profit. The booming industry segment of hormone supplements prospers because of our quest for a better life, but too often we don't get what we pay for.

## Rejuvenators or False Hope?

The desire to remain young is as old as mankind. Although the fountain of youth may be nothing more than mist on the horizon, the discovery of

Florida by Poncé de Léon was the result of a search for the Fountain of Youth.

Today outrageous claims attract highly educated people who should know better than to believe the impossible. Not long ago several hundred people responded to an advertisement in a bodybuilding publication for giant arctic albino wolverine extract. The fact that the post office box was in rural Sweden and that there is no such thing as a giant arctic albino wolverine didn't deter them. Neither did the total lack of any scientific studies or the placement of the "advertisement" in the humor section of the magazine flash a warning in their minds. It may have been a joke as far as the editors were concerned, but readers were dead serious and wanted to know more.

Desperation is the name of the game for those who live for their sports triumphs. Athletes and bodybuilders want a competitive advantage more than anything else and will take almost any supplement to boost their chances. They know that winners are separated from losers by a few thousandths of a second or a hundredth of a point, and attempt almost anything that may have a chance of maximizing their performance plus the earnings tied to success.

A researcher surveyed athletes hoping to compete in the Olympics about their willingness to take an illegal drug if they were certain it would bring them success. Almost all of them said they would take the drug, and half of them said they'd take it for at least five years—even if it were killing them. For them, life has no meaning aside from winning.

This all-consuming drive to get the "edge" is probably as old as mankind. Students of antiquity tell us that Greek athletes swallowed hallucinogenic mushrooms and morphine to improve their performance, and gladiators took ephedra and other herbs that had a stimulating effect before fighting for the roaring crowds in the Roman Coliseum.

Today we continue the tradition of seeing sports heroes as superstars. The amount and type of body-boosting medications athletes seek depends on their sport as well as their goals. Some want to build better heart and lung performance for endurance competition. Others are looking for muscles and strength. Still others strive to compete on the basis of speed and agility. Whatever their desire, a product is waiting for them. Some products promising stronger and faster bodies may contain hormones or substances mimicking hormones.

The well-documented hormonal effects on motivation and physical performance cannot be ignored. In recognition of their power and their interdependence, hormones are labeled as potentially harmful drugs. All androgenic (male sex) hormones including testosterone, growth hormone or any other anabolic substance are regulated as controlled medications by the FDA and are not legally available in the US without a prescription.

Sometimes those who purchase protein supplements that are advertised for their bodybuilding qualities get more than they bargain for. Athletes, especially football players, often test positive for prescription anabolic steroids after consuming over-the-counter protein powders. When accused of drug abuse, they protest that they've done nothing illegal. In most cases they did not realize that the innocent-looking powders they were taking were laced with microscopic amounts of bodybuilding hormones.

The manufacturers added these illegal compounds in order to magnify the positive results and build brand loyalty. Once the product was established in the marketplace, the illegal hormones were removed from the ingredients. Combining the expectation that the product would work with the time-honored placebo effect (see page 45), users continued to believe they worked wonders, when nothing of note was included in the mix.

Athletes represent just the tip of the iceberg for the nutrition industry. The huge wave of baby boomers constitutes the biggest market for anti-aging drugs. Unlike world-class athletes, these youth seekers have no way of knowing what they take. The sad truth is that vitamins and herbal concoctions to lengthen life, pills and creams to increase penis length are nothing but advertising gimmicks no better than the snake oils of the past.

The pitches for these products continue to escalate. People spend billions of dollars chasing hyped-up claims and because of coincidence or the placebo effect; initially they may actually enjoy some of the benefits they seek. In the end, most of them have wasted their money rarely asking the companies to fulfill their money-back guarantee. Companies constantly change the names and bring out new products to keep profits high.

## Growing Old in Spite of Human Growth Hormone

The aura surrounding human growth hormone (HGH) is a classic example of how unscrupulous marketers mix desire, misinformation, and exaggerated claims. Middle-aged people desperate to avoid aging, experiment with human growth hormone, the most advertised anti-aging drug on the Internet. We keep searching for anything with a promise of improved vitality.

Scientific studies demonstrate that in youth HGH is critical for maintaining youthful strength and vitality. Growth hormone levels decline with age but this may be due to decreases in the hypothalamic growth hormone regulators. Older adults with extremely low levels do develop flabbier midsections, and weaker muscles. However, patients with human growth deficiency who use HGH therapy experience a significant increase in lean body mass, heightened exercise performance, improved cholesterol levels and spinal bone density. A quick look at these facts may lead to the conclusion that growth hormone therapy could be an ideal way to turn back the clock. Alas, it is not so!

Although patients with a true growth hormone deficiency will develop more muscle and less fat with hormone replacement, we lack scientific proof that they will live longer or suffer less illness. Much more research is still needed, and the use of growth hormone is still being investigated.

Pharmaceutical grade HGH is not available in a pill you can buy at the local drug store. Like most hormones, HGH is classified as a drug and regulated by the FDA. You may find advertisements about nasal sprays containing human growth hormone, but these substances contain a few micrograms, if any, of the hormone. They do not have enough HGH in them to come under FDA scrutiny. Not only that, but human growth hormone is such a large molecule that it cannot be absorbed through the mouth or nose. The acids in the digestive system dissolve the molecule, making it impossible for it to function. Only injectable growth hormone available from your pharmacy has any biological activity in the human body.

Several marketing companies on the Web sell capsules or liquids that supposedly stimulate the pituitary to release the growth hormone. These substances are known as “secretogogues” because they stimulate the pituitary and other organs of the body to release—secrete—hormones.

Arginine, for example, is an amino acid that helps synthesize nitric oxide, the substance that regulates blood flow to the penis and vagina during sexual intercourse. That makes it fit into the secretogogue category. But how arginine is delivered can make all the difference in the world. Arginine injected into a vein into may stimulate the pituitary to secret human growth hormone for forty-five minutes or so, but an arginine capsule or tablet does not have that effect.

A researcher at Johns Hopkins Medical School conducted trial studies over twenty-six weeks and found that growth hormone does seem to increase lean body mass and decrease fat in elderly individuals. Unfortunately, adverse effects were frequent, including diabetes, swelling, and finger numbness. Until the results confirm the safety of any HGH product, treatment of the elderly with human growth hormone should be limited to controlled experimental studies. Proper balancing of hormones seems to be much safer than injecting the growth hormone on a daily basis.

## IGF-1—Mankind's Gift from Human Growth Hormone

So far we have looked at many of the ways that hormones interact to keep our bodies functioning normally, but there is so much more to explore. Consider the relationship between growth, aging, and eating, for example. We know that children eat to grow, and that youngsters going through puberty need more food than at other times of their lives. We are just beginning to understand some of the intricate and delicate relationships between calorie intake, growth, and aging in relation to human growth hormone.

Our search for more knowledge leads us to the insulin-like growth factor known in medical circles as IGF-1, a component of life that is taking center stage in multiple medical research projects seeking to explain the aging process. Technically speaking, IGF-1, also known as somatomedin-C, is not a hormone at all, but merely a molecule produced in the liver that acts like a hormone by influencing growth, reproduction and other biological activities.

A powerful molecule, IGF-1 sets changes such as uterine cell growth, in motion during puberty. By attaching to muscle cells, the insulin-like growth factor increases their size—not by metabolizing more protein as testosterones does, but by acting directly on the cells. The insulin-like growth factor regulates cell death, tooth development, and hair growth acting both as a hormone and as a regulating protein. The studies below show that the effects of IGF-I on the pituitary cause the inhibition of growth hormone. The release and production of growth hormone by the insulin-like growth factor probably reflects a negative feedback loop for maintaining tight control over growth hormone cell function. These findings further indicate that the insulin-like growth factor also has potent effects in regulating growth hormone.

Around the age of three, children have higher levels of this growth factor than before, and by the age of ten to twelve they reach adult levels. A high level of the insulin-like growth factor at puberty stimulates growth and sexual maturity. In clinical studies, girls at all age levels have been found to have higher levels of the insulin-like growth factor than boys of the same age, possibly explaining why girls mature earlier.

After adolescence, individuals gradually lose the amount of the insulin-like growth factor circulating in their bloodstream and ultimately reach very low levels in their old age. A decline of the growth hormone-IGF-1 axis is probably caused by altered hypothalamic regulation with a decrease in the growth hormone releasing hormone and an increase in somatostatin. Both these compounds regulate our concentrations of the insulin-like growth factor. Somotostatin blocks the action of growth hormone and increases with age. Again we can see how complex our endocrine system can seem, but if we listen we can begin to hear that there are ways to balance our hormones.

All of our hormones change as we age. For example, our pituitary gland releases less and less growth hormone after we become adults during the phenomenon called "the somatopause." The cause of the somatopause is complicated by several factors that contribute to the age-related decline in growth hormone secretion. Tests of aging men show that growth hormone secretion declines by fifty percent every seven years after age twenty-five.

The primary cause of declining growth hormone levels is therefore probably aging. Obesity, falling levels of testosterone in men and estrogens in women, along with decreased physical fitness affect our growth hormone secretion. Because growth hormone secretion occurs predominantly during slow-wave sleep, levels of the growth hormone can by affected by altered sleep patterns. Since we know that declining levels of IGF-I affect actions of the growth hormone, it could be that somatopause is part of normal aging rather than a disease.

The manipulation of hormones and genes to slow the aging process may soon lead to amazing outcomes in the field of longevity. A much simpler method to add years of healthy living to your life, advocated by some physicians, is simply to cut your daily calorie load to about 1,000 or 1,200 for women and about 1,500 or 1,750 for men. Before you conclude that semi-starvation may not be the easiest way to live longer, consider the following.

As early as 1935 lifespan enhancement was reported in rodents, flies, fish and worms, by reducing the number of calories consumed. Laboratory rats and squirrel monkeys under caloric restriction also seem to age more slowly. In humans, only observational studies are available. Japanese living in Okinawa where a low-calorie diet is typical, "have a forty-fold increase in odds of becoming centenarians," according to Chris Vojta, a fellow at the Institute on Aging, at the University of Pennsylvania. It could be as straightforward as this: fewer calories mean lower levels of circulating blood sugar or glucose, insulin and cholesterol. A decreased rate of cell division and free radical damage plus a lower fat mass and a more robust immune system may be responsible for this effect. Diets, including vegan (plant-based) proteins, have been shown to lower elevated cholesterol levels and decrease circulating levels of the insulin-like growth factor activity lengthening both the average and maximal lifespan.

In fact, vegans tend to have lower blood fats, leaner physiques, slower growth and maturation in children, and decreased risk for certain prominent "Western" cancers; a vegan diet has documented effectiveness in rheumatoid arthritis. Low-fat vegan diets may be especially protective in regard to cancers linked to insulin resistance—namely, breast and colon cancer—as well as prostate cancer. However, according to Dr. Vojta, "the long-term effect of decreases in body temperature, metabolic rate and the size of most major organs is still unknown."

No positive association has been established between levels of the insulin-like growth factor and muscle strength, body composition, and physical functioning either. To explain this, scientists consider the possibility that the insulin-like growth factor levels do not really reflect growth hormone status or that they do not correlate with the biological activity of IGF-1. Before you sign up for supplements, you should know that there isn't enough evidence to show whether treatment with the insulin-like growth factor can either slow or reverse age-related changes in human beings. Ironically, you may accelerate your death rather than turn back the hands of time if you embark on your own hormone-replacement program. Be careful!

It's a different story with the insulin-like growth factor when we are young. Testosterone, which stimulates growth of the bones at puberty, cannot make bones grow unless there are high levels of IGF-1 present. This growth factor is therefore largely responsible for the growth spurt we see at puberty. Adding three, four, five or more inches in a year is not uncommon for adolescents. One man who reached a very tall height in a short time quipped, "I went to bed wearing trousers. I woke up wearing shorts."

Pygmies, on the other hand, grow to adulthood without achieving normal height as achieved by the majority of humans. Studies of pygmies show that they have only one-third the amount of the insulin-like growth factor compared to adults of normal height, though their levels of testosterone and human growth hormone are equal to those of normal adults. Their bodies simply stop growing at the height they reach at puberty.

Does this mean that we should consider prescribing the insulin-like growth factor to prolong life or increase height? No. The role of the insulin-like growth factor axis in growth control and cancer promotion has recently been confirmed at the University of Pennsylvania by the finding of elevated IGF-1 levels in association with three of the most prevalent cancers in the United States: prostate cancer, colorectal cancer, and lung cancer. Lower levels of the insulin-like growth factor with aging may thus prove beneficial, actually inhibiting cancer induction (as is seen in animal studies).

In a recent study of healthy older men and women, those taking growth hormone with or without sex hormones experienced increased leaner body mass and decreased fat mass. When sex steroids such as testosterone and DHT were added, increased muscle strength and lung capacity were noted in men, but not in women. These controlled studies indicate that more research is needed before growth hormone is routinely used to attempt to delay aging or increase endurance.

Another matter of concern is the potential misuse of healthcare resources. Growth hormone replacement in growth hormone–deficient adults with pituitary disease is expensive, costing up to ten thousand dollars a year. We do not know precisely how much growth hormone is prescribed for "off label" uses, but estimates suggest that one third of prescriptions for growth hormone in the United States are for indications for which it is not approved by the Food and Drug Administration.

I need to emphasize here that growth hormone therapy is *not an accepted standard of medical care* but is being promoted by anti-aging doctors who sometimes profit from sales of growth hormone to their patients. Growth hormone is just one hormone released from the pituitary that decline with increasing age. This observation, together with the changes in body composition associated with adult growth hormone deficiency, has led to the suggestion by some anti-aging physicians that all elderly people are deficient in growth hormone and may benefit from human growth hormone therapy. These physicians should also tell their patients that taking human growth hormone also increases estrogen and testosterone levels.

In summary, taking extra human growth hormone by injection may be a proven, safe therapy for children and adults who are markedly deficient in the hormone. Until studies prove its value in elderly persons, a better course would be enjoying the natural benefits of human growth hormone with exercise, nutrition and restful sleep. Exercise that produces sweating and rapid heart rates for short bursts of time has been scientifically proven, along with food reduction, to increase longevity.

Take time to listen to your hormones, ask for testing by your doctor, and request replacement therapy with testosterone, DHEA, estrogen, progesterone, melatonin or whatever hormones are found deficient after testing. This is the safest and most sensible approach to treat the ravages of time and live at peace with our hormones.

## Should Aging be Treated as a Disease?

Why do we suffer from such dread of aging? After all, aging is a natural phenomenon, not a disease. Many folks in their eighties are still totally competent and physically functional. *Vintage People,* written by Dr. Jerry Old, celebrates the successful aging of many Americans, with stories of remarkable people in their eighties and nineties who maintain a vigorous and upbeat lifestyle.

So far the mortality rate of the human race is running at one hundred percent, but that doesn't mean we have to look forward to our final years in the throes of pain and disease. At the close of the century there were 77,000 people one hundred years and up in the US, and statisticians predict that the number of centenarians is expected to double with each decade for the foreseeable future.

Since certain hormones decline with the aging process, it is only logical to assume that restoring these hormones to younger levels should slow the aging process. Total testosterone, for example, declines at the rate of 110 nanograms per deciliter every year after age forty. Levels of bioavailable testosterone fall off much more dramatically. Binding with the sex hormone binding globulin (SHBG) increases with the aging process and thus decreases the available free testosterone. Healthy men and women with low testosterone levels enjoy a positive effect when testosterone is administered. Benefits include leaner body composition, stronger muscles, better brain function, and heightened sexual drive.

Little is known about the effectiveness of substances that are being promoted to consumers as "anti-aging" therapies. Hormones such as DHEA, human growth hormone, melatonin and testosterone do decline with aging, but that does not prove that replacing them to normal levels will reverse the aging process. Such conclusions are only theoretical at this time and must be substantiated by large-scale controlled clinical trials before being accepted.

Your primary care physician ought to offer anti-aging therapy as nothing more or less than the practice of good medicine. Your doctor should know that diet and moderate exercise are the essential building blocks of a healthy body and that the best source of nutrients is a balanced diet—although some older patients may benefit from Vitamins C, A, D, E and supplements of organic phytonutrients from fruits and vegetables.

As mentioned, in laboratory tests a low-calorie-diet without starvation doubles and triples the lifespan of simple creatures like earthworms and fruit flies. In more sophisticated animals such as mice, monkeys and dogs, decreasing calories increases the lifespan dramatically but these animals are observed in a laboratory setting. Those who consume fewer calories seem to build up less resistance to insulin and increase their supply of DHEA. Insulin resistance is a major factor in adult-onset diabetes, and while it is not a wonder drug that will prolong life indefinitely, the hormone DHEA has a beneficial effect on the function of the heart, the brain and the immune system.

So is it calories, hormones, lifestyle, or exercise that makes some people age better than others? The answer may surprise you. The ability to maintain active and independent lifestyles for as long as possible is almost certainly not related to medical care, diets or hormones. When centenarians (people living to one hundred years of age) are asked for their "secrets of good health," the most important factor contributing to longevity is always *genetics*. Investigators studying the habitability of lifespan have concluded that up to thirty-five percent of the variation is due to genetics. These "Methuselah" patients simply had long-lived relatives and healthy families. Most of them also refrained from use of alcohol and tobacco. Assume for a moment that lucky genes are the sole reason for a long and healthy life. What determines these genetic factors? The answer, of course is "our hormones."

Since the decoding of the human genome early in 2003, mankind has come a step closer to determining some of the genetic factors that may one day unlock secrets of the aging process. The future may yield a wealth of information and medical techniques for modifying genes and slowing the aging process. Choosing parents with exemplary health would be the best way to guarantee a long and healthy life, but there are realistic steps you can take at whatever age you may be. Meanwhile we know that quality of life is much more important than quantity. Finding life pleasurable involves the enjoyment of sex, hobbies, friends, relatives, and the avoidance of disease and infirmity.

In his book, *The Evolution of Aging,* Theodore Goldsmith observes that while there are reports that people who engage in sex more often live longer, it has not been established that there is a cause-and-effect relationship. After all, we can assume that people who are healthy will have a more active sex life than those who are not. Still, the increase in hormonal activity triggered by sexual relations may be a contributing factor in longevity. So "do it till you die" is still the best advice.

Medical science will continue its fascination with the human genome and the secrets it has yet to reveal. Hormone replacement therapies will transform over time, and many more uses will be found for hormones. Our search for immortality will take new directions.

Aging is still a natural phenomenon. To treat aging as a disease is not medically sound, but to put off the ravages of time by restoring hormones to optimum levels is simply good preventive medicine.

You can follow preventive guidelines to help you avoid disease, keep alert, and incorporate positive lifestyle changes in your life. You can adopt a healthier life style by giving up cigarettes and drinking alcoholic beverages only with meals. Wellness is improved by eating more nutritional food, and by avoiding the use of illicit drugs. These simple steps won't guarantee you a long and active life, but they are essential in building a healthy mind and body for your final years.

When we look at problems associated with aging in our society, we can see that adopting healthful strategies such as these should reduce medical and social costs as well as pain and suffering as we age. An increase in the quality of life of the elderly enables them to remain productive and to contribute to the well being of society. In light of these facts, public awareness needs to be increased, and basic research in slowing aging should be intensified.

## How Nutrients Affect Aging

Yes, we all get old—*if we're able to survive* the risks of living in a fast-paced world. But have you ever wondered why some people age gracefully with a sharp mind and physical fitness while others become crippled and lose their memory?

Nutrition could be another important reason why some get along better than others in their advancing years. In elderly patients in whom nutrition may be a problem, measurement of zinc levels is important. Zinc has anti-aromatase action and can be used to treat hypogonadism. Older people are often deficient in essential vitamins such as A, C, E and D, and key minerals such as calcium, zinc, magnesium, iron, chromium and selenium. Enzymes like Coenzyme Q10 and gingko, ginseng and grapeseed have all been used as anti-aging therapies. Eating fruits, vegetables, and grains (a plant-based diet) will provide all these essential nutrients while avoiding excess proteins that are bad for the heart, according to nutrition expert Dr. Dean Ornish.

While most of our body's functions continue to operate into old age at almost seventy-five percent of their youthful level, our digestive system doesn't fare that well. As we age, our taste buds, the concentration of our stomach acid, our thirst sensitivity, and our elimination system become far less efficient. As a result, we do not absorb all the vitamins and other nutrients. We have to take extra steps to be sure we have enough of these valuable substances in our bodies. Many people complain about taking pills but swallow dozens of vitamins daily. There must be an easier way to get all the nutrients you need for optimum health.

With aging, our hormones gradually lose their ability to deliver their marvelous benefit. It works like this. As we grow older, we seem to have more fat and less muscle. Our kidneys don't eliminate toxic substances as efficiently, and our livers lose some of their filtering capabilities. All these factors add up to a less effective delivery system for the hormones that need to circulate freely through our body for the best of health. Because of declining efficiencies, aging people may therefore become dehydrated without being thirsty, malnourished without feeling hungry, or constipated without being aware of an urge to have a bowel movement. These changes can greatly affect the quality of your life. Your moods, appetite, energy, and the absorption of medications are all adversely affected.

Of course, not all elderly people respond identically to hormones or nutrients. Assimilation can be affected by over-the-counter medications like antihistamines or antacids that interfere with absorption by the body. Drug-to-drug or drug-to-food interactions further contribute to problems that arise in the improper dosing and use of medications in the elderly.

Another problem with hormones or prescribed medicines used by older people is that with aging, the human body produces less of the proteins such as globulins and albumin that bind to medications. Drugs that are not bound up with blood proteins can reach higher than desired levels in the bloodstream. The opposite effect occurs with hormones because the sex hormone binding globulin increases with aging, lowering levels of existing hormones. An unnecessarily high intake of the essential amino acids—as is found in animal meats relative to total dietary protein—may prove to be as serious a risk factor for degenerative diseases as is excessive fat intake. Lower protein intake as we age has been shown to improve health and decrease the toxic load on our kidneys.

## Sex after Seventy

Misconceptions are plentiful regarding what is normal aging and what is a sign of disease. We do know that aging is much more complex than a simple hormone deficiency. We also know that the best anti-aging medicine is talking to your doctor about nutrition, preventive medicine, stress reduction and enjoyable sexual communication with your partner. Be sure to ask your doctor about any problems you have with your sex life. It may not be easy because these problems are often masked by other disorders. In addition, many patients have difficulty discussing these personal problems openly. Make the effort to be open about all matters related to your sexual experience regardless of your age.

Many Americans still think that losing their sex drive is a natural part of growing old. We expect sexual function in older Americans to decrease as they age until sooner or later sex becomes nothing more than a memory. The truth is, you don’t have to give up sex because you’re past sixty.

Dropping hormone levels, reduced sexual activity, and decreased sexual interest are related to the aging process, but they do not completely account for age-related changes in sexuality. Your doctor must consider all aspects of your emotional and physical health before concluding that aging is to blame for a lack of sexual interest. Stress, cancer, debilitating diseases, and many other conditions sometimes make their presence known first through a loss of sexual desire.

Sexual activity helps us cope with stress. The discharge of "natural opiates" plus the bonding that come with a positive sexual experience brings a touch of peace into our sometime chaotic lives. But healthy sexual functioning requires both an adequate hormonal balance and appropriate neurotransmitter levels. Either of these factors can be affected by medications used by many aged folks.

Medicines to improve our mental or emotional state are among the most frequently prescribed medications in this country, and the elderly receive a major portion of these drugs. Three out of four drugs prescribed in nursing homes are tranquilizers, according to a 1986 study. Other popular medicines that work on the mind are known collectively as psychotropic medications and include tranquilizers, antidepressants, antipsychotics and stimulants. Most of these psychotropic drugs destroy sexual urges and performance. The reality is that sexual passion, physical enjoyment, a normal sex drive, and thoughts of love are more important in overall life satisfaction than erections or the physical performance of the sex act. Whereas most men consider the physical act of making love as a sign of their virility instead of a form of communicating love, women are much more involved with the emotional aspects of sex. Women, in point of fact, suffer from sexual dysfunction more than men but they are less likely to discuss it with their male doctors.

Hormone deficiencies are an unfortunate side effect of growing older, but by taking steps to improve your hormonal balance, and discussing these problems with your personal physician, you can function at optimal levels well into your golden years. We should all be able to enjoy sex and continue to do it till we die!

## Memory and Intelligence–Hormones in Your Brain

Depression is associated with high cortisol levels caused by higher amounts of the cortisol releasing-hormone than are needed. The symptoms of depression can result from constant stress, which is accompanied by low levels of growth hormone and testosterone along with elevated levels of cortisol. Too much cortisol has been shown to result in shallow sleep, bad moods, carbohydrate cravings and loss of memory in individuals with depression.

High cortisol levels (see page 58) and sleep deprivation can both alter our moods and erode our short-term memory as well. Back in Chapter Two, we looked at ways that melatonin, regulated by light, triggers sleep and our body rhythms. Years of research by Dr. Axel Steiger at the Max Planck Institute in Germany have shown that the growth hormone-releasing hormone (GHRH) and the corticotropin releasing-hormone (CRF) also participate in sleep regulation and the increased memory retention.

The growth hormone-releasing hormone (GHRH) works like this. The hormone regulates the release of growth hormone to the body during the night. Deep, dream-filled, slow wave sleep (REM sleep) is essential for normal memory and good health and the avoidance of depression. Hormones including growth hormone, prolactin, cortisol, estradiol and melatonin blend into this complex balance to induce refreshing sleep. As we have just noted, raised levels of cortisol impair sleep while GHRH enhances the slow wave sleep by increasing growth hormone. Note that hormones can antagonize each other as well as provide balance for optimum function.

In a study involving healthy volunteers, GHRH increased slow wave sleep (REM) and growth hormone (GH) secretion while blunting cortisol release. The combination of these effects tends to de-stress an individual during sleep allowing the brain to retain and store complex memories. Normal sleep requires a balance of brain hormones and leads to improved memory.

An entire new class of memory drugs is being developed to take advantage of this research. Antidepressants based on cortisol-releasing hormone blockers, which will reverse the cortisol excess that is so destructive in the body and the brain, are part of this new drug pipeline. Agents that have a dual action, affecting both serotonin and norepinephrine are being perfected as sleep-inducing pills. Memory enhancing drugs are also being developed to treat Alzheimer's disease.

Restful sleep is essential for optimal functioning of our brains. During sleep our brains and bodies recharge, providing energy for daily tasks and a retentive memory to get everything we want accomplished. Unfortunately, lower levels of the growth hormone releasing hormone and melatonin occur with aging, affecting normal sleep. Can anything be done to "slow down aging" and maintain our hormonal balance?

Yes, but it's not exciting or earth-shattering news. It comes down to proper diet and exercise. The growth hormone inhibitor somatostatin can be blocked with a healthy diet containing adequate amounts of arginine, ornithine, glutamine and other essential amino acids. You won't find these nutrients listed on the ingredient list because they are naturally occurring protein components found in plants that have evolved with humans to provide all the essential nutrients needed for optimal health. Watching the amount of food you eat and decreasing IGF-1 with calorie restriction seems to stimulate DHEA, in addition to reducing cortisol production. On top of this, pregnenolone used as a food supplement seems to improve memory.

The preventive approach is simple: a healthy diet coupled with regular, moderately intense exercise increases the release of the helpful growth hormone during the night and decreases the release of cortisol. A good night's sleep guarantees improved mental functioning.

## Modifying Your Food Choices

The dramatic rise in youngsters who are hyperactive or suffer from Attention Deficit Disorder is a puzzle begging to be solved. Christine Wood, M.D., a pediatrician and author of *How to Get Kids to Eat Great!* says we need look no further than the food our children are eating. She cites more than a dozen studies showing that when children with behavior problems eat less sugar and fewer refined foods, they are able to concentrate better and experience far fewer incidents of disruptive behavior. It may seem like a leap of faith to link mood disorders in our children with their diet, but Neurophysiologist William Calvin in his book, *How Brains Think,* gives his perspective on how our brain developed intelligence and why we eat the way we do. Calvin feels that our ancestors led the way in adopting "basic searching moves" because they had to become omnivores and "switch between many different food sources. They need more sensory templates, mental search images of things such as foods and the predators for which they are on the lookout."

By matching these mental images with the behavior required to obtain the food they were seeking, our human ancestors were able to adapt to their world. That was the past but now we worry more about obesity than starving to death. Family eating patterns help mold our likes and dislikes. As children we pretty much eat what our parents feed us until we're old enough to forage for food on our own. All mammals go through a period as playful juveniles to learn the skills they need to survive as adults. For apes and humans this learning time is much longer and aids in the development of greater intelligence.

As soon as we're old enough to make our own choices, we modify our food choices and try new things to eat. Calvin points out that a long life promotes versatility and adaptation to change by giving us more opportunities to discover new behaviors and adapt to them. Another advantage to a long life is that the longer we live, the more we can use our intelligence for our own benefit and enjoyment. This equips us with brainpower we can use to choose a calorie-reduced, toxin-avoiding, plant-based diet as a means of slowing the process of aging and the deterioration of our brains. Recognizing that a low-fat diet of whole foods can cut the harmful effects of dioxin, we can make the choices that bring our behavior into harmony with our knowledge and prolong our health and vitality. An active social life also prolongs life.

You can operate a knife, fork, and spoon whether anyone else is with you or not and enjoy a good meal, but for most of us, a meal shared with others is more rewarding. The reality is that eating gives human beings a welcome opportunity for social interaction. As we observe what other people are eating and how they relate to their food, we have new chances to follow their example and take advantage of useful discoveries they have made. You might never enjoy peanut butter on a stalk of celery, for example, if you didn't see your father-in-law enjoying this treat. Fried green tomatoes, onion-seasoned popcorn, or muffins smothered in pizza sauce may not sound appetizing until you taste a sample at a social gathering of some kind.

Besides introducing us to varied foods, a rich social life gives us the challenge of solving interpersonal problems that go well beyond the usual environmental challenges for basic survival and reproduction of the species. Think about the last time your family—including in-laws, cousins, aunts, uncles, and grandparents—got together for a celebration. At such gatherings children quickly learn by the behavior of adults which members of the family demand respect, which ones test the limits of acceptability, and which relatives bring special talents to the experience—from strumming a guitar to story-telling to baking a tasty home-made apple pie.

We know intuitively that food is essential for life. A newborn baby has no way to avoid starving to death without a nursing mother, and the infant turns instinctively to its mother for all the nutrients needed to survive and grow.

If the mother of the newborn is not able to supply milk from her breast, baby formulas have been developed in an attempt by the food industry to match the nutritious value of breast milk. The reality is that while packaged baby food may contain the required amount of carbohydrates, fat, protein, and vitamins, only human milk contains the antibodies essential to establish a strong immune system in the baby. Not only that, but prepared foods introduce the infant to environmental toxins and harmful components programmed into processed food. Most baby foods are simply ground-up adult food mixed with lots of sugar and salt.

The shocking reality in our rapidly changing world is that breast milk of mothers in every industrialized country today contains dioxin residues. In 1998, studies of Swedish breast milk showed that levels of flame-retardants were doubling every two to five years. Another study of twenty first-time mothers found considerably higher flame retardant levels in American women than those recorded in Sweden. Biomonitoring has become a necessary tool in medicine for detecting the degree of human exposure to synthetic chemicals. We need to be on the lookout for the link between industrial chemicals and human ailments.

Like the animals of the plains or the jungle, we humans are always on the lookout for food. Ironically, the search is the problem in America because food is everywhere. Close by is corner market or a huge supermarket loaded with thousands of brands of food, not to mention ice cream shops, restaurants representing a vast array of cuisines, and vending machines. We have an abundance of food of every type and description, far more than we need. Worse, most of the food is loaded with fat, sugar, and more protein than we need.

Food companies know that people are highly susceptible to food-related advertising in the mass media. They spend more than seven billion dollars a year on advertising telling us what they'd like us to eat. Of course we do not have to eat everything we see on television or in restaurants, and we should not let commercial messages paid for by manufacturers of processed food determine what we eat.

We should make our own food choices using the intelligence we have developed over the eons and stop giving into the constant temptation of food promoted in our culture. Listening to your hormones is safer than absorbing the advertising messages of the processed food industry.

As we become more sophisticated about food's effect on our lifelong health and environment, we are learning to rely less on animal fat and more on whole grains, fruits, and vegetable. The notion that meat is essential for health is outdated and just plain wrong. We should accept the fact that high quality protein with all the essential amino acids needed for hormonal balance is readily available with a vegetarian diet. Furthermore, we are learning that relying on plant foods for our nutrition is far more economical than raising and slaughtering animals. When you become conscious of these basic facts of nutrition, you have made a giant step along the evolutionary process.

"Progress comes from the intelligent use of experience."
—Elbert Hubbard.

## Americans Deserve Good Health

Many doctors focus on treating symptoms and spend very little time helping Americans enjoy their right to health or their healthright. We'll talk more about this in the last chapter of the book. The majority of deaths in the USA are self-inflicted. From cancer and diabetes to heart disease and infection, diseases can be prevented. Following health-building guidelines can improve our quality of life and help us avoid chronic disease. In spite of the value of preventing disease, preventive medical care is not available to most of our population.

For the most part Americans with jobs receive shoddy care from their medical care health plans. Diet and environmental pollution are not addressed by many managed health plans, and welfare programs inadequately support the poor and unemployed in North America.

PCBs and dioxins poison the nervous systems of infants leading to sexual dysfunction in many Americans, due to hidden dangers in our air, water and food from environmental poisons. "We all have these compounds in our body," according to the Linda Birnbaum. The call to alarm concerning dioxin and its harmful effects has begun to make a difference in the amount of this pollutant in our systems, but researchers continue to report high levels in people who have been exposed to dioxin released in forest fires and other activity.

What can the average American do?

Promoting health and longevity is not a priority of our government. The extent of our country's national offense against disease is collecting taxes on alcohol and tobacco and restricting some forms of tobacco and alcohol advertising. Cost cutting to deliver higher profits are driving our health care system. Whether non-profit organizations or not, hospitals exist for the sole purpose of making money. Their goal is to maximize the surplus of income over expenses. Those in need are cut out of the system if they can't pay the full price. Write-offs for care to the poor are not charity but debts the hospital is unable to collect after following every possible means to extract the money from the person requiring surgical or medical care. For underinsured or uninsured individuals, a major episode of illness requiring hospitalization almost inevitably leads to bankruptcy or seizure of their assets.

In American supermarkets today you see more consumers picking up containers and carefully reading the labels. Unfortunately, warning labels haven't kept us from the consequences of alcohol or tobacco abuse. Approximately twenty-six million Americans drink to excess, and over thirty-four million smoke cigarettes. One fifth of our nation's people are drug dependent. Very few people over the age of eighty-five smoke or drink because those who do live fewer years.

Good medical care has increased the length of time we can live, adding about thirty years to our lifespan over the past century. We are encouraged to follow diets and to exercise more to answer our health problems, but this is not enough for many elderly Americans. In the US today, over six out of ten people are obese. Despite the popularity of fitness centers and diet books, out of every one hundred dieters who lose weight, all but five will gain it back within five years.

The leading causes of death and the actual causes of death are not the same, as the table on the following page shows. It is clear that the way we treat our bodies affects our health and the length of our life.

More than 190 million people in the United States will soon be over sixty-five, and half of them have lost their sexual drive by that age. Aging is influenced by multiple hormone deficiencies, genetic predisposition for certain diseases and environmental hazards, which are probably destroying our reproductive and sexual abilities.

| Leading Causes of Death United States 2000 | | Actual Causes of Death United States 2000 | |
|---|---|---|---|
| Heart Disease | 30% | Tobacco | 18.1% |
| Cancer | 23% | Poor diet/physical inactivity | 16.1% |
| Stroke | 7% | Alcohol consumption | 3.5% |
| Chronic lower respiratory disease | 5% | Microbial agents (influenza, pneumonia etc.) | 3.1% |
| Unintentional injuries | 4% | Toxic agents (pollutants etc.) | 2.3% |
| Diabetes | 3% | Motor vehicles | 1.8% |
| Pneumonia/influenza | 3% | Firearms | 1.2% |
| Alzheimer's Disease | 2% | Sexual behavior | 0.8% |
| Kidney disease | 2% | Illicit drug abuse | 0.7% |

Source: Centers for Disease Control and Prevention

The gap is widening between the cost of health care and the degree of health attained by the American public. The US ranks twenty-fourth in the world in the quality of health care. The importance of exercise, proper diet, and appropriate nutritional supplements cannot be over-emphasized. Not all factors that cause disease and death can be easily eliminated. Banning toxic substances, for example, is not feasible. In the words of Linda Birnbaum, "What are you going to ban? We don't even know where half this stuff is coming from."

We need to rely more on common sense methods of avoiding disease through sensible eating of a near-vegetarian diet and regular exercise rather than taking medicine or herbal supplements to relieve symptoms.

Doctors with patients who would benefit from hormone replacement therapy should prescribe hormones as appropriate, including hormone rebalancing to help offset some of the worst effects of dioxin poisoning.

Hormones have been proven safe and effective over decades of use. Side effects are minimal and can usually be eliminated by reducing the dose. Most negative effects are reversible and mild. Hormone replacement can make a huge difference in the health and functioning of many patients at a reasonable cost.

Too often the patients must lead the advance by educating their doctors about the best means of treatment for the hormone-related problems.

Scott wrote to me that he was getting weary of wasting time and energy looking for a doctor to help him. "All I hear is, 'But your test results are within normal range,' or 'Since you can still get an erection you don't need testosterone.' Too many docs tell me that testosterone replacement would give me prostate cancer and make my good cholesterol go to zero. They say I need to stay on cholesterol drugs to lower those triglycerides, that testosterone will only make it worse. Most shocking to me, I hear this: "There is no need to test you for high estrogen levels because your breasts aren't enlarged enough."

He continued, "It's like these guys haven't read a thing since they got out of medical school. They have this attitude, 'I know what's right so please don't try to confuse me with facts or new information.'"

Scott's doctor did not listen to his patients or did not want to spend carefully budgeted managed care dollars pursuing his patient's concerns. Like most health care providers, Scott's doctor was probably just too busy to learn about the new uses and benefits of hormones and other anti-aging therapies.

Meanwhile the rich and famous are benefiting from hormone therapy. They can afford to search for doctors who are highly qualified and will listen to them. This is not right. No one should be denied access to care or information about treatments that can improve life.

A change in how doctors view patients and their problems is slowly taking place in our medical system. From bitter experience of anguished patients we are learning that limiting medical care by basing it on cost-saving principles is neither practical nor in our patients' best interests. We are beginning to promote the concept that all Americans have a "right to health."

The only way to improve our chances of a long and healthy life is to deliver this right. Our physicians should share the knowledge they have as physicians and listen to their patients' complaints. Doctors need to involve patients in their own care. They need to give them feedback about their own ideas and thoughts and encourage them to participate in planning for their treatment and recovery. This is a better way.

Following a healthy diet, exercising regularly and avoiding poisons and toxins will help anyone earn a right to health. Running to the doctor for a symptom reliever whenever a cold or flu strikes doesn't do it. Doctors need to work with their patients to educate them and to help diagnose their sexual problems. Quality of life will be improved considerably by making headway in preventing sexual dysfunction and related problems.

Androgen replacement therapy has been found effective in multiple medical conditions including anemia, wasting diseases such as cancer or AIDS, impotence, hypogonadism, prostate enlargement and pituitary deficiency. Prescriptions for either transdermal testosterone or DHT should mimic the natural cycles of hormones, for example, causing an increase of testosterone in the early mornings, and a corresponding decrease of estrogen and prolactin during that same time period. Turning off the lights should create an increase in melatonin at midnight.

You can restore passion and vitality to your love life. Your doctor can help you attain your healthright—the right to accurate and easy-to-understand information about your body and how it works and the right to high quality medical care as a United States citizen. Just as the inalienable rights to freedom, liberty and the pursuit of happiness are ingrained in our constitution, the right to health can become a critical part of our lifestyle.

Our hormones are talking to us whether we are awake or asleep. They tell us about our bodies, our brains, and our emotions. They send signals to us twenty-four hours a day, seven days a week, about how well they're able to work for us. They give us up-to-date information about deficiencies, declining levels, and hormonal imbalance.

When we think about the possibility of enjoying optimal health throughout our maturing years, "old" thinking too often gets in the way of the messages our hormones are sending us. "The chains of habit," as Samuel Johnson observed, "are too weak to be felt until they are too strong to be broken."

You don't need to be bound any longer by rumors and faulty information. Instead, you can salute the advances of modern medicine mentioned in this book and work to live full and rich lives. Knowing that new findings offer satisfying solutions to most of your hormone-related problems, you can face the future with confidence as the aging process catches up and leads you to your final years.

A slogan in my medical office reads like this: "Health is merely the slowest possible rate at which one can age." Nature dictates that as we grow older, the levels of many of our hormones slowly decline until we begin experiencing the signs and symptoms associated with aging. The only way to eliminate the aging process is to die young. And die we will, because nature has determined that death is the inevitable consequence of life.

If you are feeling the twinges of aging or are well into your "elderly" years, you would probably love to reverse or at least slow down the aging process. Millions have similar aspirations. Be careful. Plenty of enterprising businesses offer empty promises to stop aging in its tracks or help roll back the years if you buy their products.

One company, for example, offers "genuine" Romanian anti-aging tablets or injections for ten dollars a month. Another sells specially formulated creams that claim to counteract wrinkling in the skin for seventy-nine dollars for half an ounce. A company offers dietary supplements containing human growth hormone that, it says, will restore your hormones to youthful levels. Pay seventy-nine dollars and get your money back if it doesn't work.

We've talked about HGH several times in the book so far, but let's look at this hormone now in light of our quest of a sure way to turn back the clock and forestall the aging process.

## Longer Life with HGH—Myth or Reality?

An online advertisement for human growth hormone reads, "If you increase your body's level of HGH, you can reverse some aging symptoms." Another marketing statement proclaims that the "benefits of higher HGH levels include moderate weight loss, increased strength, more energy, better sleep, and enhanced sexual function." These advertising messages seem to be saying that HGH-based medications are the fountain of youth.

Watch out. Deception runs rampant, and you need to arm yourself with the facts in order to keep from being disappointed, or worse.

First of all, be aware that it is illegal to sell medically effective HGH in the US without a prescription. To get your attention, marketers claim that the tiny amounts of the hormone in their product are sufficient to add muscle power and revive your sex life.

The reality is that by law, any "real" human growth hormone in non-prescription pills or patches can be no more than the amount you would absorb from eating meat from an animal that consumed hormones while being fattened for the market.

Though it is possible that microscopic amounts of HGH could be included in medicines you can buy without a prescription, they are not the same as the HGH your body produces. Scientists use human growth hormone produced through genetic manipulation of yeast cells in their research. This type of human growth hormone cannot be obtained legally without a prescription. Any manufacturer or seller who tells you its HGH pills have the same amount of human growth hormone as the injections of natural HGH prescribed by a doctor is not telling a true story.

Another ploy for selling commercial human growth hormone products on the web is the announcement that the substances contain a hormone "releaser." The idea is that the "releaser" will trigger the delivery of therapeutic amounts of human growth hormone in your body. Not true. These releaser products contain amino acids that are part of the building blocks of human growth hormone, but they don't become HGH. Before they can be part of human growth hormone, the amino acids must undergo a chemical transformation in the body, and this change cannot occur from taking releaser pills.

Some manufacturers sell a product that claims to boost production of human growth hormone by including ingredients that raise the body's level of the insulin-like growth factor (IGF-1). These products usually include tiny amounts of human growth hormone and IGF-1 as well as releaser compounds. (See page 198 for more details about IGF-1.)

Other companies claim that enzymes in their capsules or liquids stimulate the pituitary gland to release human growth hormone. The enzyme in these products is an amino acid called arginine that helps synthesize nitric oxide, the substance that regulates blood flow to the penis and vagina during sexual intercourse. A shot of arginine in the vein might stimulate the pituitary to secrete human growth hormone for as much as an hour, but a pill with arginine in it has no such effect. Researcher Mary Lee Vance, MD, has commented that taking a pill with arginine as an ingredient delivers as much growth hormone as eating a steak.

Mouth or nose sprays offered without a prescription as human growth hormone products contain at most a few micrograms of the hormone. If they did include measurable levels of HGH, the molecules of this chemical are so large that they cannot be absorbed through the mouth or nose. Instead, the acids in the digestive system dissolve the molecule, rendering it totally ineffective in the body. Only injectable growth hormone has any biological activity in the human body.

You may have heard of 1990 studies reported in the *New England Journal of Medicine* showing some benefits reported by twelve older men who took human growth hormone for six months. The editors of the journal state emphatically that the study was inconclusive at best and should not be used as the basis for a costly self-administered therapy with HGH.

Speaking of human growth hormone products sold on the web, editor Jeffrey M. Dazen, a physician, is quoted as saying that "they're just a waste of money, and you're better off spending your time in the gym." HGH without a prescription has been dubbed pure quackery. The millions of dollars spent on bogus human growth hormone products would be better spent on research for ways to modify the aging process. Why all the fuss about HGH? Is the stampede for human growth hormone giving positive results?

## The Quest for Long Life

With all the struggles of pain, suffering, and financial woes we human beings confront, we have to wonder why most people seem to want to live a long life. Do they just want to go on with the hope that things will get better and better?

You may want to live well into your eighties and nineties and beyond, but you probably wouldn't choose long life unless you could also have good health. The best of all worlds would be to stay active and healthy so that we could enjoy the pleasures of youth along with the rewards of maturity.

Anti-aging has become a huge industry and is growing rapidly. Thousands of products and treatments are offered today to slow the aging process. Costly anti-aging medications have emerged in the marketplace to give people the illusion that they can buy longevity—if they have enough money. They are assured that by injecting themselves every day with a human-like growth hormone, they will enjoy longer life.

Even without miracle hormones, we are already living longer than our forefathers. The elderly population is growing so fast that before long they'll be the majority. For thirty years starting in 1970 life expectancy worldwide grew four months for every year. New forecasts project that halfway through the twenty-first century the median life expectancy will surpass previous estimates by 1.3 to 8.0 years.

The number of persons sixty-five and older will increase by eighty-two percent from 2000 to 2025 although the birth rate will increase by only three percent. World population may actually decline in the foreseeable future, with a higher percentage of individuals in their older years. Imagine the impact this will have on the global economy.

Citizens of the seven most highly developed countries (G-7) will live to the following ages, on average, by 2050:

| | |
|---|---|
| Canada | 85.26 years |
| France | 87.81 years |
| Germany | 83.12 years |
| Italy | 86.26 years |
| Japan | 90.91 years |
| UK | 83.79 years |
| US | 82.91 years |

The US comes in dead last in the list. Still, a lifespan of just under eighty-three years is remarkable compared with a life expectancy of only fifty-seven years three quarters of a century earlier. The fact that it is not uncommon these days for people to live one hundred or more years should assure us that we all have the potential for living that long.

The oldest documented human in recent times is a 122-year-old French woman who smoked and drank during the last twenty years of her life. Did smoking and drinking encourage her longevity? Not at all! Studies of centenarians show that people living over one hundred have only one factor in common—a genetic trait. They had long-lived grandparents, brothers, and other family members. Genetics is the secret to long life. You, too, could live to be one hundred if you could choose your relatives.

We now believe that the maximum possible lifespan for humans may be as much as 150 years. In the future humans may be able to live closer to their maximum lifespan thanks to genetic engineering, a more abundant supply of organs for transplants, and medical discoveries that will make replacement parts common. With such a long lifespan, people may choose to retire at age one hundred. The difficulty in surviving will no longer be avoiding chronic diseases, but living for more than a century without being bored.

We aren't there thus far, but we do know that with advancing age, production of certain hormones declines, including human growth hormone, DHEA, oxytocin, melatonin and, of particular interest, testosterone. We have to ask: Is the decline of these hormones a natural consequence of aging, or are we dying prematurely?

The manipulation of hormones to slow the aging process could lead to amazing strides in the road to greater longevity. In the last chapter we discussed the promise of growth hormone supplements as an anti-aging agent, only to reach the conclusion that lower levels of these potent hormones are healthier than higher ones. The addition of specific antioxidants plus the use of sun block to minimize the photo aging of the skin is all we can do at this time to avoid aging.

At the same time I must report that my experience in administering growth hormone to elderly people who are very deficient in this hormone has been nothing short of miraculous. I have seen these patients enjoy improved heart function, decreased pain and weakness, better motivation, and more joy in living. Therapy with human growth hormone can be rejuvenating. This is far different from pushing normal HGH levels into abnormal ranges and risking serious side effects.

In the 1800s Voltaire said, "Doctors are men who prescribe medications of which they know little, to cure diseases of which they know less, in human beings of whom they know nothing." We have come a long way since then in achieving medical breakthroughs, but we have much to learn. We are still on the frontier of knowledge about many areas of health, especially regarding aging and new discoveries about how hormones affect the changing human condition.

That doesn't stop the parade of "anti-aging" drugs. I continue to be amazed by the variety of drugs you can purchase on the Internet without a prescription. Marketers currently promote both HGH and IGF-1 as anabolic hormones you can simply spray up your nose and benefit from their life-prolonging effects. Do they work? Or are these drugs another cruel hoax thrust upon an unwary population looking for a longer, healthier life? Read on.

# 10

# Anabolic Steroids and Testosterone Myths

## Boosting our Hormones

The flow of life depends on a complex set of body parts made out of chemicals, enzymes, and molecules working in harmony to bring us satisfaction and good health. Our hormones are by far the most interesting of these microscopic components of life because of their incredible power, flexibility, and uncanny ability to regulate other hormones as well as entire body processes. Hormones of the precise composition and strength we need for life hover in our parent cells at conception and stay with us until our last heartbeat.

Some men have attempted to harness this power in the quest of the perfect body or the strength of Hercules. Boosting their hormones artificially they have created an aura of myth and invented new uses and a new language for the Big T. In this chapter I provide a general overview of the abuse of anabolic steroids—not only for this generation but also for generations to come.

## Anabolic Steroids and the Perfect Body

We have seen that hormones are affected by light, age, and imbalances in the way our neurotransmitters work. We have discussed feedback systems that our hormones use to regulate the activities of other hormones circulating in our bloodstream. What happens if we overdose on these wonderful hormones? Embracing the "more is better" concept, some individuals experiment on themselves without physician supervision or any kind of monitoring. These people are determined to possess a perfectly developed body, but too often their dreams never come true.

Before we find out what goes wrong with a program of self-administered steroids, let's look at some of the ways these hormones affect our muscles and physical strength.

Anabolic (body-building) steroids are derivatives of testosterone that treat a variety of medical conditions, including muscle wasting or severe anemia. Today they are popular in enhancing athletic performance and muscular development. To achieve this purpose testosterone must be chemically modified to enhance its anabolic, or bodybuilding, effects rather than its androgenic, or masculinizing, actions.

The resulting anabolic steroids boost nitrogen levels in the body, which promotes protein synthesis, muscle growth and the multiplication of red blood cells. An abundance of nitrogen allows the cells to hang on to extra nitrogen that is needed to form the amino acids that are the building blocks of protein. This effect, combined with a high intake of high-calorie and high-protein foods, causes muscle tissue to grow in size. Muscles grow stronger and bigger as a result of increased hormonal activity.

Many body builders fail to understand that they are merely increasing muscle size and not the number of muscle cells when they take anabolic steroids. They also ignore the possibility of severe side effects from excessive use of steroids—hypertension, acne, hardening of the arteries, increased blood clotting, jaundice, liver cancer, tendon damage, loss of fertility, and psychological problems. Additional complications for men include reduced fertility, shrinkage of sex organs, and breast enlargement or gynecomastia. Women taking steroids can develop masculine characteristics such as deep voices.

The opposite of anabolic or bodybuilding steroid is catabolic or destructive. For example, when we exercise strenuously, tissue breaks down, and we call this breakdown of tissue catabolism. Other catabolic states include cancer, malnutrition, AIDS Wasting Syndrome, and muscle wasting conditions such as muscular dystrophy or multiple sclerosis. Anabolic steroids can block the breakdown of tissue and reverse undesirable weight loss or wasting syndromes.

The major muscles of our arms, legs, and back are the same ones we had when we were thirteen; they are just bigger. Bodybuilders may measure their muscle power in pounds, but strength comes from the anabolic (bodybuilding) effect of testosterone on muscles, tendons, and ligaments.

Anabolic steroids stimulate the formation of additional protein within the cell. They provide enough building blocks to the cells so that they double or triple their size in a short time. Testosterone and its steroid derivative promote rapid healing of muscles, ligaments and tendons. Instead of feeling soreness and aching in their joints and muscles after a workout, men using anabolic androgenic steroids have a shorter recovery time. They can return to the gym the next day feeling rejuvenated and ready for more intense exercise. No wonder their muscles get so much bigger.

The strengthening effect of testosterone supplements can help older men with hypogonadism overcome muscle weakness. By following a carefully managed program involving diet, hormone supplementation and exercise, these men can enjoy testosterone's anabolic effects and watch their muscles grow in size and strength.

This may tempt you to try to treat yourself with steroids. Don't listen to your gym buddy or be taken in by advertising. The stakes are too high. Don't go there.

Hormones running amok can sabotage your self-regulating endocrine system, leading to erectile dysfunction, heart disease, hypertension, and sudden cardiac death. Anabolic steroids, for example, especially testosterone, the primary hormone affecting androgen receptors in heart muscle, increases the size of the heart muscle, leading to irregular heart rates and serious problems.

Have you ever wondered why women don't build big muscles when they exercise? The main reason is that they possess much lower testosterone levels—approximately one tenth those of men. Women can firm and tone their muscles by lifting weights, and their lean body mass will increase slightly. If they use anabolic steroids, however, the anabolic qualities of these steroids will develop their muscles just as it does for men. Yes, women can "bulk up"—just like men.

Women using powerful anabolic steroids may feel good about increasing their muscle mass, but it startles the rest of us when we notice hair growing on their faces and chest. Their breasts shrink, and they develop a deep, masculine voice. These are the masculinizing (androgenic) effects of testosterone, and they are *not* reversible.

An average teenage girl naturally produces somewhere around one half milligram (0.5 mg) of testosterone a day. At one time East German sports authorities routinely prescribed steroids to young adolescent girls in doses of up to 35 milligrams a day—*seventy times* the normal amount. After the fall of the Berlin Wall, an investigation into former female athletes found that most retained masculinized physiques and voices years after stopping their steroid therapy.

Other side effects were far more serious. Women came forward with tales of deformed babies, inexplicable tumors, liver dysfunction, internal bleeding, and depression—but only after *stopping* their steroids. It was as if their systems suddenly went haywire.

I often get letters from young men who are experimenting with self-injection of anabolic steroids. Here's a typical one.

A young patient I'll call Mark told me that he had taken blood tests and had managed to buy injectable testosterone in Mexico. Mark read the numbers wrong and assumed the concentration was half what it was. As a result he gave himself a double dose.

After self-injecting 600 milligrams of the product, Mark saw his test measurements jump sky high. A normal reading of DHT (dihydrotestosterone) for an adult male is 30 to 85. Mark's level thirty-six hours after the injection was 5,023, and his free testosterone and total testosterone levels were also off the charts. Mark was concerned about the effect of this super dose on his testicles and liver—as he should have been.

However, he should have been more concerned about becoming addicted to his high levels of testosterone and DHT, an ever-increasing problem for users of injectable steroids.

Evidence has surfaced showing that testosterone and steroid hormones such as oxytocin can produce beta-endorphins, the brain's own morphine-like compounds. These chemicals can alter the perception of pain and pleasure. Normally only opioid substances can affect these pain receptors, but anabolic steroids can mimic some of their opioid actions. Feelings of power and euphoria induced by super high levels of steroids contribute to addiction.

Alcohol is well known for its sedative effect and the way it relieves people from their inhibitions. Anabolic steroids can block these effects and alter behavior by increasing the pleasure of dopamine-dominant behavior while decreasing the sedative effects of serotonin. This effect means that men using steroids can "hold their liquor," giving them the feeling they are not drunk, so they imagine they can drive safely while under the influence, but they often end up as roadway fatalities.

The sport of bodybuilding abounds with statistics and stories of premature deaths from steroid abuse. Nonetheless, body builders are not criminals and should not be prosecuted for trying to improve themselves with drugs. They would not need to resort to such measures if doctors would be more available to diagnose and treat men who feel they cannot develop sufficient muscle mass.

Steve, an email friend of mine, explained it to me like this. "It's amazing how big you can look with the right lighting, a good tan and a clean shave," he said. "By the way, I meant to ask you, do your patients stay on testosterone cream year round? Do they cycle it? Do they need any kind of drug to restart natural testosterone production? You must have been thrilled to see the recent press coverage on testosterone supplementation. I would not be surprised if steroids were taken off the Schedule 3 list in a couple of years. I would hope that if the mass audience gets interested in testosterone supplementation and people want it, lawmakers would reconsider and accept the wonderful benefits of testosterone supplementation in appropriate dosages. What do you think?"

My answer to Steve is that anabolic steroids will never be taken off the controlled substance list. Some bodybuilders feel a need for steroids—or more steroids if they're already taking them—to grow bigger after they have reached their goals. Remember, however, that anabolic hormones only increase protein metabolism and speed recovery. Neither testosterone nor DHT can give you a muscular body unless you work hard. Only the effort involved in weight-bearing exercises can cause muscle tissue and its supporting structure, collagen, to grow. Testosterone simply makes it less painful to gain more muscle mass.

Many athletes lift far more weight than is necessary to develop a muscular physique. Remember that muscles grow in response to the stimulation of supporting tissue in the presence of adequate testosterone or the more anabolic DHT.

A complex interaction of diet, hormones and exercise plus the anabolic effects of testosterone makes muscles grow. At the risk of repeating myself, let me emphasize that hormones, especially androgenic anabolic steroids (AAS), affect many organ systems and should not be used without medical supervision.

Hormones such as testosterone directly affect physical characteristics in powerful ways. Professional athletes, men who are active in gyms, and the average Joe should have access to testing to see if their testosterone levels are adequate for normal functioning. In order to avoid common problems of overdosing such as abscesses, acne, swelling breast tissue, and small testicles, a physician should supervise all restorative efforts.

Of course it won't be that easy. An estimated one million individuals in the United States are current or past users of anabolic steroids. In the United States fifty percent of anabolic steroid users self-administer their compounds by an injection into the muscle tissue. Twenty-five percent of adolescent anabolic-androgenic steroid users share needles, placing them at risk for sharing HIV and hepatitis infections with other users.

The only safe way to have your hormones tested and any deficiencies treated is to find a qualified physician who will explain to you how your body is using hormones and will carefully monitor any supplementation program supported by your tests results.

## Testosterone: The Misunderstood Hormone

Numerous men—and women, to a lesser extent—suffer needlessly because their bodies no longer produce enough testosterone. It's time for us to listen to the king of all hormones.

We have always assumed that testosterone enables the brain to tolerate risk and peril and that testosterone levels are closely related to the realization of risky objectives. Our primitive forefathers leading the hunt were probably the dominant males with the highest testosterone.

Our definition of danger has escalated beyond chasing buffalo or fighting off wild elephants to include binge drinking, drunk driving and risky sex. These forms of risk and danger do not require testosterone, and it is wrong to assume that high levels of testosterone motivate today's risky behavior in the same way that they did during the days of old.

Make no mistake. Testosterone is the most important male hormone, responsible for the development of male sexuality and "manliness."

Men with high testosterone levels are often successful, highly motivated men while those with low testosterone levels are far more likely to be moody and insecure with higher than normal levels of estrogen and cortisol. To compensate for their low self-esteem, men with low testosterone levels seem to look to physical and emotional excitement to stimulate them. They then seek out dangerous behaviors such as drug abuse, sex with multiple partners, and bungee jumping, skydiving and other high-risk sports.

Another wrong belief about testosterone is that it causes prostate cancer or increases the risk of this common form of cancer. As we point out on page 147, there is no evidence to support a link between high testosterone levels and prostate cancer. In fact the link seems to be stronger between low levels of testosterone and prostate cancer, at least in families where someone has died from this disease.

Fear of testosterone as a dangerous drug is based on misconceptions about the role of this hormone in our bodies. Of course we know that testosterone is a powerful substance and that its misuse can lead to serious disorders. Nevertheless, for men with a testosterone deficiency, medically sound supplementation offers such a range of definite benefits that it cannot possibly be considered "dangerous."

## The Truth about Testosterone and Motivation

As I mentioned in the last section, the need to survive has influenced our biology from the time that men first evolved as hunters. Dangerous, sensation-seeking behavior was essential on a daily basis to bring in game from the hunt. Testosterone enabled the brain to tolerate risk and peril. Cavemen leaders and chieftains probably had the highest testosterone levels in their tribes.

In our society today, the "common wisdom" is that binge drinking, drunk driving, and risky sex, are dangerous activities resulting from very high levels of testosterone. This is not true. Levels of cortisone and estrogen seem to be much more of a factor in sensation seeking than are testosterone levels.

We now have abundant evidence that testosterone is not the primary factor in risky behavior. A research team led by Dr. J. C. Rosenblitt at Florida State University studied college students and found that, contrary to popular belief, a positive relationship between testosterone and sensation-seeking behavior does *not* exist in this population.

Robert suffered from testosterone deficiency-induced mood disorder with irritation, anger, and muscular weakness. These are symptoms of a high cortisol level in the brain as well as a low testosterone level.

He was married and had two young children—an eleven-month old and a two-and-a-half year old. "It seemed they were always getting to me," Robert said. "I was always angry about something. In addition, I did not have morning erections for a year and a half or longer." Rob realized something was wrong; his marriage was falling apart, and his children were no longer a joy to him. He understood that he had to change something to get rid of his unhappiness.

Finally Robert got some testosterone cream. "I was told to rub this into my biceps, a soft tissue absorption area. I did, and I am telling you this for a fact," he said. "After one week of using this cream, I had a full hard erection in the morning and have had one every morning for the past three months or so. My wife is pissed off, for now I always want more sex—a good thing to us men, but bad for the women!"

Robert also felt more pleasant and relaxed about the things that bothered him before. "My wife also saw this and made many comments about the difference."

Three months later Robert went back to his doctor and was tested for testosterone. His levels were in the high 800s. As early as one week after taking the testosterone therapy, Robert said, he had "the energy level of my younger days, doing much more work, and feeling almost no fatigue or laziness. I started lifting weights again. I'd been busy spending time with my two children and didn't have time for much else. But I was ready to lift and train again, with unlimited possibilities."

Fortunately, Robert's doctor was astute enough to prescribe transdermal testosterone, and Robert started working out again, dieting and put on more muscle mass. Three months later he sent me this report:

"I have put on some new muscle," he said, "and I started a diet, a major one, because, I said to myself, this time at forty-four years of age may be my last chance to get in shape. So I went to the limit and worked very hard at lifting and now dieting. I am determined to diet till my abs come out, no matter how long it takes. To make a long story short, I started at 250 pounds, and looked good and big. Now after six months, I am at 223 pounds, but I have I lost very little muscle mass. I was about twenty-four percent body fat before; now I am thirteen percent."

Robert is enthusiastic about his experience. "I realize that all of these benefits were not from testosterone," he told me, "but I could not have gotten where I am at here without it. Believe me, you can be all you want to be. If dieting and getting in shape is what you want, then, by God, set your mind and do it, but you cannot do it as a hypogonadal male. I tried it!"

Robert got a few local doctors interested in the testosterone cream and persuaded several of his friends who did not know they had low testosterone levels to be tested. "I feel that hormone replacement is the best thing for many males. I'm using it daily and will for the rest of my life. If I had not used a testosterone product, I would have gone to the gym and got almost no result because of my low T level, and I could not grow anymore. Testosterone provided a double benefit for me. I am a lifter and bodybuilder, and now I can do all I wanted to with unlimited results!

Eventually Robert went on to win second place as "World's Strongest Man 2002" by throwing around 700-pound tractor tires in a local contest.

Over the past decade, I have been prescribing hormone replacement in various forms to men like Robert who are suffering from a hormonal deficiency. Many people have sent me positive letters regarding their experience with the transdermal testosterone products. These men generally feel better, happier, calmer, more motivated, and they say they are enjoying life. They tell me that they now awaken with early morning erections after years of erectile problems.

Women suffering with low energy, obesity and hot flashes have seen pounds melt away and their sexual energy return with bioidentical hormone replacement therapy (BHRT). (This is *not* the same as HRT with Premarin and Provera.)

Hormone supplementation can make a huge difference in people's lives, restoring their self-control and optimizing their sexual functions.

Not all of us come with a perfectly balanced supply of hormones performing their hormone-related functions flawlessly, and very few of us will maintain that ideal state throughout our lifetimes. Any time we come up short in the hormone department, we experience a less-than-ideal life whether it's in the area of aging, sex and libido, raw physical strength, or mental capacity.

We still need to learn much more about how to live happily with the hormones we have been given. Future studies will add new information to the store of knowledge, and within a decade or two we will be able to enjoy a better life with the prudent use of hormone supplements.

Let's not cast doubt on progress made so far. In an idealistic sense it could be said that this is the golden age of hormones. Men are learning for the first time that they can enjoy the same benefits of hormone replacement therapy that women have enjoyed for decades but without the risks of excess estrogen and progesterone. Women are discovering hormone replacement therapy that is safe and affordable. Natural bioidentical hormones are emerging as a safe and effective alternative to synthetic hormones, which are being tossed aside as dangerous and cancer promoting.

An exciting future is unfolding. Our goal as we delve into the exploding world of rapidly changing information is to seek ways to live our lives with determination. As the nineteenth century biologist Thomas Henry Huxley put it, "The great end of life is not knowledge but action."

## Love, Libido and Hormones

The release of oxytocin is triggered by cells in the hypothalamus, as a result of changes in light intensity either due to the changing seasons or artificial lighting. Melatonin, the "night hormone," activates the receptor site in the brain. Oxytocin is also involved in the production of sperm and in the ejaculation response. Oxytocin can reverse the delay in ejaculation caused by certain antidepressants and may thus have a potential role as an option in patients who have sexual side effects such as delay in orgasm from the use of SRIs.

Most physicians are not aware that the association between testosterone and oxytocin can be tapped therapeutically for treating difficulties in human sexuality. Having postulated that oxytocin might be the elusive "love hormone," I decided to test this theory with a few patient volunteers. I conducted a small study to determine if "loving feelings" in men might be related to oxytocin stimulation in the brain. I wanted to see if there was a hormonal component to "falling in love."

I was not treating any illness, and I soon learned that finding "lovesick" volunteers for the study was impossible since, by definition, people who are lovesick do not want any treatment. As the poet Samuel Daniel stated, "Love is a sickness full of woes, all remedies refusing." So we told the men in the trial that the purpose of the study was to measure the volume of ejaculate before and after oxytocin use. Scientific literature indicated that there would be an increase of ejaculate in men using oxytocin, and I told the volunteers that I wanted to see if this was true. Side effects are mild, if any, so we both felt that it was worth a try. Informed consent was first obtained from the volunteers.

However, the hypothesis we were actually testing was that love is merely affection with intense bonding following orgasm. In other words, we were testing the idea that love is a direct emotional response resulting from sexual intercourse (ejaculation and orgasm) that makes two people feel closer. The underlying question of the study was, "Does a man's orgasm create the bond he feels with his mate, or is the effect due to oxytocin increases that correspond to feelings of love?"

We tested this theory in patient volunteers using a diluted oxytocin formula delivered by nasal spray. The nasal spray deposits the hormone directly at the base of the "olfactory" brain (via nasal mucous membranes). From there it diffuses to the hypothalamus. You may recall that this region also contains our biologic clock. Each of the men involved in our small clinical study had used a transdermal testosterone replacement program for at least six months prior to the study. Each volunteer complained of the loss of the spark he used to feel when making love with his wife. No placebo drug was used. The two patients each believed that oxytocin served primarily as a stimulant for increasing their ejaculate volume. When used prior to intercourse, oxytocin elicited the following reports:

Roger said that oxytocin affected the emotional aspect of the sex. "I did not notice the orgasm as stronger physically, but it was stronger emotionally," he said. Roger felt that oxytocin was rather like the emotional counterpart to testosterone. "I felt my wife had a prettier face when I had sex using oxytocin," he said. "I also felt the act of sex was a bit more sacred. I cannot say that I feel more monogamous since I am always monogamous except occasionally fantasizing about what girls' butts would look like naked when I see a young woman rated eight to ten. My sex drive remains extreme, and I honestly feel that in another time and place I could have easily been a great lover."

Another trial volunteer who used the oxytocin nasal spray did not have the same experience that Roger did. Mark said, "Doc, that OXY stuff is fantastic! I will not try to describe the events. All I can say is Wow! I felt like a young man again. The amount of sperm or whatever just kept on coming. The orgasm, if that is what you call an orgasm, lasted twice as long as it usually does, but the amount of stuff was incredible! My partner and I both felt we experienced the best sex ever and fell asleep in each other's arms. When we awoke, we made love again."

I was not surprised by this response because oxytocin has been found to facilitate reproduction in all vertebrates at several levels and seems to be intimately involved in sexual relations. Oxytocin acts on the brain as well as the uterus, testes, heart, thymus, kidney and pancreas in response to a variety of stimuli such as sucking, birthing and ejaculation.

John had a different response to oxytocin. "I've already used the oxytocin twelve times," he wrote, "and it looks like there's quite a bit left in the bottle—more than the fifteen total doses you said were in the bottle. The results have been mixed. Sometimes I ejaculate the original baseline amount, sometimes twice as much and sometimes three times as much. I'm sure there are other factors at work, like how excited I am at the time of ejaculation and how long a period of foreplay precedes the orgasm. The orgasms are noticeably more intense, which is great. We're going to try for a pregnancy again (seriously this time), as soon as I finish the oxytocin experiment."

This limited study showed us that while multiple chemical brain mediators and other factors induce the dazzling "feelings of love," oxytocin definitely plays a role in this complex process. In our uncontrolled study the use of oxytocin as a nasal spray doubled the volume of ejaculate for all of the men. Of course, a few anecdotal cases do not make for breakthrough science, and their over-interpretation should be resisted. Scientists prefer to rely on double-blind studies, where neither the patient nor the researcher knows who is using the effective drug, for acceptable evidence of a drug's effectiveness.

A few promising studies involving oxytocin have been conducted. Early in the 1970s reports began to appear showing that mating increases blood oxytocin concentrations in animals and humans. A compound that blocks the action of oxytocin seemed to reduce sexual responsiveness in rats after they were given estrogen and progesterone, two hormones that usually promote responsiveness. Similar but less convincing studies found male rats displaying more mounting behavior when oxytocin was delivered to their hypothalamus. Results of other animal studies suggest that oxytocin promotes bonding and directs female nursing and birthing behaviors. We have seen that androgens and oxytocin work together in human sexuality, and doctors may one day prescribe oxytocin for persons with orgasm or ejaculation problems.

My personal belief is that the role of oxytocin as a sex hormone and a key player in the behavior we call "love" will become more evident as research in sexual dysfunction progresses. Furthermore, I believe that sexual dysfunction may be shown to be the direct result of a hormone deficiency. To me it's not a big reach to believe that hormones are responsible for some of the emotional component of lovemaking. Bonding supplies the behavior humans need to be successful moms and dads for their children, and oxytocin stimulates the mechanisms that help us adapt to our parental roles. Apparently oxytocin unleashes a chemical that signals endorphins and dopamine receptors in the brain. Responding to the oxytocin, the brain translates the secret code.

More doctors are taking advanced courses and studying new developments in the field of sex medicine to learn how to help people with sexual problems. A new medical specialty has risen from this interest. Meanwhile, there are signs that the age of the medical manipulation of human sexuality in all its aspects has already begun. Erection enhancers, and drugs to stimulate sexual arousal are only the beginning. In the next section we will discuss melanocyte stimulating hormone or alpha-MSH, a hormone that scientists now believe plays a key role in preparing us physically, emotionally, and mentally for the sex act.

## Can You Restore Passion to Your Love Life?

Too many couples complain, "The passion has gone from our lives." For some that may be true, but it does not have to stay that way.

Could hormones provide the "passion trigger" that couples need after years of familiarity? Passion can be defined as "intense or overpowering emotion; ardent affection for one of the opposite sex or love." Passion is an essential component of all sexual relationships. Passion is present where there is enthusiasm, love, or desire, and in the opposite sense when there is anger, jealousy, or violence.

In a good sense emotionally positive passion provides the essence of sexual responsiveness, including arousal, pleasure, and orgasm. Unfortunately, passion sometimes converts to a negative emotion, "a fit of intense and furious anger; rage; a strong impulse tending to physical indulgence; the endurance of some painful infliction; suffering." Negative passion can often be associated with the destruction of relationships and the loss of life. Most homicides are committed under the influence of passion gone astray. In spite of that fact, without passion people feel as if an important element of their life has been lost. For millions of people the loss of passion or loss of love is blamed on various life stresses, when the true culprit is probably a hormonal imbalance.

Several hormones and brain chemicals play an essential role in the interconnected feelings of sex, love and passion. Most of these biological compounds are themselves interrelated. We have already discussed oxytocin and testosterone. The melanocortins are a newly discovered group of sex hormones. This tiny army of small protein hormones includes the andrenocorticotropic hormone (ACTH) that regulates the release of the hormone cortisol from the adrenals. (See page 58 for more about the effects of cortisol in the human body). The half dozen or so hormones in the melanocortin system play a key role in regulating our appetite and body weight as well as a variety of human conditions such as the color of our skin, how readily we digest fat, how much food we eat, our body's temperature, how our body responds to an inflammation, and our memory. One of these regulating hormones, alpha-melanocyte stimulating hormone or *a*-MSH, triggers physical responses such as grooming, stretching, yawning, and penile erection. Quite an interesting array of behaviors!

In her book, *Why We Love,* Helen Fisher expresses her belief that passion is a human drive as fundamental as hunger for food. Using Magnetic Resonance Imaging she recorded brain activity of people "in love." She concluded that romantic love is "deeply embedded in the architecture and chemistry of the human brain." She believes that knowing more about how the brain functions in areas of love and passion can help us understand divorce, stalking behavior, and criminal behavior.

A sexual problem should not automatically be assumed to be psychological in nature.

With proper hormonal balance, sexual arousal, orgasms and passion can return to your sex life. From my perspective, love and sex are considered complementary and essential for normal intimacy and positive passion is essential for the enjoyment of life! Listening to your hormones will help you hear what you need to do to restore that passion for life and love!

## Is Our Environment Spoiling Our Food?

In his book, *Total Health, The Next Level*, Peter Burwash states that animal protein is responsible for most of the diseases we suffer, as we grow older. He blames a diet heavy in meat for heart disease, kidney problems, colon cancer, and liver disorders. He believes that our internal environment becomes contaminated from obtaining protein from meat instead of other sources to build muscle mass. An athlete as well as a writer, Burwash is convinced that these problems will accelerate until our society learns to eat healthfully avoiding animal meat.

The fact that animals have become the route by which environmental toxins become incorporated into our body is indisputable. Chemicals embedded in animal fats damage our sex lives, our health, our hormonal balance and, ultimately, our minds. The combined action of estrogens, dioxins, PCBs, and heavy metals like lead and mercury transferred from our environment to our bodies can be subtle but deadly. For example, increased levels of PCBs and dioxin residues in animal fats are highly toxic interfering in brain and immune function. Excellent commentaries on the subject have been written by Dr. Andrew Weil in *Optimum Health Eating* and John Robbins in *Diet for A New America.*

The poisons that contaminate the animal products that we consume cannot be removed unless we change the way animals are fed. The diet of the animals we eat for food today does not even remotely resemble the food their ancestors ate when they fed on grasses and grazed free in the fields. As a result, the meat from beef, sheep, pigs, and chickens does not contain any of the essential fatty acids that were a major component of meat from range-fed animals. Commercially produced meat is not only lacking healthful components, but is tainted with chemicals such as bovine growth hormone, which is unsafe for human consumption. As we discussed in Chapter Four, human health is not a priority for the meat and dairy industry when compared to increased production and higher profits.

I believe that the debate about animal protein as an essential part of our diet will fade away when people realize what great foods are available to us without eating the flesh of dead animals. Rising levels of PCBs and dioxin residues in animal fats interfere with our bodies' ability to regulate our hormones and our immune system to work effectively. Meat substitutes such as soy, eggs, whey, seeds, and nuts deliver high-quality protein. Gains such as rye, oats, quinoa, and legumes such as amaranth, lentils, and beans are healthier, cheaper, cleaner, and easier to digest than meat. When prepared properly they taste better too.

The chorus is growing in volume. Contemporary health writers such as Andrew Weil, Peter Burwash and John Robbins voice their concerns, deploring the view that animal meat is part of a "healthy" diet. They point out that animals not only absorb environmental estrogens, but also concentrate these substances in their bodies passing them on to humans in dangerously high doses. They emphasize that animal protein containing low levels of dioxin is responsible for many our Western world diseases.

What chance do we have to restore the balance?

Listening to our hormones is a good place to start. Once we understand what they are telling us, then we can educate others about contaminants in our food that are interfering with the way our hormones can help us enjoy health. We need an abundance of clear thinking bolstered by accurate facts. This information should persuade people to lobby our government to promote clean air, water and food for all Americans rather than to subsidize our dairy and meat industries.

We are starting to pay the price for our wasteful and ignorant eating habits. Our diet makes us fat because we eat more food than we need and because the food we eat has too much fat in it. Half of our calories come from fat instead of the thirty percent recommended for good health. We don't have to eat like this. We can enjoy a wide variety of healthy foods. Choices for organically grown food are on the rise in this country. In the future meat could start to reflect its true environmental costs and at that time it could become such an expensive delicacy that it won't be eaten on a daily basis. Once you wake up to this reality, the desire to make healthier food choices will occur spontaneously. At that time, the health of all Americans can actually improve.

# 11

# The Future is Now...

## It's Not Too Late

Prediction is very difficult, especially of the future." It wasn't Yogi Berra who said that, but Niels Bohr, winner of the 1922 Nobel Prize in physics. Our most brilliant scientists continue to stumble over contradictions and puzzlements as they attempt to understand how the universe functions and how mankind fits into the entire cosmic picture.

As you think about what the future holds, take a moment to imagine you are living in our scientifically advanced society fifty or a hundred years from now. What do you see as you look far into the future down the horizon of time?

You might see infertility threatening the very existence of our once vital American culture. Pregnancies have become rare among married couples, and many men and women have lost their sexual desire by the age of forty. Sexual problems and infertility are common too early in life. Mid-life crises occur in the middle thirties as lifespans shrink year by year. Male pattern baldness strikes twenty-year-olds, and "old age" now begins in the mid-thirties. The enthusiasm for sex is all but gone. Our vibrant population is weakening.

As we continue to look into this far-away time zone, we foresee a polluted environment stirring up harmful hormone-like chemicals that wreak havoc on bodies and minds. Around us thousands of men and women are weakened and dying prematurely from hormone-related cancer, and cancer is now the leading cause of death, claiming the lives of half of all Americans. The combination of lower birthrates and early death from disease and premature aging threatens our very survival. Our passion for love has all but disappeared. Our once robust men are being chemically castrated without their consent. Artificial insemination seems to be the only option for the survival of the human race.

In this not-distant world scientists are working day and night to find a cure for this epidemic of sexual apathy. They suspect that an unknown hazard may be destroying the fertility of the human race. They are exploring probable causes of this grave condition affecting most of the Western world.

How frightening! But there's good news. The bright side of the picture is that by reading this book and taking steps to put what you have learned into action, you can help stop this awful scenario from occurring. You can make a difference in *your* life and in the lives of those close to you. You can begin to change your future for the better by recognizing the importance of hormones in the unfolding drama of your daily existence. As you learn about the ways your hormones have influenced your life from birth, your knowledge gives you the power to control the foods you choose to eat and many aspects of your health. Small decisions you make daily have huge effects on your well-being.

Beginning today you can check your hormone levels and work with a doctor to obtain the supplements you need for a healthy hormone balance. You can proclaim the dangers of hormones found in our food and the environment. You can help your neighbors and friends reach the goal of clean living. It is time for you to now come into the story with your own perspective.

In the final pages of this book I leave you with five valuable messages about our hormones. These final statements may give you some idea of what it takes to enjoy life to its fullest. At the same time, be aware that we haven't discovered all of the secrets of our hormones, how they work in our bodies and how to harness them for the healthiest results.

It is true that many techniques try to stop us from growing old, but no proven therapies turn back the hands of time, even on a temporary basis, without unwanted side effects. By restoring your hormones to more youthful levels through the use of natural bioidentical hormones, you can improve the quality of your life.

Briefly, here are five assumptions I hope will help you listen to our hormones.

## 1. The 'sexy trio' can renew youthfulness

The "sexy trio"—testosterone, DHT, and estrogen—combine to assure vigorous sexual functioning in both sexes. Besides a heightened sexual drive, people with balanced levels of these three hormones have a leaner, younger-looking body, stronger muscles, and tougher bones. In addition, testosterone promotes healthy hearts by helping to prevent hardening of the arteries and weakening of the heart muscle. Elderly people with higher levels of free testosterone have improved memories and less age-related senility.

Estrogen once promised "eternal youth" to women, only to fail miserably to live up to its promise—although we shouldn't overlook estrogen's positive effects on skin, hair, and bones. Move over estrogen. Make way for testosterone, the hormone that now takes credit for helping women live longer than men.

Slowing down the aging process has been a goal of modern medicine since its inception. As we roll through the first years of the new millennium, slowing down the aging process is high on the wish list of baby boomers, including doctors, who are now looking at their retirement years. Thousands of doctors now offer pills, creams, powders, surgery, and dozens of regimens promising to block the ravages of time.

Doesn't this sound to you like a better way to age?

It's true we can look younger if our hormones are released at "youthful" levels. By now you know that reaching those levels does not happen by taking more hormones. You should be aware that other factors play important roles in fine-tuning our personal hormone system.

Besides the "sexy trio" of hormones, proteins such as the sex hormone binding globulin (SHBG) can also function as hormone regulators in the brain. According to research by Jack Caldwell at the University of Illinois College of Medicine, SHBG acts like a switch that can turn sex hormones off and on in the blood stream, and also stimulate sexual arousability receptors in the hypothalamus. Prior to Caldwell's work, we believed that only free or bioavailable hormones (which are weakly bound to albumin) could exert beneficial effects in the body, certainly not those bound with SHBG.

We need to do more than merely identify hormone deficiencies. We need to measure SHBG levels so that we can determine the amount of active hormone available to the body. We also need to know more about the role of the body's hormone delivery system in determining the final availability of a hormone to its receptor. The genetic structure of our hormones is only part of the picture. We need to understand that our hormones are controlled on a day-to-day basis by the brain's action on the hypothalamus and the pituitary gland. Our nervous system continually modifies the delivery of our hormones, responding to changes in our internal environment through the natural processes of growth, maturity and aging.

Because of extremes in hormone levels after an injection, shots are not always the best way to deliver hormones. Testosterone or estrogen delivered by injection can result in dangerously high levels immediately following the injection, with rapid declines afterwards. Pills are not much better, carrying the risk of serious liver damage, blood clots, and other problems. Patches and gels that administer hormones through the skin are more efficient than pills or injections and have fewer side effects. Delivering hormones directly into the blood stream through the skin seems to come closer to duplicating the natural action of the endocrine system than do other methods of delivery.

You are fortunate if you reach the stage in your doctor's office where you are discussing the method of testosterone delivery. Often the discussion ends prematurely because doctors are nervous about prescribing testosterone for men. They subscribe to the myth that testosterone may cause prostate cancer; though numerous research studies (see references on page 298) show that estrogen plays a more significant role as an initiator of prostate cancer than testosterone. Most doctors are also unaware that there is simply no scientific evidence that testosterone supplementation alone increases the risk of prostate cancer.

Various factors including SHBG, DHT and estradiol have been implicated in prostate cancer. Diets high in soybeans, fruits and vegetables containing all the essential vitamins and minerals you need to stay healthy, helping to SHBG levels under control. Zinc and selenium, and the Vitamin E complex of alpha and gamma tocopherols may block the conversion of testosterone to estrogen. These helpful phytochemicals are found in seeds, nuts, and avocados—which also provide essential fatty acids similar to those in fish oils. Such compounds not only help maintain prostate health but also help tilt the ratio in favor of optimum cholesterol and free testosterone levels. Sometimes these agents can help to prevent the occurrence of prostate cancer. Testosterone applied through the skin also helps to delay osteoporosis, senility, and loss of motivation. The accumulation of excess fat that is so common in elderly men shrinks with testosterone stimulation.

Avoid traditional American diets that are high in protein and fat that contribute to an elevated level of SHBG (sex hormone binding globulin), which reduces the amount of testosterone available to your body. Our favorite American foods, especially those we buy at fast food restaurants and in the prepared-food section of the supermarket, may contain environmental toxins, which exert estrogen-like effects increasing SHBG and contributing to heart disease, diabetes, obesity, and cancer.

A healthy diet is not enough to make it possible for you to maintain high levels of bioavailable testosterone forever. Inevitably the relative amount of SHBG-bound testosterone increases so that less testosterone is available to strengthen your bones and muscles. When your available testosterone reaches low levels, you will probably find that taking appropriate testosterone supplements will improve your libido and reverse many of the devastating effects of frailty, associated with old age. As a man you should be able to achieve and maintain a healthy erection well into your nineties with hormone replacement therapy.

## 2. You don't have to wait for your doctor to diagnose hypogonadism

Good news! You don't have to wait for your doctor to screen you. You can first determine your own hormone levels by salivary hormone testing and then work with a doctor to correct any deficiencies or take simple steps to boost your own hormones. Regular high-intensity exercise and an active sex life, for example, have been shown to contribute to keeping testosterone at optimal levels.

Take these steps to assure that you do not suffer from hypogonadism. Begin by asking your doctor to increase your testosterone levels if they are lower than they should be or you are suffering from sexual problems such as lack of libido.

All of us need to stop avoiding the fact that much of the sexual dysfunction we experience is related to low testosterone levels. Probably more than forty million women and thirty million men have an unsatisfactory sex life because they don't have enough testosterone in their systems.

Six million men in the US suffer from hypogonadism, or extremely low levels of testosterone. The numbers for women are undoubtedly higher because when a woman's ovaries are removed in a total hysterectomy, they automatically become deficient in testosterone. I believe that further research will demonstrate that inadequate testosterone levels in the citizens of industrialized nations are linked to declines in birthrate and lower sexual drives.

Heavy exercise does boost testosterone levels, and some men spend a lot of time working out at the gym to improve their physical performance. If you are healthy and have a testosterone deficiency, you'll be more likely to restore normal levels with a transdermal (applied to the skin) testosterone supplement than with hours in the gym.

For the most part, our physicians are blind to the benefits of appropriate testosterone therapy in men and women whose sex life, mental health, and general health are woefully lacking as a result of low testosterone levels. Most look the other way and try to pacify their patients with vague assurances that they're "normal." Others might prescribe testosterone for conditions other than hypogonadism.

The Institute of Medicine report says that more than 1.75 million testosterone prescriptions were written in 2002, up from 648,000 in 1999. Researchers at the National Institute on Aging were concerned that the testosterone boom was a public health issue and wanted a large clinical trial.

Those at the National Cancer Institute worried about giving healthy men testosterone in such a study when it might fuel the growth of prostate cancer. The heads of the two institutes asked the Institute of Medicine for help. Dr. Dan G. Blazer, a professor of psychiatry and behavioral sciences at Duke University and chairman of the Institute of Medicine's committee set to work. The report of the WHI was on everyone's mind. "No one wanted to repeat that experience with testosterone," Dr. Blazer said. On the other hand, he said, testosterone may well be effective and the published studies do not show it is harmful. The committee searched for evidence that testosterone helped aging men.

We all need to stop and listen to the messages testosterone and its active products are sending through our bodies. We should not hold back from taking medically advised steps to correct any sexual dysfunction we may suffer because we do not have enough sex hormones in our systems. Ask your doctor to test your hormone levels; you may both be surprised at the results.

## 3. Toxic chemicals lead to testosterone deficiency (hypogonadism)

Almost every day we hear about another way our world has become contaminated with our humanity. Toxins are continually released into our environment from industrial wastes, auto fumes, landfill breakdowns and drugs we flush down the toilet. Ironically, as we bring improved products and systems to the marketplace we suffer from the by-products of innovation.

Polluting chemicals can interfere with the function of our endocrine system. Evidence from ongoing research passes a good share of the blame for disease, weakened immune systems, and a premature decline in testosterone to these poisons. One alarming effect caused by the onslaught of estrogens from the environment is the tilt of the ratio of testosterone to estrogen in favor of estrogen dominance. As I have pointed out many times in this book, too much estrogen is bad for both men and women. An excess of estrogen creates a lowered sex drive, an increased risk of various types of cancer, or chemical castration.

Pollution is the price we must pay for human progress. However, we must work tirelessly to support policies at the local, regional and national level for more reasonable use of nature's resources. We must appeal to our government for clean air and water rather than supporting beef and dairy and oil and coal industries with costly subsidies.

We should also clean up our own backyards. Becoming vegetarian or following a plant-based (vegan) diet by avoiding meat and animal products involves simple steps all Americans can take toward improving their health. Choose from the abundance of low carbohydrate, non-meat foods that give you high quality protein and are still available at reasonable prices at your grocery store. At the very least, grow salad greens and other vegetables in your own garden or a planter or window box. *The Food Revolution* by John Robbins extols the health virtues of avoiding meat and following a vegan-type diet. He also points out the environmental hazards created by raising animals for food. The contamination of our water supply by animal pollution is a big factor

Don't hesitate to demand accountability from your elected representatives for the quality of your water supply. As a nation we must stop the contamination of our rivers and streams with drug-laden animal manures, environmental estrogens and toxic wastes. Our environment is too precious to waste on breeding organisms that are resistant to antibiotics and multiplying hybrid polluting chemicals that can destroy our future, our fertility—and inevitably our lives.

## 4. Bioidentical, natural hormones are more potent

What is DHT anyway? As noted earlier, DHT is an abbreviation for dihydrotestosterone, the most important metabolic product of testosterone for men and women. This hormone plays a crucial role in sex drive and the development of our sexual organs during puberty. Regrettably, it may be linked to acne, hair loss and increased prostate size.

You may hear the comment that DHT just makes our prostates balloon up and our hair fall out. Not true. DHT is a beneficial hormone that can help combat environmental contamination and build muscles. As mentioned earlier, boosting levels of this hormone can reduce the toxicity of dioxin-laden animal fats. DHT, not testosterone, carries androgenic (male) signals throughout the body. When it reaches an androgen receptor, DHT can bind to the receptor with three to five times the strength of testosterone. This superior binding strength gives it the deserved reputation for having more power than any synthetic anabolic steroid.

Because DHT has more than twice the power of testosterone as an anabolic (growth promoting and bodybuilding) steroid, it has been used for years in Europe as a potent topical agent for treating erectile dysfunction and prostate enlargement. Topical DHT could soon be available in the US to help shrink the prostate and to stimulate sexual drive in the elderly.

Hormones such as DHT may also be able to reverse some of the toxic effects of dioxin on the human body. Research from Germany, UK, Canada and Japan indicates that adequate DHT levels could offset some of dioxin's harmful effects. DHT gels are being studied for their ability to prevent prostate cancer and breast cancer and will soon be available in the US. DHT has also been used in London and Israel to successfully promote penis growth in infants and children with abnormally small penises.

How can one hormone have so many good and bad effects? The answer is not easy to understand. My theory is that the two forms of the 5-AR enzyme that are present at all androgen receptors produce two functionally dissimilar types of DHT, which act in a mutually inhibitory fashion. In other words, each hormone's form can regulate and obstruct the activity of the other.

The two forms of this hormone are called DHT-1 and DHT-2. The form known as DHT-1 is found in skin, hair and bone, and is responsible for blocking the action of DHT-2. An opposing role may be played by DHT-2, which is found primarily in the prostate, scalp and the penis, and works to increase hair growth and organ size at puberty by limiting the activity of DHT-1.

Other important hormones from the brain such as oxytocin and SHBG, which we have already discussed, can affect the conversion of testosterone to DHT. Jack Caldwell states that DHT can inhibit SHBG binding in the brain, affecting female arousability. This outcome involves oxytocin action in the hypothalamus.

Studies show that hair follicles on top of a man's head contain more receptor sites for DHT. This could explain why men with high levels of DHT-2 are likely to become prematurely bald. Another consequence of too much DHT-2 in men is benign prostate hyperplasia, or an enlarged prostate gland—a condition we've discussed earlier in the book (See page 128). Super-high levels of DHT can also cause acne because of the hormone's effect on the development of the oil glands in the skin.

Responding to some of these observed effects, pharmaceutical companies are promoting highly effective DHT-blocking products, including Proscar®, Propecia®, and Avodart®.

The danger of focusing on the negative action of this hormone is in ignoring the positive way it works with testosterone within our bodies. Not all DHT is bad. Correctly understood, DHT can become an ally for healthy prostates and strong sexual drives.

The secret to living in harmony with all of the hormones our body produces is the magic word, "balance." This includes DHT. If your levels are below normal and you experience lackluster sexual performance but still show normal testosterone levels, don't hesitate to discuss your concerns with your doctor. Instead of avoiding DHT at all costs, you might benefit from bringing those below normal levels into balance with your other hormones. Sexual arousability, sexual preference and sex drive may be closely linked to levels of this hormone.

Much of this book has targeted sex and the wide variety of its expressions among humans. Sexuality encompasses a broad spectrum of preferences from heterosexual to homosexual and everything in between.

Many people are offended for religious or other reasons about homosexuality. They ascribe criminal or psychological intent to homosexual people and see them as a risk to society, often quoting Scripture to justify their judgments. I am not advocating a homosexual lifestyle for anyone. What I do suggest is a careful consideration of relevant information about the influence of hormones and human genes on sexual orientation. After all, from three to five percent of our population is homosexual, and there is strong evidence that this has always been the case.

Is sexual preference a choice that people make?

We are talking about men and women whose bodies are normal for their physical gender. They are male or female, but instead of falling in love with someone of the opposite sex, they are physically and emotionally drawn to others of their sex. How does this happen? The study of how the mind develops is fascinating. We know that the mind continues to develop from the first brain tissue formed from by rapidly dividing cells in the unborn infant on through childhood and adolescence. New evidence suggests that the brain is very plastic and can continue to grow and adapt throughout life.

Other recent research indicates that levels of free testosterone in the body and levels of dihydrotestosterone (DHT) in the developing hypothalamus somehow play a deciding role in determining the mindset for sexual preference. At the time of puberty a burst of DHT not only drives the growth of sex organs but also the individual's sexual attraction towards people of the same or opposite sex.

The way our genetic code is programmed determines the rate at which free testosterone converts to DHT or estradiol from birth to old age. In other words, our genes determine this rate of conversion. An individual's testosterone-to-DHT ratio is under genetic control. For this reason, it remains constant throughout life regardless of any hormone replacement method used. The enzyme 5-AR, 5-alpha reductase which we discussed earlier, regulates how much and how rapidly free testosterone is converted to DHT.

In my medical practice approximately ten percent of my patients show much higher testosterone levels than normal. They are considered "testosterone dominant." Many of these patients, male or female, tend toward homosexuality or bisexuality in their sexual orientation. The ratio of testosterone to DHT for these individuals is three to six times higher than for other patients when these levels are measured in the blood and up to fourteen times higher than others when measured in saliva.

Why is this significant?

The direct effects of DHT and free testosterone on the androgen (male) receptors of the brain are powerful. They determine attitudes, aggression, and various behaviors. Studies indicate that levels of free testosterone and DHT are significantly higher in male homosexuals than in heterosexuals of similar age. Scientists in Canada, the UK, and the US have reported an interesting observation. As we pointed out in our section on sexual preference in Chapter Six, the difference in the lengths of the second and fourth finger length seem to vary among people according to their sexual orientation. The theory that explains this phenomenon again relates to the action of DHT during adolescence. Unequal finger-length ratios can be interpreted as an example of the physical differences between males and females caused by the effect of free or bioavailable testosterone and DHT on bone growth.

Since 1973 the American Psychiatric Association has officially considered homosexuality as an expression of sexual orientation and not as a mental disorder. This perspective is supported by the American Academy of Pediatrics, which states that while we do not know with certainty the cause of homosexuality, "the current literature and the vast majority of scholars in this field state that one's sexual orientation is not a choice" and that "individuals no more choose to be homosexual than heterosexual."

To me the logical assumption is that people are born gay rather than choosing to adopt this lifestyle. Theories about sexual preference are only that—theories. Science has not provided conclusive evidence about its cause, although biological influences do seem to play a greater role than once thought. A genetic condition does not excuse us from taking responsibility for the consequences of our choices, but we need to stop blaming other people for feeling a sexual preference they did not choose. As mothers and fathers we should show compassion for boys and girls caught in the trap of sexual ambiguity and not punish or ostracize them for it.

## 5. Oxytocin plays a vital role in sexual arousal and much more

Oxytocin has cast a magic spell on lovers through the centuries. Today the bewildering, seductive powers of oxytocin continue to guide us relentlessly through the stages of arousal, orgasm and ejaculation. Can a biological chemical really create feelings of love? Certain pharmaceutical companies want you to think so. You can buy dozens of products sold with the promise that their use will bring you more love and sexual fulfillment.

If you've ever been in love, you've experienced the power of oxytocin. Merely touching a woman's skin releases oxytocin and can create a desire in her to be caressed and loved. Because oxytocin depends in part on estrogen to work and because women have far more estrogen than men do, the arousal effect of touching is much greater in women than in men. Besides increasing a woman's sexual desire, oxytocin prepares her body for intercourse by increasing vaginal lubrication.

Women who are capable of experiencing multiple orgasms generally have higher than usual levels of oxytocin in their systems and experience more intense orgasms. Men also are subject to the magic of oxytocin. When a brain hormone known as the alpha melanocyte stimulating hormone (α-MSH) floods certain cells within the hypothalamus, creating feelings of intense arousal and inducing an erection. Immediately after this, the pituitary hormone vasopressin is secreted, triggering a burst of oxytocin from the paraventricular nucleus. Oxytocin is released at the exact moment of ejaculation. Once it released, oxytocin mediates satiety, suppressing further arousal.

The presence of oxytocin may reinforce monogamy—the desire for one sexual partner. One researcher, Pedersen, found that the brains of certain animals that mate with only one member of their species have higher concentrations of oxytocin than do animals with many sexual partners. Courtship and couple bonding are strengthened when sufficient oxytocin is present. Orgasms and ejaculations intensify, and the need for a monogamous relationship is assured.

According to Dr. George Gimpl at Guttenberg University in Germany, the action of oxytocin on the central nervous system includes creating and directing complex activities involved in reproduction and the care of infants. For example, oxytocin exerts potent anti-stress effects that may facilitate the bonding of male and female as well as inducing mothering and fathering behavior. The stress-reducing effects of oxytocin on both sexual and maternal behavior lead to a positive connection between mother and child and father and child. Oxytocin seems to help mothers nurture their offspring and helps intensify bonding to keep fathers in the family unit.

Oxytocin has been used for decades to help women in the birthing process and a synthetic form of the hormone, Pitocin nasal spray, is used to facilitate breast feeding in women who have trouble nursing their babies. Some researchers now believe that oxytocin regulates nursing and birthing behaviors in all animal species.

After ejaculation, oxytocin and IGF-1 trigger the pituitary to release higher levels of prolactin. The added prolactin suppresses testosterone and puts off another orgasm from occurring for up to several hours. I suppose this is one way nature helps perpetuate various species, by giving participants a welcome rest, keeping them from being worn out by the arduous work of constantly making love. Humans are the only animals that have sex for love rather than exclusively for impregnation.

Two graduate students, Cindy Meston and Penny Frohlich, found evidence that oxytocin and vasopressin when combined have a powerful effect on sexual function in humans. Their paper reports that circulating levels of oxytocin increase during sexual arousal and orgasm in both sexes. Vasopressin, on the other hand, drives sexual aggression. Female animals with high levels of oxytocin adopt postures showing their readiness for the sex act. These oxytocin activities can be shut down by SHBG. They also found that higher oxytocin levels correspond with more intense orgasmic contractions in men and women.

Physicians should consider the potential of oxytocin in treating people with sexual dysfunction. These men and women could perhaps enjoy greater sexual arousal and more intense orgasms with oxytocin nasal sprays. An added bonus for men is the increased volume and intensity of ejaculation set off by oxytocin release.

Be careful about off-label use of any hormone, including oxytocin. Men using oxytocin on a regular basis as a "sex drug," for example, may be setting themselves up for prostate enlargement and other problems. Women taking oxytocin may notice milk flowing from their breasts during sexual activity. The excess use of vasopressin sprays can upset the delicate mineral balance. The hormonal interrelationships are neither simple nor direct.

Some day we may find new formulas for sex medicines based on this intriguing hormone. In the future we may be able to buy sexual bonding and commitment in an oxytocin spray bottle. Meanwhile let's listen thoughtfully to the needs of our sexual partners who are searching for that spark to revitalize their own passion.

## Sex and Mankind

You may be wondering why much of the emphasis in this book has been about the sex drive and sexual experience of men. The first reason is that as a man I have a personal interest in this subject. Secondly, I have been treating men in my clinic for decades. I have become deeply concerned about misunderstandings and lack of information that keep men from living fulfilling sexual lives. The third reason is that I am troubled by the fact that most doctors look the other way when men seek advice about sexual dysfunction.

I do not believe that patients or doctors are willfully ignorant. It could be that men's egos are too inflated to admit to sexual inadequacy. I suspect that they are simply ignorant or influenced by a stream of self-serving information from the media or big business in search of financial rewards. Many andrologists are women, and I suspect this is because female doctors are less threatened by sexual problems than their male counterpart, so they listen more attentively to their male patients. All of us—doctors, parents, teachers, and sexual partners—are subjected to erroneous opinions about our hormones. Too often we pass on unfounded beliefs and assumptions without the filter of scientific evidence.

We can place most of the blame for the lack of adequate knowledge about sexual performance on our reluctance to deal with the facts. When it comes to sex, too often we're like the couple that married for better or worse—she couldn't have done worse, and he couldn't do better. We just shrug our shoulders and go on with life.

George Burns put our complacency about love in perspective. "Do you know what it means to come home at night to a woman who'll give you a little love, a little affection, a little tenderness?" he asked. "It means you're in the wrong house, that's what it means." We smile, but inside we know that the comedian was commenting on the emptiness of our relationships. We toss the high expectations of long-lasting passion out the window without a thought and live from day to day with scarcely a loving glance or a wink at our mates.

It's true that nobody ever died from not having sexual intercourse or a thrilling sex life. You don't have to have sexual relations to survive, and many people have lived long, satisfying lives in a celibate state. Nevertheless, I believe that a loving sexual bond and a passionate loving relationship are not considered as seriously as they should be.

Men who are earnest in their longing for a healthier sex life and improved connection with their life partner often endure less than satisfactory performance for years without complaining. By the time they muster the courage to unload their personal problem to their doctor, they are many years older than the doctor. Men past sixty who have become impotent are often reluctant to trust advice about sex and hormone-driven feelings from a young doctor.

The reality is that impotence, or the inability to achieve a hard erection, is a serious condition in the life of most men. As they age, men—and women as well—long to hold on to the passion of their earlier years. They want to retain as much as they can of the vigor and vitality of youth. The universal dream is, "if only a man could enjoy the wisdom and insights of a sixty-year-old mind in the body of a thirty-year-old." Instead, wisdom usually comes too late for us to make any practical use of it. As the famous actor John Wayne said on his deathbed, "If I had known I was going to live so long, I would have taken better care of myself."

The dream of restoring sexual vitality to our lives is not that far-fetched. Through the magic of modern medicine and the power of our human hormones, we can make great strides in maintaining enthusiasm and libido into our older years. A saying I use often in my clinical practice is, "Health is merely the slowest possible rate at which one can age." Don't accept "old age" as a sentence of impending death.

Keith, a patient of mine, suffered from a condition called unilateral cryptorchidism, or, in simple terms, the failure of one of his testicles to descend fully from the abdomen into the scrotum. "I always sensed that something wasn't quite right," Keith told me, "but for thirty-six years my doctors didn't seem to think that my condition would have any detrimental effects whatsoever."

Keith wasn't convinced. After years of going along with what the doctors told him, he decided to dig out the facts himself. From a search on the web he found out that his inability to grow a beard or hair on his chest, a lackluster libido, and a lifelong tendency to gain weight could be related to the lack of testosterone. That connection, he learned, could be that with only one testicle, his body could be producing insufficient quantities of testosterone. In clinical terms, he could be suffering from true hypogonadism.

Reading a men's health magazine, Keith came across an article about AndroGel, which had been approved by the Federal Drug Administration in July of 2000. His next step was to find a doctor who specialized in hormone replacement therapy. While he was searching the web he came across my web site, got in touch with me and made an appointment to see me. He traveled all the way from Texas. After a thorough examination and evaluation, I concluded that he would benefit most from topical testosterone, a cream compound I dubbed TestoCreme® rather than a series of self-injections with all of its attendant problems.

Keith agreed to give TestoCreme a try and took home a jar that would last him three months. The results were direct, immediate, and positive.

"Imagine having a dialogue in your mind like a tape recorder that constantly reminds you of the 'bad' things that have happened in your life,"

Keith wrote. "You can't get rid of the images of people you think you have disappointed and opportunities that you screwed up. I felt paralyzed by this constant dialogue about the past making me feel guilty, unworthy, scared and constantly feeling like a failure."

For Keith the "transformation was almost instantaneous. Now imagine the tape recorder just being turned off," he continued. "This is literally what happened in the first forty-eight hours of using your TestoCreme. I remember being on Amtrak on my way home when it happened."

Two and a half years later Keith, happily married, wrote to me, "Now I live one day at a time. No guilt and no regrets. During most of my life I have only stayed at a job until I got fed up with it. I was always unsettled. That trend has ended, and I have a very focused, confident career path now."

Some of the effects were more obvious than others. "I have experienced an increase in facial and chest hair growth," Keith said, "predictable morning erections and an increase in my libido. My lifelong inability to lose weight has been stalled. My weight has remained steady while I have increased my upper body strength and have reduced the fat in my hips dramatically."

Much more important was the improvement in Keith's ability to get a good night's sleep, something he missed for more than twenty years. "Now that I have been using TestoCreme," he wrote, "I wake up refreshed every morning." Keith has discovered the power of a new high-potency topical testosterone.

## A Trail to New Heights

This short book has led you on a journey I trust you have found interesting and informative. Now you are ready to follow a path that will take you to higher levels of personal health and vitality.

Before you even picked up this book, you probably realized the importance of hormones for a vibrant sex life. Now, I trust, you have learned that living and loving more intensely depends on more than positive relationships. Genuine concern for others as well as caring for yourself requires a balanced life. I am sure that, like most people, you want to experience the satisfaction of a well-balanced life. You realize that life is more than simply earning a living, or eating and sleeping. You should enjoy the music, smell the roses, and relish precious friendships. More than ever, you have learned that your body's hormones hold the key to the *"joi de vivre"* you desire.

Our hormones talk to us whether we are awake or asleep. They control our cycles, our brain function, and our emotions. They send us signals twenty-four hours a day, seven days a week, working for us efficiently and continuously. They give us up-to-date information about any declining levels or hormonal imbalances, if we would only listen to them.

Modern medicine offers practical solutions to most of our hormone-related problems. We need to stop paying attention to folklore and assuming that we have to put up with problems we accept as a part of growing old. In short, it's time to stop complaining about how bad it is and do something about it.The journey towards optimal health may be long and sometimes confusing, but it is always worthwhile.

Before you can listen to your hormones, you need to know what they are and how they are working in your body. I hope this book has helped you to learn more about the marvelous hormones that circulate through your body. Let's stop and listen to our hormones.

# Appendix A

# The Power of TestoCreme®

At the beginning of the era of testosterone in 1929, Carl Richard Moore, in collaboration with other scientists, succeeded in isolating the primary secretions of the testicles. Androsterone and testosterone were identified as the hormones responsible for developing the male sex organs in the unborn infant and for enhancing and maintaining the sexual functions of the male during and after puberty. This discovery opened the door for breakthrough research in understanding how our body's hormones work together.

My interest in the medical powers of testosterone began when I was a young doctor and noticed that many of my male patients were already experiencing a loss of sexual desire and were feeling "old" even though they hadn't reached their thirty-fifth birthday.

"I can't hold an erection, and I don't even want to have sex any more," John, one of my patients, told me. He was a forty-year-old firefighter, well built, handsome, happily married, and the father of five children—but as far as sex was concerned, he was hanging it up.

I wondered if John's hormone levels were falling into the lower levels of normal as are commonly found in elderly men. Sure enough, when the blood results came back, his testosterone levels were quite low. John, like many other men with similar test results, seemed to be reasonably healthy, but I could sense that he was not enjoying life to the same degree, as were men and women with normal testosterone levels. But why?

My research led me to the conclusion that the toxic pollutants we are pouring into our environment interfere with our body's intricate system of hormones, resulting in sexual and physical deterioration in many men. I found myself in agreement with leading environmental scientists and became a champion for educating doctors and the public about the hazards of dioxin and other estrogen-like chemicals that had the potential of ruining the human race.

Meanwhile I needed to take care of my patients who were losing their zest for life. Regardless of the cause of their distress, I had to find a way to give them the testosterone they needed to restore their sexual vitality.

Injections are the fastest and cheapest way to load the body with testosterone, but as I pointed out in this book, there are serious consequences from the extremely high levels that result immediately after the injection. When anabolic steroid pills are taken, the digestive tract is not able to absorb the hormones into the blood stream efficiently. To get the needed results, the person would have to take such huge quantities of testosterone pills that serious liver problems could result.

I knew that plastic testosterone patches that deliver a timed-release hormone gel when applied to the back, arms, or chest, had been around for decades. The problem with patches for most people was that they became irritating and uncomfortable.

Then I considered a cream form of testosterone therapy. Creams are much easier to apply than patches. You just rub them on the skin, and in most cases the active ingredients immediately enter the bloodstream and begin working. The problem was that only very low potency products containing one or two percent of testosterone were available from compounding pharmacies.

Back on page 46 we talked about medications that are mixed or "compounded" by trained and certified pharmacists. When I began getting excited about helping my testosterone-deficient patients with appropriate supplementation, I chose a transdermal route to deliver the testosterone. As I doctor I could prescribe any hormone supplementation I felt would be effective, and a compounding pharmacist would fill the prescription for my patients.

Of course I didn't want my patients getting sick or feeling out of control because the dosage was more than their bodies could handle. Neither did I want to prescribe medication that was so weak or ineffective that my patient wouldn't obtain any benefits with a daily application. I certainly didn't want my patients covered head to toe in cream.

Working with a local pharmacist experimenting with various strengths and absorption enhancers, we came up with a formula that worked. It was a high potency, ten percent testosterone in a soy-based cream known as an organogel. I chose the organogel because for decades this form has been used to deliver medications safely into the bloodstream. Compounding pharmacists had used organogels since the early 1990s.

The resulting product was a higher potency testosterone in a cream formulated to absorb completely into the blood stream. I called the product TestoCreme®. I registered the name and began the process of obtaining a patent. I was delighted to learn in June of 2004 that patent #6,743,448 for TestoCreme® has been granted by the US patent office.

I am not writing this to convince you to purchase this product but only to share with you my experience in developing it. TestoCreme transdermal is a prescription item used only for men with hypogonadism and not for symptoms of andropause, which is not a treatable condition at this time.

When there is enough clinical data to support TestoCreme use as a new drug, I will submit my "invention" to the FDA in a new drug application (NDA).

I do not prescribe TestoCreme or any other medication over the Internet. Every patient mentioned in this book has come to my clinic for examination and testing. A diagnosis of hypogonadism or erectile dysfunction with low DHT is necessary before any hormone treatment is prescribed.

My patients often share their experiences with me by email, and I have shared several of their communications with you throughout this book.

Following are comments by some of my patients who have made specific references to TestoCreme®, after they visited me in my office in Montery.

Andy from Michigan sent me email in 2004. "Dr. Kryger," he wrote, "have your patients who have been on TestoCreme for a while talk to you about the physical benefits of this cream? I have been on it for almost one year and I feel better now then I did last summer. Besides an erection every morning I've noticed a larger amount of ejaculation, longer orgasms and easy arousal. I used to find sex a lot of work and not enjoyable but now it is like discovering it all over again with so much pleasure. I know my problem was caused by my low levels of testosterone. I only wished a doctor would have put me on it a long time ago!"

Daniel wrote to me after returning to Georgia. "TestoCreme is amazing," he said. "I feel like I have about fifty percent more energy and feel I have the drive and energy to achieve some long-postponed goals."

For Dan in Florida it was a combination of benefits ranging from more satisfying sexual relations to better erections, more muscle mass in legs and arms, better blood pressure, and the appetite of a twenty-year-old. "I am reluctant to run out of TestoCreme," he said.

An older man who had gone through prostate surgery for an enlarged prostate told me that when he doesn't use TestoCreme it is almost impossible for him to have an erection, but he has little trouble when he uses the cream. He also likes the lower cost of the cream compared with patches.

From Texas, Dale had this to say: "Before I found out about Testo-Creme from you I had difficulty in achieving an erection that would last long enough to satisfy me or my wife. She began to think I was having an affair because of my reluctance to have sex with her. I felt tired and lethargic. When I got on the program I immediately noticed an increase in sexual desire. My wife and I went from having intercourse one or two times a month to three or four times a week. I am also more confident and energetic and have been working out on a regular basis without being worn out."

I could share positive testimonials from hundreds of other men who have followed my exact instructions for applying TestoCreme and have been delighted with the results. Not once have I heard a negative comment from any patient who has used the cream as prescribed.

In order to get marketing approval for widespread use from the FDA, I will need to conduct a double blind study with a few hundred male subjects, half of them receiving TestoCreme, and the other half a placebo, as well as an objective panel of scientific observers verifying the results. Setting up a study like that would cost hundreds of thousands, up to millions of dollars. This is why treatment with FDA-approved topical testosterones costs so much.

Instead, I merely prescribe TestoCreme as a compounded preparation exclusively for my private patients who have been diagnosed with hypogonadism. These men are carefully monitored to establish the effectiveness of the skin delivery system, which is compounded by my pharmacist. Because the high potency testosterone in TestoCreme is absorbed painlessly through the skin, there have been no allergic reactions or other side effects after nine years of use.

Like many other substances, testosterone is "big" in a negative as well as a positive sense. Too much testosterone, and you run into serious trouble. An excess of testosterone in the blood of a male can result in the creation of extra estradiol, which can cause several unwanted effects mentioned earlier.

As we have discussed in this book, knowing whether or not you have enough testosterone is not as simple as we once thought. It's too easy to reach an incorrect conclusion when the lab reports only total testosterone. All men should request that the lab measure their bioavailable or free testosterone and not merely total testosterone.

Normal ranges reported by Esoterix Laboratories are given below.

## Normal Levels of Testosterone by Age

| | | |
|---|---|---|
| **Bioavailable Testosterone** | | |
| Pre-pubertal | | <0.2 to 1.3 ng/dl |
| Adult females | | 1.1 to 14.3 ng/dl |
| Males | 20 to 39 years | 128 to 430 ng/dl |
| | 40 to 49 years | 95 to 350 ng/dl |
| | 50 to 69 years | 95 to 285 ng/dl |
| | 70 to 79 years | 60 to 240 ng/dl |
| **Serum Testosterone (total)** | | |
| Boys | <9.8 years | <3 to 10 ng/dl |
| | 9.8 to 14.5 years | 18 to 150 ng/dl |
| | 10.7 to 15.4 years | 100 to 320 ng/dl |
| | 11.8 to 16.2 years | 200 to 620 ng/dl |
| | 12.8 to 17.3 years | 350 to 970 ng/dl |
| Adult males | 20 to 50 years | 350 to 1030 ng/dl |
| Adult females | 20 to 50 years | 10 to 55 ng/dl |
| **Serum Testosterone (free)** | | |
| Adult males | 20 to 50 years | 52 to 280 pg/ml |
| Adult females | 20 to 50 years | 1.1 to 6.3 pg/ml |

Esoterix is the FDA-approved hormone testing lab.

Esoterix, Inc.
4301 Lost HIlls Road
Calabasas Hills, CA 91301
800-444-9111 www.esoterix.com

For saliva-testing—

Diagnos-Techs, Inc.
6620 South 192nd Place, Building
Kent, WA 98032
800 878-3787
diagnos@diagnostechs.com www.diagnostechs.com

# Appendix B

# Your Healthright: Why Americans Deserve Good Health

In antiquity a birthright was a precious treasure passed on the oldest child in the family as a way of preserving wealth and family tradition. Whether property, leadership, money—or all of these—a birthright was highly valued and helped preserve a sense of belonging.

I would like to propose that regardless of our heritage or our financial capabilities, we are born in this country with the right to enjoy good health. It is our healthright. I believe that from our earliest years we have the right—and the responsibility—to discover our own path to our highest possible level of health. As parents, teachers, and role models, we are duty-bound to guide others in discovering their own healthright and making it real in their lives.

Instead, we spend far too much time thinking about our symptoms and too little time learning how to enjoy our right to health. Most physicians fall into the same trap and do little to help their patients avoid disease. Lacking access to preventive medical care, our citizens end up dying from diseases that could be eliminated or postponed if prevention were a higher priority. At the lowest end of the health care spectrum, families caught in the welfare net have almost no effective support for learning the principles of healthful living.

Whether we are wealthy or poor, pollutants feed deadly substances into our bodies, putting our health at risk. Meat, processed foods, water, and the air we breathe are often tainted with environmental toxins. We pollute our internal environment by eating too much, exercising too little, and using harmful drugs because they make us feel good. The statistics are alarming. One fifth of our nation's people are drug dependent, and six out of ten are obese. Newspapers, magazines, and all the electronic media, encourage us to follow "healthy" diets and to exercise more, but we ignore the message.

Nearly half of the 190 million people in the United States over age sixty-five lost their sexual drive by their sixty-fifth birthday. Multiple hormone deficiencies, genetic predisposition for certain diseases and environmental hazards are affecting our reproductive and sexual abilities in negative ways. Although doctors prescribe medications in quantities never approached in the past, the majority of older Americans suffer with various illnesses leading to hormonal deficiencies and depression.

Doctors need to prescribe hormone placement therapy for their patients who would benefit from this type of care. Hormones have proved safe and effective over decades of use. Side effects are minimal and can usually be eliminated by reducing the dose. Hormone replacement can make a huge difference in the health and functioning of many patients at a reasonable cost. In spite of the facts, doctors are often reluctant to use hormones for their hypogonadal patients.

This puts the problem at the feet of patients like you who must take the lead in educating your doctors about treatment for their hormone-related problems. Most men are told by their doctors, "But your test results are within normal range" or, "Since you can still get an erection you don't need testosterone."

The lucky ones who can afford to search for doctors who are highly qualified in hormone replacement therapy will receive the care they need. The others will go without. In my opinion, no one should be denied access to care or information about treatments that can improve their life. One bottleneck in the provision of effective hormones as part of your healthright is built-in redundancy in the testing of new pharmaceuticals. Another is difficulty in licensing cheaper derivatives of successful drugs. Many of these hormones are controlled drugs subject to government policing, which further drives up the cost. Add to this pharmacy charges and super budgets for advertising, research, and product development budget, and hormone medication costs are escalating faster than the cost of living.

I see light at the end of the tunnel. A change in how doctors view patients and their problems is slowly taking place with concierge, VIP, or "fee for service" medicine emerging as an alternate to traditional managed health care. Those who can afford the price can pay doctors a "retainer" fee and receive unlimited access to the best medical care. But this is only a right for the rich, not a health right for all Americans.

We need to take necessary steps to deliver the right optimal health to every citizen. Physicians should freely share knowledge with their patients, listen carefully to their complaints, and involve them in their own care. Patients who share ideas and thoughts about their treatment and recovery with their private physician and receive thoughtful feedback will be empowered to build their own healthright.

Doctors need to look beyond physical diagnosis and treatment and work to educate their patients to assist in the diagnosis of their medical, psychological or sexual problems. For our part, we need to stop running to our doctor for relief from symptoms whenever a cold or ache strikes, and think instead of the doctor as a coach or adviser to show the way to better overall health. Following a healthy diet, exercising regularly and avoiding poisons and toxins will help a person make great strides towards earning the right to health.

The rewards of your healthright are a greatly improved quality of life along with access to techniques for detecting health problems early and treating them before they become serious.

Consider this book as one doctor's invitation to help you improve your health and add high-quality years to your life. Your own doctor can help you attain your "healthright"—the right to accurate and easy-to-understand medical information about your body and how it works so that you can prevent disease and postpone aging. Your right to preventive health care must take its place along with the inalienable rights to freedom, liberty and the pursuit of happiness that are ingrained in our constitution.

It's your healthright.

# Glossary

A quick survey of this book will tell you that hormones are powerful chemical messengers in the human body, but you may be wondering exactly how they originate, what they do, and what makes them so powerful. The following glossary should be helpful to you.

**5-AR.** 5-alpha reductase. An enzyme involved in producing DHT, concentrated in the skin, hair, and genital organs and four times higher in balding areas than in the back of the scalp. Without this enzyme it's impossible to become bald or have a sex drive.

**ACTH.** Adrenocorticotropic hormone. ACTH is a releasing hormone from the pituitary that increases production of adrenal steroids and plays a major role in stress.

**ADH.** Anti-diuretic hormone. See vasopressin. Stops nighttime urination.

**Adrenaline**. A chemical transmitter originating in the adrenal gland and causing the "flight or fight" reaction. Also called epinephrine. Used to reverse severe allergic reactions.

**aldosterone**. A salt-regulating hormone that comes from the adrenal gland and affects the functioning of the kidney. It interacts with progesterone and affects blood pressure.

**Alzheimer's Disease.** A degenerative brain disease which strikes older people and is associated with dementia or loss of memory. Named for a Dr. Alzheimer who first described the disease in his wife but he could not find a cure. The disease seems to have a hereditary component,

**anabolic (bodybuilding) steroids.** Synthetic derivatives of testosterone originally developed to treat a variety of medical conditions and used today to enhance athletic performance and muscular development. Also called "roids" or "juice" by the bodybuilding community.

**Androderm®.** A skin patch delivering testosterone and used for two decades without negative effects other than occasional skin reactions. A similar product is TestoDerm® by Alza Pharmaceuticals. These plastic patches deliver about 5 milligrams of testosterone daily. Manufactured by Watson.

**AndroGel®.** The first 1% testosterone gel on the market. Manufactured by Unimed, a subsidiary of Solvay pharmaceuticals and approved by the FDA in 2000. Requires one 5-gram packet to deliver about 5 milligrams of testosterone into the blood stream.

**androgens.** Male hormones such as testosterone or dihydrotestosterone. (Andros means "man" in Greek.) These hormones control sex drives in both men and women.

**andropause.**The male equivalent of menopause. Associated with declining hormone levels in men 55 to 70 years of age. Not recognized by the American Medical Association.

**androstenedione.**A precursor hormone of testosterone. Has a potent action in women and can directly convert to estrogen form called Estrone (E1). Sold for years over-the-counter as food supplement and used by young men to try to increase testosterone but instead increases estrogen. Removed from the market by the FDA in March, 2004.

**androsterone.** The definitive male sex hormone discovered in the testicles in 1931. The first "steroid" hormone known to man.

**ANS.** Autonomic nervous system. Also known as the visceral or automatic system. The ANS transmits impulses from the blood vessels, heart, and primary organs to the brain, which simulates mostly automatic or reflex actions such as digestion and childbirth.

**anti-androgen.** A substance working in opposition to male hormones and interfering with the actions of testosterone. Estrogen, for example, is an anti-androgen.

**antigens.** Substances such as invading viruses or bacteria that are recognized as "foreign" by the immune system, which subsequently produces antibodies to destroy them.

**aromatase.** An enzyme complex responsible for the conversion of testosterone to the form of estrogen known as estradiol. Anti-aromatase drugs, such as Tamoxifen®, interfere with the formation of estradiol are used in treating breast cancer.

**ART. Androgen replacement therapy.** A program of male hormone supplementation, effective in treating anemia, wasting diseases such as cancer and AIDS, impotence, hypogonadism, prostrate enlargement and pituitary deficiency. Not yet an accepted therapy.

**BGH. Bovine growth hormone.** A growth hormone produced in cows and used as a supplement to increase the size of cattle. Present in milk and beef but considered "safe for human consumption." There is some evidence that it may be involved in prostate cancer.

**BPH. Benign prostatic hyperplasia.** Non-cancerous enlargement of the prostate gland, which increases with aging in men and is affected by both estrogen and DHT. Causes men to wake up more than once during the night to urinate and can be treated by 5-AR blockers.

**catabolic.** Characteristic of tissue breakdown. Catabolic states including cancer, malnutrition, AIDS, and multiple sclerosis and are treated with anabolic (bodybuilding) steroids.

**Cialis®.**Tadalafil, a new erection enhancer, which is supposed to last thirty-six hours, compared to Viagra, which lasts four to six hours. Dubbed the "weekend pill," Cialis has become a popular sex drug. Manufactured by Lilly/Icos.

**cortical.** Related to the cortex, the outer part or "rind" of the brain, including multiple lobes and areas involved in integrating information received from our senses. The cortex or cortical brain controls emotions and holds memories and thoughts and is destroyed in Alzheimer's Disease.

**cortisol.** A major hormone released by the adrenal glands whenever we feel anxious or stressed or allergic. Regulates our fuel source, blood sugar (glucose), and converts proteins to glucose during times of stress to give us energy to deal with the stressful situation. Too much cortisol can cause confusion and weight gain; too little makes it difficult to handle stress.

**CRH. Cortisol releasing hormone.** A hormone that is released from the pituitary to regulate the production of cortisol by the adrenal glands. CRH blockers are being studied as future antidepressants.

**daidzein.** An isoflavone found mostly in soybeans, legumes, and peas. Daidzein has been shown to have a beneficial effect on some types of cancer and bone health. Daidzein inhibited prostate cancer cell growth without causing DNA damage and may also protect against breast cancer.

**DDT. Dichlorodiphenyltrichloroethylene.** An insecticide (bug killer) that is highly toxic to both animals and humans. The most widely used insecticide until it was banned in the US in 1972. Still used in Mexico and South America as well as in Africa.

**DEA. Drug Enforcement Agency.** The policing arm of the Federal Drug Administration, involved in preventing abuse and illegal marketing of drugs in the US.

**depo-testosterone.** Testosterone enanthate, a long-acting synthetic testosterone injected once every two weeks in men who are testosterone deficient. Often diverted to black market.

**DES. Diethylstilbestrol.** The first synthetic estrogen developed for treating animals. When prescribed for pregnant women, DES created estrogen levels hundreds to thousands of times more potent than estrogen produced naturally by the body. As a result babies were born with severe deformities and ambiguous sexual preference.

**DHEA. Dehydroepiandrosterone.** The primary steroid secreted from the adrenal gland. The DHEA steroid has a positive effect on the central nervous system and is being investigated as a future medication for treating, depression, obesity, heart disease and immune deficiency.

**DHT. Dihydrotestosterone.** A metabolite of testosterone involved in regulating sexual drive and the development of sexual organs. Essential for normal growth and development, normal sexual arousal, and expansion of muscular tissue. Involved in hair and prostate growth. Found in skin, gums, hair follicles, prostate and the brain. Works the same way in men and women.

**dioxin.** A herbicide (kills plants). Also called Agent Orange in the Vietnam War. Produced as a by-product when chlorinated materials such as plastics are burned. Toxic at a dilution of less than one part per trillion. A proven cause of cancer, not merely statistically linked to a higher risk of cancer. A powerful hormone-disrupting chemical associated with a small penis size, lower sperm count, miscarriages, and reproductive disorders including infertility.

**DNA. Deoxyribonucleic acid.** The stuff of life. The coded information or blueprint for every living thing. A molecule of DNA in which nucleic acids are coiled in a helical structure has the ability to reproduce itself within the cell. Toxins, UV light, vitamin deficiencies and radiation can alter DNA. Several sections of the molecule have regulatory functions that can turn genes off and on.

**dopamine.** The pleasure chemical that is able to bridge the gap (synapse) between neurons (nerve cells) and send signals from one neuron to another. Dopamine is essential for feeling pleasure. Insufficient amounts of dopamine can cause chronic fatigue, stimulate the appetite, and interfere with concentration. Too much dopamine can produce hallucinations, aggressive behavior, and excessive libido. Nicotine and testosterone both increase dopamine.

**E2 or Estradiol.** The "active" female estrogen. Secreted by the ovaries, testicles and adrenal glands. E2 is present in all birth control pills, female hormone supplements.

**endorphins.** Natural morphine-like (opioid) chemicals in the brain. Can decrease the perception of pain, creating a state of euphoria, or feeling "high." They can be triggered by hormones, narcotics and exercise as well as by intense pain or pleasure.

**environmental estrogens.** Toxic compounds formed in the environment that mimic the function of the body's natural estrogen compounds and are blamed for the deterioration and decrease in the number of human sperm, the decrease in reproduction of salmon, alligators, birds and other wildlife. Also called xenoestrogens.

**erogenous zones**. Those parts of the body such nipples that respond to sexual stimulation by becoming engorged with blood.

**Estratest®.** A combination estrogen-testosterone pill for women, which entered the market twenty years ago although the FDA never approved it. Manufactured by Solvay, Belgium.

**estrogens.** Female sex hormones. The three types, E1, E2 and E3, are known collectively as conjugated estrogens. In a healthy young adult female, the typical mix of these hormones is 10 to 20 percent estrone (E1), 10 to 20 percent estradiol (E2), and 60 to 80 percent estriol (E3). Estrogen stimulates the ovaries to produce mature eggs and the testicles to make sperm. Estrogen promotes networking between brain cells by encouraging nerve growth and blood flow to the brain.

**enzymes.** Proteins produced by genes which act as biological catalysts to create various bodily compounds. Enzymes are used for digestion, hormone conversion and tissue destruction. Some enzymes are triggered by light.

**epinephrine.** Also known as adrenaline. Epinephrine is a powerful stimulant of female sexual arousal and increases heart rate, breathing and muscular strength.

**FDA. Food and Drug Administration.** A government agency that regulates the use and safety of medicine. The FDA allows drugs to come to market but does not approve them.

**FSD. Female sexual disorder.** A new term for women who cannot achieve orgasm or have satisfactory sexual relations. Affects over 40 million women in the US.

**FSH. Follicle stimulating hormone.** A hormone that stimulates the developing egg and triggers its release from the ovary. At the same time it increases a woman's estrogen production it is involved in triggering the male testicles to grow.

**GHRH. Growth hormone releasing hormone.** A hormone originating in the hypothalamus, which regulates the secretion of the growth hormone during the night. It is only effective during deep rapid-eye-movement (REM) sleep.

**glycogen.** A form of reserve of fat and muscle-stored sugars. Also found in the liver. Can be converted to glucose when energy is needed due to the action of a hormone in the pancreas.

**gynecomastia.** Breast enlargement in males, usually occurring in adolescent males or in men using excess estrogen. Also called man boobs, bitch tits or breast buds.

**HCG. Human chorionic gonadotropin.** A hormone produced early in pregnancy. Resembles LH in structure and so it can increase testosterone production by the cells in the testicles.

**HGH. Human growth hormone.** Short for recombinant human growth hormone. A protein molecule containing more than 190 amino acids which varies from species to species but is responsible for growth of muscle, bone and organs in all mammals. HGH levels peak in young adulthood and gradually taper off but are being sought after as an "anti-aging" drug.

**HPA. Hypothalamus-pituitary-adrenal.** The regulating system in the brain, located between the hypothalamus and the pituitary gland. The love triangle of hormone interrelationships, the HPA begins to function poorly after a few months of constant stress.

**HRT. Hormone replacement therapy.** Synthetic hormones, usually estrogen and progesterone, given to most women after menopause to replace hormones no longer produced by their body.

**hypogonadism.** Extremely low levels of testosterone, especially in the male. Can be treated with testosterone replacement therapy if detected early. Usually refers to total testosterone levels of less than 300 nanograms per deciliter.

**hypothalamus.** The hypothalamus is the seat of emotional expression and regulates everything from fear to aggression to sex drive. In addition to controlling hormonal functions, the body's water and salt balances, blood pressure, sugar and fat metabolism.

**IGF-1. Insulin-like growth factor.** A protein that regulates the secretion of GH and mimics the effect of insulin on the human body, making muscles more sensitive to the insulin effect. Circulating IGF-I levels increase at puberty to cause growth spurts and sex organ growth and then decrease to very low levels in the elderly.

**isoflavones.** Hormone-like compounds found in soybeans. The main isoflavones are geneistin and daidzein. Isoflavones are a class of Phytoestrogens that are concentrated in soybeans. Soy isoflavones are also free radical scavengers (potent antioxidants) and are antiangiogenic (they interfere with unwanted blood vessel growth in disease states).

**Levitra®.** Vardenafil. A new erection enhancing medication whose manufacturers claim has fewer side effects than Viagra. Levitra comes in 5, 10, 20 mg and enhances erections for about 4-6 hours. Manufactured by Bayer.

**LH. Luteinizing hormone.** A hormone secreted by the pituitary gland to regulate the testicular production of testosterone and the ovarian production of progesterone or testosterone. LH may also be involved in regulating other hormonal releasing factors such as FSH and SHBG.

**Lipitor®.** Pfizer's best-selling anticholesterol agent. It regulates the liver's production of cholesterol and is used as a cholesterol-lowering drug for anyone with high cholesterol not responding to diet or hormone replacement.

**lithium.** A very common basic element that is used as a mood stabilizer in persons with bipolar depression. Lithium can affect the thyroid gland and is effective in boosting the action of any antidepressant even in persons without bipolar depression.

**lycopenes.** Antioxidants found in watermelon, grapes, tomatoes and some shellfish, released only by cooking the food. Lycopenes are one class of 650 carotenoids found in high concentrations in the testicles of normal males and in low levels in infertile males. Used to help treat dioxin-induced infertility in men.

**Mediterranean diet.** A diet that eliminates red meat and uses large servings of fish, fresh vegetables, olive oil and pasta to control heart disease and reduce high cholesterol levels.

**melatonin.** A hormone regulator released by the pineal gland in the brain, causing sleepiness and enabling one to fall asleep when it gets dark at night. Regulates the body's internal clock and the cycles of other hormones. Melatonin also regulates the action of other hormones.

**muscle dysmorphia.** An obsession with muscular development of the human body. Men with this condition think they are never "big enough" regardless of how much muscle mass they develop. This condition can lead to anabolic steroid abuse, obesity and premature death.

**Muse®.** A prostaglandin derivative inserted into the end of the penis to induce an erection. Obviously, though it worked, it never became very popular.

**Natural opioids.** Naturally occurring substances, which affect the brain's receptors for pain and pleasure. Steroid hormones can induce beta-endorphins, the brain's own morphine-like compounds. These compounds can alter the perception of pain and pleasure. Opioid substances derived from the opium poppy can block these pain receptors.

**neurosteroids or neurohormones.** Neurohormones are a fascinating class of hormones that are produced in your brain's control center and serve as signaling, transmitting, and switching devices. These chemical messengers are secreted from nerve cells or neurons. Neurosteroids are made in the brain from progesterone or pregnenolone. They can circulate in the blood stream or work locally on other brain cells.

**neurotransmitters.** Molecules of proteins which carry the message from one nerve to another across a space called a "synapse" in the brain or spinal cord. They can also act as hormones and trigger the release of brain hormones. Neurotransmitters regulate our moods, our appetite, our sleeping, dreaming, impulses, energy levels and perception of pain.

**NO. Nitric oxide.** A gas that changes the walls of the blood vessels, swelling the arteries so that blood can fill the blood vessels. NO allows blood to flow into the penis and is increased by erections enhances like Viagra, Levitra and Cialis.

**norepinephrine.** A precursor of dopamine and an essential brain and spinal cord neurotransmitter. Norepinephrine (NE) is crucial for nerves to communicate and triggers arousal in men. NE can act as a hormone in the brain triggering other hormones involved in arousal.

**oxytocin.** A sex hormone secreted by the pituitary, testicles, ovaries and the brain. Directs female nursing and birthing plus bonding behaviors in many animal species. May even play an important role in ejaculation, orgasm and sexual preference.

**PASAS. Post anabolic steroid abuse syndrome.** Symptoms that occur in men who have been self-medicating with anabolic steroids and then suddenly stop. Loss of erections is the first sign of PASAS. This syndrome is not recognized by the AMA.

**pheromones.** Humans use pheromones—odorless, chemical messages that we continuously emit through our skin—to communicate, protect our children, and recognize and connect with each other, on what feels like an "intuitive" level. Pheromones may even explain why we feel comfortable with some people and have virtually nothing to say to other people; why we're attracted to some people and repulsed by others. They are totally different chemical compounds in men and women, and companies have been unsuccessful in manufacturing them.

**phthalates.** Dioxin-like chemicals routinely used in soaps, shampoos, and nail polish and in medical products like tubing and plastics to keep them soft and flexible. Phthalates and dioxin exposure can have devastating effects on the developing sex organs of men and women.

**phytochemicals.** Beneficial antioxidants and other plant-based compounds. Vitamins C and E used in conjunction with the beneficial bioflavinoids from fresh fruits, seeds, nuts and vegetables can remove bioactive compounds which can cause the DNA and tissue damage.

**phytoestrogens.** Plant-based compounds that can bind to the estrogen receptor without generating estrogen activity. By blocking this receptor they stop the occurrence of hot flashes, decrease bone loss and reduce the risk of breast cancer in some women. Phytoestrogens are hormone-like bioregulators that come from plants, without the harmful side effects related to some estrogens.

**pregnenolone.** The most abundant hormone in the brain. The second step in formation of all hormones from cholesterol. Pregnenolone is a precursor for every other hormones. When used as a supplement, it seems to work as a neurotransmitter to clarify thinking, promote concentration and prevent memory loss.

**Premarin®.** A popular estrogen used in estrogen replacement programs. Derived from pregnant mare's urine (PREgnant MARe's urINe). The most popular conjugated estrogen in the world.

**progesterone.** A hormone best known for its role in preparing the lining of the uterus to secure the placement of the fertilized egg, is also involved in the production of important hormones for both men and women. Progesterone naturally opposes the action of estrogen in women just as testosterone opposes estrogen excess in men. It seems to affect SHBG levels and sexual drive in women and can convert easily to testosterone.

**progestins.** Sex hormones that are synthetic versions of progesterone, made in labs to last at least 24 hours in the body. Commonly combined with Premarin as Provera®.

**prolactin.** A hormone secreted by the pituitary gland. In women prolactin regulates the flow of milk from the breasts of nursing mothers; in men prolactin secreted after male ejaculation brings about a refractory period that prevents another erection for at least one half hour. Prolactin inhibits sexual desire in men and prolactin also causes women to feel less sexual desire after giving birth.

**Prometrium®.** A natural progesterone form that is available in vaginal cream or oil filled capsule for women needing bioidentical progesterone supplementation. Manufactured by Solvay.

**prostaglandin.** Discovered in the prostate glands of sheep in 1982, they played a role in testosterone regulation through feedback to the pituitary gland. Injected directly into the penis of impotent men prostaglandins (Caverjet®) produce an immediate firm erection. Topical forms of Alprostadil® or Alprox® and Topiglan® are being developed by pharmaceutical companies.

**Provera®.** A synthetic progesterone or progestin. May be the culprit in causing breast cancer and the multiple side effects seen with hormone replacement therapy. Manufactured by Wyeth.

**Provigil®.** Modafinil. An alertness drug that activates the brain's histamine system. Recently approved for jet lag and shift workers as well as for narcolepsy and sleep disorders. Manufactured by Cephalon.

**psychotropic medications.** Medicines that work in the mind such as tranquilizers, antidepressants, antipsychotics and stimulants, including street drugs like cocaine, speed, methamphetamine and crack as well as legal drugs such as caffeine and nicotine.

**PVN. Paraventricular nucleus.** Located next to the hypothalamus. Produces oxytocin during sexual arousal.

**SCN. Suprachiasmatic nucleus.** The body's clock processing light signals and determining how much melatonin the pineal gland should release. Located in the brain inside the hypothalamus and produces vasopressin. The SCN may be the site of the sexually dimorphic nucleus, which determines sexual preference. The SCN is also loaded with receptors that are stimulated by oxytocin, which is released during ejaculation and orgasm.

**secondary hypogonadism.** A condition of testosterone deficiency, which occurs later in life when the pituitary does not respond to low levels of testosterone by increasing LH production.

**secretogogues.** Amino acids that stimulate the pituitary and other organs of the body to release (secrete) hormones. An example is arginine, an amino acid that helps synthesize nitric oxide. L-arginine can stimulate the pituitary to secret human growth hormone for forty-five minutes or so, but a pill with arginine in it has no such effect.

**Serotonin syndrome.** An overdose of serotonin (5-HT) can cause vomiting, loss of orientation, and possibly death.

**SHBG. Sex hormone binding globulin.** SHBG increases with age, binding up more hormones and causing lower concentrations of biologically available testosterone. Also acts as a regulator of arousability in the hypothalamus and can turn sex hormones off and on.

**SRIs. Serotonin re-uptake inhibitors.** Also called SSRIs. A popular class of antidepressants including Prozac, Paxil®, Zoloft®, Lexapro® and Celexa® used in treating severe premenstrual conditions.

**somatopause.** A time from early adulthood onward when our pituitary gland releases less and less growth hormone, so we stop growing and start aging. Freud said that at age 35 we become aware of our own mortality; somatopause occurs much earlier.

**somatostatin.** A natural blocker of the growth hormone or growth hormone inhibiting hormone (GHIH). Blocks the pituitary production of HGH and increases with aging.

**steroids.** Compounds based on the "sterol" molecule from cholesterol. Also a common term referring to anabolic hormones that can increase muscle mass and are used by many bodybuilders to boost the size of their muscles. All hormones are actually steroids.

**T4. Thyroxine.** The main hormone secreted by the thyroid gland. Thyroxine contains 4 iodine molecules and is converted to T3, the active form of thyroid hormone in the thyroid gland.

**TCDD. Tetrachloro-dibenzo-dioxin.** The most toxic dioxin found into the environment. As little as 5 parts per trillion can be lethal.

**Testim®.** A new 1% testosterone gel, manufactured by Auxillium; released to market by the FDA in 2003. Auxillium claims that it is more potent than AndroGel.

**TestoDerm®.** The first testosterone transdermal plastic patch applied to the scrotum. Although extremely effective it has been discontinued by Alza Pharmaceuticals, which was taken over by Johnson and Johnson, since it was too large and uncomfortable and did not sell well. No other testosterone product has been approved for application to the scrotum.

**testosterone.** The most important of all male hormones. A molecule originating in male and female sexual organs, circulating at different levels in men and women, normal total testosterone levels for adult males range from 300 to 1,100 ng/dl or nanograms per deciliter. Testosterone influences men's ability to perform different types of tasks involving spatial memory, motivational tasks and is responsible for dominant behavior.

**testosterone cypionate.** An injectable testosterone that lasts about 4 to 9 days. It is a moderately long-acting testosterone mixed with peanut oil for injection into the muscle.

**Tribulus.** An over-the-counter, so-called testosterone stimulant, an herbal preparation. Tribulus has been found scientifically to have minimal effects on testosterone production.

**TRT. Testosterone replacement therapy.** A program of daily testosterone supplementation designed to improve man's sexual drive and moods as well as the firmness of the penis during sexual intercourse.

**TSH. Thyroid stimulating hormone.** TSH is released from the pituitary to make the thyroid secrete thyroxine or T4. TSH has also been found to affect the formation of bone.

**vasopressin (VP).** Also called anti-diuretic hormone or ADH. A neurohormone that originates in the pituitary gland and is involved in controlling nighttime urine production, sexual arousal and aggression and regulating the fluid volume of the body.

**Wellbutrin®.** An antidepressant used as a dopamine stimulant to help smokers quit smoking, decrease weight and increase sexual drive in women. Available in a new XL or long-lasting form. Manufactured by Galaxo.

**WHI. Women's Health Initiative.** An organization that put traditional hormone replacement therapy in a very bad light. Based on long-term studies over a quarter of a century involving thousands of women, the organization reported that equine (horse) estrogens and synthetic progestins like Provera did not protect women against heart disease but actually increase the risk of cancer, dementia and heart attacks. However, it found that HRT did prevent osteoporosis and skin wrinkling.

**WHO. World Health Organization.** A global nonprofit organization that promotes sanitation, health initiatives, and education for nutrition and physical health.

**xenoestrogens.** (Xeno is Greek for "stranger") Estrogens derived from the environment and concentrated in the fat of animals used for food. These environmental estrogens, are affecting the fertility and sexual functions of all Americans.

**yohimbine.** A receptor blocker that comes from the bark of a tree from Africa. Used by tribal witch doctors as a treatment for sexual problems. Once available as an over-the-counter male product, but now available only by prescription as Yocon®. Yocon is believed to work as a libido enhancer but studies using high doses have not confirmed this claim.

# Recommended Resources

## Books

The following books were written for ordinary people who want to know more about their hormones. I do not necessarily agree with everything in these books, but I think they are important for a solid background in the field of hormones affecting sex, love, and longevity.


Archer, J., & Lloyd, B. *Sex and Gender* (2nd ed.). New York: Cambridge University Press. 2002.7

Berman J, Berman L. *For Women Only: A Revolutionary Guide to Overcoming Sexual Dysfunction and Reclaiming Your Sex Life.* Henry Holt and Company. 2001

Blasius, M. (Ed.). *Sexual Identities, Queer Politics*. Princeton, NJ: Princeton University Press. 2001

Burwash, P. *Total Health The Next Level: A Simple Guide for Taking Control of Your Health and Happiness Now!* Torchlight Publishing. 1997

Cadbury D, *The Estrogen Effect: How Chemical Pollution is Threatening Our survival.* St. Martin's Press, NY. 1997).

Calvin, William H.*: How Brains Think; Evolving Intelligence, Then and Now.* HarperCollins Publishers Inc. 1996.

Carruthers M. *The Testosterone Revolution.* Thorsons. 2000. Originally published as *The Male Menopause,* HarperCollins, 1996

Colborn T, Dumanoski D, Myers JP. *Our Stolen Future, Are We Threatening Our Fertility, Intelligence, and Survival? A Scientific Detective Story.* Plum (Penguin) 1997.

D'Augelli, A. R., & Patterson, C. J. (Eds.). *Lesbian, Gay, and Bisexual Identities and Youth: Psychological Perspectives.* New York: Oxford University Press.2001

Dean, T. *Beyond Sexuality.* Chicago: University of Chicago Press.2000

Diamond J. *Surviving Male Menopause: A Guide for Women and Men.* Sourcebooks, Inc. 2000

Diamond J. *The Warrior's Journey Home.* New Harbinger Publications Inc. 1994

Diamond J. *Male Menopause.* Sourcebooks, Inc. 1997

Esterberg, K. G. *Lesbian and Bisexual Identities: Constructing Communities, Constructing Selves.* Philadelphia, PA: Temple University Press.1997

Fisher H. *Why We Love. The Nature and Future of Romantic Love*. Henry Holt and Co. Inc. 2004

Hakim L, *The Couple's Disease: Finding a Cure for your Lost Love Life.* DHP Publishers, 2002

Kahn, Carol. *Beyond the Double Helix: DNA and the Quest for Longevity,* Times Books, 1985

Krimsky S.Hormonal Chaos: The Scientific and Social Origins of the Environmental Endocrine Hypothesis. The Johns Hopkins University Press. 2000

Kryger M.H. *The Woman's Guide to Sleep Disorders.* The McGraw-Hill Companies. 2004

Malesky, G. Kittel, M. *The Hormone Connection: Revolutionary Discoveries Linking Hormones and Women's Health Problems.* Prevention Health Books for Women. Rodale Inc. 2001

Manning, J. *Digit Ratio:* A Pointer to Fertility, Behavior and Health. Rutgers University Press, New Jersey 2002

Old, J. *Vintage People: The Secrets of Successful Aging.* Pathway Publications. 2000

Patterson C. *Eternal Treblinka: Our Treatment of Animals and the Holocaust,* Lantern Books, NY 2002

Quinn, D. M. *Same-sex Dynamics Among Nineteenth-Century Americans: A Mormon Example.* Urbana, IL: University of Illinois Press.1996

Rako, S. *The Hormone of Desire.* Three Rivers Press, NY. 1996.

Reid, DP. *The Tao of Health, Sex and Longevity: A Modern Practical Guide to the Ancient Way.* Fireside. 1989

Reiss, I. L., Ellis, A. *At the Dawn of the Sexual Revolution: Reflections on a Dialogue.* Walnut Creek, CA: Altamira Press.2002

Richardson, D. *Rethinking Sexuality.* London: Sage Publications.2000

Richardson, D., & Seidman, S. (Eds.). *Handbook of Lesbian and Gay Studies.* London: Sage Publications. 2002

Robbins J. *Diet for A New America: How Your Food Choices Affect your Health, Happiness, and the Future of Life on Earth.* HJ Kramer. 1987

Robbins, John. *The Food Revolution: How Your Diet Can Help Save Your Life and the World.* Conari Press, Berkeley, California. 2001

Robbins, J. *Reclaiming Our Health: Exploding the Medical Myth and Embracing the Source of True Healing.* HJ Kramer Inc. 1996

Schechter A, Gasiewicz TA. *Dioxins and Health,* second edition. John Wiley &Sons, 2003

Shippen G, Fryer W. *The Testosterone Syndrome. The Critical Factor For Energy, Health, & Sexuality: Reversing The Male Menopause.* M. Evans and Company. 1998

Somers S. *The Sexy Years: Discover The Hormone Connection.* Crown Publishers, NY. 2004

Thomas, C. (Ed.). *Straight with a Twist: Queer theory and the Subject of Heterosexuality.* Urbana, IL: University of Illinois Press. 2000

Thornton J. *Pandora's Poison: Chlorine, Health, and a New Environmental Strategy.* MIT Press. 2000.

Townsend, J. M. *What Women Want, What Men Want: Why the Sexes Still See Love and Commitment so Differently.* New York: Oxford University Press.1998

Veldhuis J, Iranmanesh A, Mulligan T. *Toward a Healthier Old Age: Biomedical Advances from Basic Research to Clinical Science.* Barcelona, Spain: Prous Science Publishers. 1999

## Helpful Information from the Worldwide Web

Adult Growth Hormone Replacement. Key points by the Society of Endocrinology on diagnosing and treating adults with a deficiency of somatrophin, at www.endocrinology.org/SFE/gh.htm.

American Association of Clinical Endocrinologists (AACE). For press releases on professional meetings, new studies, and reports on research in the field of endocrinology, go to www.aace.com/pub/press/releases. For current guidelines regarding medication and other treatment of hormone-related disorders, go to www.aace.com/clin/guidelines.

Andropause. Information by the Canadian Andropause Society, at www.andropause.com.

Anabolic Steroid Abuse. National Institute on Drug Abuse. A government program dealing with problems and solutions involving the misuse of steroids, www.steroidabuse.org.

Androglogy Database: Normal ranges for animals and humans, www.il-st-acad-sc.org/data3.html.

Cannabis. Health Aspects and changes in male sex hormones. A 1986 paper provided by the American Society of Pharmacology and Experimental Therapies, users.lycaeum.org/~painter/ENDWAR/marij1.html.

Control of Endocrine Activity. An illustrated presentation from Colorado State University on how the body regulates the supply and delivery of hormones, arbl.cvmbs.colostate.edu/hbooks/pathphys/endocrine/basics/control.html.

Endocrine System Topics. For comprehensive reports from the National Institutes of health, go to the following URL and enter the word or words in the search box at the top of the page. www.nlm.nih.gov/medicineplus/search.html.

Endocrinology of Aging. Easy to understand discussion of current thinking on aging and hormones. The report was financed by Soreno, a leading biotech research firm. Go to www.medscape.com/viewarticle/407921_1.

Endocrinology Glossary. The medical school at the University of Maryland has prepared a readable glossary of key terms related to hormones, at www.umm.edu/endocrin/glossary.htm.

Estradiol. The Laboratory Corporation of America gives normal levels of this hormone in males and females at www.labcorp.com/datasets/labcorp/html/chapter/mono/ri003600.htm.

Estrogen Evolution. The Hormone Foundation, a public education organization of the Endocrine Society, provides helpful links about the use and misuse of hormones. Go to the home page at www.hormone.org and enter "estrogen" in the search box at the top of the screen.

FDA CenterWatch. Drugs Approved by the FDA (search by name). www.centerwatch.com.

Genetic Testing and Counseling. Enter key words in the search box for pages on this topic, provided by the National Institutes of Health, at www.nlm.nih.gov.

GH Use in Adults and Children. Guidelines for prescribing growth hormone, from the American Association of Clinical Endocrinologists, at www.aace.com/clin/guidelines/hgh.pdf.

Growth Hormone (GH) Replacement in Older Men. Comprehensive information by eMedicine, at www.emedicine.com/med/topic3178.htm.

Hormone Chemistry and Synthesis. Good textbook explanation provided by Colorado State University of how hormones work in the human body, at arbl.cvmbs.colostate.edu/hbooks/pathphys/endocrine/basics/chem.html.

Hormone Rhythms. Brief patient information on topics selected by the Endocrine Society. Go to www.endo-society.org/pubrelations/news.cfm and enter "hormone rhythms" in the search box.

Hormones of the Reproductive System. A comprehensive illustrated discussion of hormones of the reproductive system, at users.rcn.com/jkimball.ma.ultranet/BiologyPages/S/SexHormones.html.

Hormones, Receptors and Target Cells. Easy to understand information from Colorado State University. Go to arbl.cvmbs.colostate.edu/hbooks/pathphys/endocrine/basics/hormones.html.

Male Hormones Linked to Prostate Cancer. Personal MD offers information to the general public on a variety of topics. Enter key words in the search box at www.personalmd.com.

Mechanisms of Hormone Action. Great textbook discussion by Colorado State University at arbl.cvmbs.colostate.edu/hbooks/pathphys/endocrine/moaction/index.html.

Menopausal Hormone Replacement Therapy (HRT). Provided for the general public at by the National Cancer Institute www.meb.uni-bonn.de/cancernet/600310.html.

Menopause Online. Information for the general public on the menopause at www.menopause-online.com.

Neuroendocrine System: Pituitary and Hypothalamus. Illustrated textbook information by Colorado State University, at arbl.cvmbs.colostate.edu/hbooks/pathphys/endocrine/hypopit/overview.html.

Pituitary Axis. Information about the hypothalamus and pituitary gland by Colorado State University at arbl.cvmbs.colostate.edu/hbooks/pathphys/endocrine/hypopit/index.html.

Sex Hormone Tests. HealthyMe gives normal levels of all sex hormones www.ahealthyme.com/topic/topic100587459.

Sexual Reproduction in Humans. Full-color illustrations and text, at users.rcn.com/jkimball.ma.ultranet/BiologyPages/S/Sexual_Reproduction.html#Spermatogenesis.

Sexual Preference. Go to psychology professor Daryl Bem's home page at www.dbem.ws and click on "abstracts and articles available online," and then choose "articles on sexual orientation."

Testosterone, Free and Weakly Bound: Serum Measurements. Technical data by the Laboratory Corporation of America, at www.labcorp.com/datasets/labcorp/html/chapter/mono/sr016000.htm.

U.S. Food and Drug Administration (FDA). Information about how the FDA regulates drugs in the US, at www.fda.gov/cder/drug/default.htm.

Women's Health Initiative (WHI). Details about the Women's Health Initiative research project about the use of estrogen in hormone replacement therapy. Go to www.whi.org.

## Videos and Books on Tape

Klapper, Michael K. Pregnancy, *Children and the Vegan Diet. Vegan Nutrition. A Diet for All Reasons* (video) www.Earth Save.com. 1996.

Robbins, John. Diet for a New America. (video). Available at www. foodrevolution.org

Weil, Andrew. *Eating Well For Optimum Health: The Essential Guide to Bringing Health and Pleasure Back to Eating* (Audio-Unabridged). 1998.

## Products and Services Mentioned in this Book

Aiello Grapeseed Oil
Nicola International Inc.
Los Angeles, CA 90039

Email Consultation Service
A. Kryger, MD, DMD
Confidential and secure email consultations on any medical subject $35
www.kryger.medem.com

Full Spectrum Light Box
Northern Light Technologies
8971 Henri-Bourassa W.
Montreal, Canada H4S 1P7
800 263 0066
www.northernlight-tech.com

Gourmet Mushrooms, Inc.
2901 Granvenstein Highway North
Sebastopol, California 95472
707 823-1743 Fax: 707-823-1507
www.mycopia.com

Immune Stimulating Mushrooms
Mycology Research Labs
Brough, East Yorkshire
United Kingdom HU15 1EF
http://mycologyresearch.com or www.aneid.com

Juice Plus+
NSA
Memphis TN, 38118
www.juiceplus.com/+ak87117

Nordic Naturals Inc.
Omega Fish Liver Oils
Watsonville, California
831 724 6200
www.nordicnaturals.com

Pure Grapeseed Oil
Soofer Company, Inc.
Los Angeles Calif. 90058
800 852-4050 extension 120
www.sadaf.com

Smart Balance Tasty Butter Substitute
GFA Brands Inc.
Heart Beat Foods Division
PO Box 397
Cresskill, NJ 07626
www.smartbalance.com

Testocreme®
Website for information about testosterone cream: www.Testocreme.com

WellnessMD Publications
1084 Cass Street
Monterey, California. 93940
831 373-4406
Fax 831 373-4481
www.WellnessMD.com
www.sexloveandhormones.com
wellnessmd@earthlink.net

# Sources for Information Included in this Book

The following medical and scientific resources were valuable to me in preparing this book. You will find them of special interest if you are familiar with medical research and literature. Below are the topics covered in this bibliography.

## Athletes, Anabolics and Testosterone


Boyadjiev NP, Georgieva KN, Massaldjieva RI, Gueorguiev SI. Reversible hypogonadism and azoospermia as a result of anabolic-androgenic steroid use in a bodybuilder with personality disorder. A case report. J Sports Med Phys Fitness 2000 Sep;40(3):271-4

Brower KJ. Anabolic steroid abuse and dependence. Current Psychiatry Rep. 2002 Oct;4(5):377-87.

Cooper CJ, Noakes TD, Dunne T, Lambert MI, Rochford K A high prevalence of abnormal personality traits in chronic users of anabolic-androgenic steroids. British J Sports Med 1996 Sep;30(3):246-50.

Daly RC, Su TP, Schmidt PJ, Pagliaro M, Pickar D, Rubinow DR. Neuroendocrine and behavioral effects of high-dose anabolic steroid administration in male normal volunteers. Psychoneuroendocrinology. 2003 Apr;28(3):317-31.

Di Bello V, et al. Effects of anabolic-androgenic steroids on weight-lifters [myocardium: an ultrasonic videodensitometric study.] Med Sci Sports Exerc 1999 Apr;31(4):514-21

Fauner M, Kisling A, Nielsen SL. [Estimated consumption of anabolic steroids among athletes in Denmark.] Nordic Medicine. 1995;110(1):23-5.

Inigo MA, Arrimadas E, Arroyo D. [43 cycles of anabolic steroid treatment studied in athletes: the uses and secondary effects.] Review Clinico Espanol 2000 Mar;200(3):133-8.

Johansson P, Lindqvist A, Nyberg F, Fahlke C. Anabolic androgenic steroids affects alcohol intake, defensive behaviors and brain opioid peptides in the rat.: Pharmacology of Biochemical Behavior 2000 Oct;67(2):271-9.

Kanayama G, Cohane GH, Weiss RD, Pope HG. Past anabolic-androgenic steroid use among men admitted for substance abuse treatment: an under recognized problem? J Clin Psychiatry. 2003 Feb;64(2):156-60.

Kochakian CD. History, chemistry and pharmacodynamics of anabolic-androgenic steroids. Wien Med Wochenschr. 1993. 143: 359-63.

Lindqvist AS, Johansson-Steensland P, Nyberg F, Fahlke C. Anabolic androgenic steroid affects competitive behaviour, behavioural response to ethanol and brain serotonin levels. Behav Brain Res 2002 Jun 15;133(1):21-9.

McGinnis MY, Lumia AR, Breuer ME, Possidente B. Physical provocation potentiates aggression in male rats receiving anabolic androgenic steroids. Horm Behav 2002 Feb;41(1):101-10.

Midgley SJ, Heather N, Davies JB. Levels of aggression among a group of anabolic-androgenic steroid users. Med Sci Law 2001 Oct;41(4):309-14

Midgley SJ, Heather N, Best D, Henderson D, McCarthy S, Davies JB Risk behaviors for HIV and hepatitis infection among anabolic-androgenic steroid users. AIDS Care 2000 Apr;12(2):163-70

Morley JE. Orexigenic and anabolic agents. Clin Geriatric Med 2002 Nov;18(4):853-66

Mottram DR, George AJ. Anabolic steroids. Baillieres Best Pract Res Clin Endocrinol Metab 2000 Mar;14(1):55-69

Parssinen M, Karila T, Kovanen V, Seppala T. The effect of supraphysiological doses of anabolic androgenic steroids on collagen metabolism. Int J Sports Med 2000 Aug;21(6):406-11

Prendergast HM, Bannen T, Erickson TB, Honore KR. The toxic torch of the modern Olympic Games. Vet Hum Toxicol. 2003 Mar;45(2):97-102.

Rich JD, Dickinson BP, Feller A, Pugatch D, Mylonakis E. The infectious complications of anabolic-androgenic steroid injection. Int J Sports Med 1999 Nov;20(8):563-6

Ritsch M, Musshoff F. [Dangers and risks of black market anabolic steroid abuse in sports—gas chromatography-mass spectrometry analyses.] Sportverletz Sportschaden 2000 Mar;14(1):1-11

Salazar E, Torres JA, Avila A, Andrade A. Hyperplastic Changes and Recpetor Status in the Breast Tissue of Bodybuilders Under Anabolic–Androgenic Steroid Stimulation. Archives of Andrology 2000; 45:1-7

Street C, Antonio J, Cudlipp D. Androgen use by athletes: a reevaluation of the health risks. Can J Appl Physiol 1996 Dec;21(6):421-40

Thiblin I, Runeson B, Rajs J. Anabolic androgenic steroids and suicide. Ann Clin Psychiatry 1999 Dec;11(4):223-31

Thiblin I, Lindquist O, Rajs J. Cause and manner of death among users of anabolic androgenic steroids. J Forensic Sci 2000 Jan;45(1):16-23

Tischer KH, Heyny-Von Haussen R, Mall G, Doenecke P. [Coronary thrombosis and ectasia of coronary arteries after long-term use of anabolic steroids] [Article in German] Z Kardiol. 2003 Apr;92(4):326-31.

Wu FC. Endocrine aspects of anabolic steroids. Department of Medicine, University of Manchester, UK. Frederick.Wu@man.ac.uk

## Baldness and Testosterone

Bartosova L. Biology of hair growth. Curr Probl Dermatology 1984;12:1-58.

Bingham KD, Shaw DA. The metabolism of testosterone by human male scalp skin. J Endocrinology.1973;57:111-21

Billoni N, et al. Thyroid hormone receptor beta 1 is expressed in the human hair follicle. British J Dermatology. 2000 Apr;142(4):645-52.

Daniel HJ, Chamberlain, M. Male Pattern Baldness. Southern Medical J 2000; 93(7):657-662

Ishino A, Uzuka M, Tsuji Y, et al: Progressive decrease in hair diameter in Japanese with male pattern baldness. J Dermatol 1997; 24:758-764

Kyung-Ho Kim, et al. The influence of testosterone propionate on the expression of several growth factors in scalp dermal papilla cell. (communication) Department of Dermatology, Chungnam National University, College of Medicine, Daejeon, Korea.

Rushton DH, Ramsay ID, Norris MJ, et al: Natural progression of male pattern baldness in young men. Clin Exp Dermatol 1991; 16:88-92

Safer JD, Fraser LM, Ray S, Holick MF.Topical triiodothyronine stimulates epidermal proliferation, dermal thickening, and hair growth in mice and rats. Thyroid. 2001 Aug;11(8):717-24.

Setty LR: Hair pattern of the scalp of white and Negro males. American J Phys Anthropol 1970; 33:40-55

Whiting DA: Diagnostic and predictive value of horizontal sections of scalp biopsy specimens in male pattern androgenetic alopecia. J Am Acad Dermatol 1993; 128:755-763

## Depression, Stress and Testosterone

Boschert S. Approvals Near for New Antidepressant Therapies. Family Practice News. Dec 1, 2002; 49

Booth A, Johnson DR, Granger DA. Testosterone and men's depression: the role of social behavior. J Health Soc Behav 1999 Jun;40(2):130-40

Carmin CN, Klocek JW. To screen or not to screen: symptoms identifying primary care medical patients in need of screening for depression. Int J Psychiatry Med 1998;28(3):293-302

Charmandari E, Kino T, Souvatzoglou E, Chrousos GP. Pediatric stress: hormonal mediators and human development. Horm Res 2003;59(4):161-79

Consoli SM. [Depression and associated organic pathologies, a still under-estimated comorbidity. Results of the DIALOGUE study] [Article in French] Presse Med 2003 Jan 11;32(1):10-21)

deKloet ER. Stress in the brain. Eur J Pharm 2000,Sep 29;405:1-3; 187-98

Goodyer IM, Park RJ, Netherton CM, Herbert J. Possible role of cortisol and dehydroepiandrosterone in human development and psychopathology. Br J Psychiatry 2001 Sep;179:243-9

Goodyer IM, Herbert J, Tamplin A, Altham PM. First-episode major depression in adolescents. Affective, cognitive and endocrine characteristics of risk status and predictors of onset. Br J Psychiatry 2000 Feb;176:142-9

Grossi AM, Zajecka J. *Critical Breakthroughs* in the Advancement of Depression Treatment. Quarter Four 2002.

Harris TO, et al. Morning cortisol as a risk factor for subsequent major depressive disorder in adult women. Br J Psychiatry 2000 Dec;177:505-10

Herbert J. Neurosteroids, brain damage, and mental illness. Exp Gerontology.1998 Nov-Dec;33(7-8):713-27

Hirschfeld RM, Lewis L, Vornik LA. Perceptions and impact of bipolar disorder: how far have we really come? Results of the national depressive and manic-depressive association 2000 survey of individuals with bipolar disorder. J Clin Psychiatry 2003 Feb;64(2):161-74

Hunt PJ, et al. Improvement in mood and fatigue after dehydroepiandrosterone replacement in Addison's disease in a randomized, double blind trial. J Clin Endocrinol Metab 2000 Dec;85(12):4650-6

Kuhn KU, et al. Chronic course and psychosocial disability caused by depressive illnesses in general practice patients during a one year period.

Michael A, Jenaway A, Paykel ES, Herbert J. Altered salivary dehydroepiandrosterone levels in major depression in adults. Biol Psychiatry 2000 Nov 15;48(10):989-95

Narrow WE, Rae DS, Robins LN, et al. Revised prevalence estimates of mental disorders in the US: using a clinical significance criterion to reconcile two survey's estimates. Arch Gen Psychiatry 2002;62(6):5-9)

Ohata H, Arai K, Shibasaki T. Effect of chronic administration of a CRF(1) receptor antagonist, CRA1000, on locomotor activity and endocrine responses to stress. Eur J Pharmacol 2002 Dec 20;457(2-3):201-6

Osran H, Reist C, Chen CC, Lifrak ET, Chicz-DeMet A, Parker LN.Adrenal androgens and cortisol in major depression. Am J Psychiatry 1993 May;150(5):806-9

Pope HG Jr, Cohane GH, Kanayama G, Siegel AJ, Hudson JI. Testosterone gel supplementation for men with refractory depression: a randomized, placebo-controlled trial. Am J Psychiatry 2003 Jan;160(1):105-11)

Rothermund K, Brandtstadter J. Depression in later life: cross-sequential patterns and possible determinants. Psychol Aging 2003 Mar;18(1):80-90

Sapolsky R. Why Stress Is Bad for Your Brain. 1999 Personal communication from Department of Biological Sciences, Stanford University, Stanford, CA 94305, USA.

Schweiger U, et al. Testosterone, Gonadotropin, and Cortisol Secretion in Male Patients With Major Depression. Psychosomatic Medicine 1999; 61:292-296

Seidman SN, Spatz E, Rizzo C, Roose SP. Testosterone replacement therapy for hypogonadal men with major depressive disorder: a randomized, placebo-controlled clinical trial. J Clin Psychiatry 2001 Jun;62(6):406-12

Serby M, Yu M. Overview: depression in the elderly. Mt Sinai J Med 2003 Jan;70(1):38-44

Shors TJ, Leuner B. Estrogen-mediated effects on depression and memory formation in females. J Affect Disord 2003 Mar;74(1):85-96

Singh RB, Kartik C, Otsuka K, Pella D, Pella J. Brain-heart connection and the risk of heart attack. Biomed Pharmacother 2002;56: 2:257-65.

Stamp J, Herbert J. Corticosterone modulates autonomic responses and adaptation of central immediate-early gene expression to repeated restraint stress. Neuroscience 2001;107(3):465-79

Thapar A, McGuffin P. A twin study of depressive symptoms in childhood. Br J Psychiatry 1994 Aug;165(2):259-65

van Niekerk JK, Huppert FA, Herbert J. Salivary cortisol and DHEA: association with measures of cognition and well-being in normal older men, and effects of three months of DHEA supplementation. Psychoneuroendocrinology 2001 Aug;26(6):591-612

Viau V, Meaney MJ. The inhibitory effect of testosterone on hypothalamic-pituitary-adrenal responses to stress is mediated by the medial preoptic area. Neurosci 1996 Mar 1;16(5):1866-76.

Wolkowitz OM, et.al. Double-blind treatment of major depression with DHEA or dehydroepiandrosterone. Am J Psychiatry 1999 Apr;156(4):646-9.

Weiller E, Lecrubier Y, Maier W, Ustun TB. The relevance of recurrent brief depression in primary care. A report from the WHO project on Psychological Problems in General Health Care conducted in 14 countries. Eur Arch Psychiatry Clin Neurosci 1994;244(4):182-9

## Drugs and Testosterone

English KM, Pugh PJ, Parry H, Scutt NE, Channer KS, Jones The effect of cigarette smoking on levels of bioavailable testosterone in healthy men. Clin Sci (Lond) 2001 Jun;100(6):661-5

Fazio SB, Mukamal, KJ. Alcohol Consumption and Coronary Heart Disease: What Do the Lessons of Hormone Replacement Therapy Teach Us? Journal COM 2002 Dec;9(12):691-95

Field AE, Colditz GA, Willett WC, Longcope C, McKinlay JB. The relation of smoking, age, relative weight, and dietary intake to serum adrenal steroids, sex hormones, and sex hormone-binding globulin in middle-aged men. J Clin Endocrinol Metab 1994 Nov;79(5):1310-6

Finch PM, et al. Hypogonadism in patients treated with intrathecal morphine. Clin J Pain 2000 Sep;16(3):251-4

Iribarren C. Cigars pose serious risks; Modern Medicine 1998, April (66); 11

Kovacs EJ, Messingham KA. Influence of alcohol and gender on immune response. Alcohol Res Health. 2002;26(4):257-63.

Purohit V, Ahluwahlia BS, Vigersky RA. Marihuana inhibits dihydrotestosterone binding to the androgen receptor. Endocrinology 1980 Sep;107(3):848-50

Roberts LJ, Finch PM, Pullan PT, Bhagat CI, Price LM. Sex hormone suppression by intrathecal opioids: a prospective study. Clin J Pain 2002 May-Jun;18(3):144-8

Sauer WH, et al. Cigarette yield and the risk of myocardial infarction in smokers. Arch Intern Med 2002;162:300-306

Sparrow D, Bosse R, Rowe JW. The influence of age, alcohol consumption, and body build on gonadal function in men. J Clin Endocrinol Metab 1980 Sep;51(3):508-12

Trueb RM. Association between Smoking and Hair Loss: Another Opportunity for Health Education against Smoking? Dermatology 2003;206(3):189-91

## Females, DHEA and Testosterone

Arlt W, et. al. Dehydroepiandrosterone replacement in women with adrenal insufficiency. N Engl J Med 1999 Sep 30;341(14):1013-20

Bachmann G, et al. Female androgen insufficiency: the Princeton consensus statement on definition, classification, and assessment. Fertil Steril. 2002 Apr;77(4):660-5.

Bancroft J, Davidson DW, Warner P, Tyrer G. Androgens and sexual behaviour in women using oral contraceptives. Clinical Endocrinology. 1980;12:327-40.

Boehnert CE, Alberts RA. Seasonal Affective Disorder in Women: How to identify and treat. Postgraduate Medicine. 2003 Jan; 6 (1): 32-36.

Davis SR. Recent advances in female sexual dysfunction. Current Psychiatry Rep 2000 Jun;2(3):211-4

Davis S. Testosterone deficiency in women. J Reprod Med 2001 Mar;46(3):291-6. Suedavis@netlink.com.au

Labrie F, Belanger A, Cusan L, Candas B . Physiological changes in DHEA (dehydroepiandrosterone) are not reflected by serum levels of active androgens and estrogens but of their metabolites: intracrinology. J Clin Endocrinol Metab 1997 Aug;82(8):2403-9

Maleskey Gale, Kittel Mary. *The Hormone Connection:Revolutionary Discoveries Linking Hormones and Women's Health Problems*. Rodale Inc. St. Martin's Press. 2001

Morales AJ, Nolan JJ, et al. Effects of replacement dose of DHEA in men and women of advancing age. Journal of Clinical Endocrinology & Metabolism.1994;78:1360 7.

Rako S.Testosterone supplemental therapy after hysterectomy with or without concomitant oophorectomy: estrogen alone is not enough. J Womens Health Gend Based Med. 2000 Oct;9(8):917-23. Susanrako@aol.com

Rako S.Testosterone deficiency: a key factor in the increased cardiovascular risk to women following hysterectomy or with natural aging? J Womens Health. 1998 Sep;7(7):825-9.

Rako S. Testosterone deficiency and supplementation for women: What do we need to know? Menopause Management, September/October. GCS Press, LLC. 1996;5:10-15.

Randolph, JF Jr, MD, Dennerstein, L. Female Androgen Deficiency Syndrome: A Hard Look at a Sexy Issue. Medscape Women's Health 6(2), 2001. 2001 Medscape, Inc

Sherwin BB, Gelland MM, Brender W. Androgen enhances sexual motivation in females: a prospective cross-over study of sex steroid administration in the surgical menopause. Psychosomatic Med 1985;47:339- 51

Shifren JL. Androgen deficiency in the oophorectomized woman. Fertil Steril. 2002 Apr;77 Suppl 4:S60-2.

Silva PD, Gentzschein EE, Lobo RA. Androstenedione may be a more important precursor of tissue dihydrotestosterone than testosterone in women. Fertility & Sterility 1987 Sep;48(3):419-22

Van Goozen SH, Wiegant VM, Endert E, Helmond FA, Van de Poll NE. Psychoendocrinological assessment of the menstrual cycle: the relationship between hormones, sexuality, and mood. Arch Sex Behav 1997 Aug;26(4):359-82

Zofkova I, Zajickova K, Hill M, Horinek A. Apolipoprotein E gene determines serum testosterone and dehydroepiandrosterone levels in postmenopausal women. Eur J Endocrinol 2001 Feb;147(4):503-506

## Growth Hormone Information

Allen NE, et al. The associations of diet with serum insulin-like growth factor I and its main binding proteins in 292 women meat-eaters, vegetarians, and vegans. Cancer Epidemiol Biomarkers Prev. 2002 Nov;11(11):1441-8.

Aimaretti G, Corneli G, Razzore P, et al. Comparison between insulin-induced hypoglycemia and growth hormone (GH)-releasing hormone + Arginine as provocative tests for the diagnosis of GH deficiency in adults. J Clin Endocrinol Metab 1998;83:1615

Appleby PN, Davey GK, Key TJ. Hypertension and blood pressure among meat eaters, fish eaters, vegetarians and vegans in EPIC-Oxford. Public Health Nutr. 2002 Oct;5(5):645-54.

Bhasin S, et al. Hormonal effects of GnRH agonist in the human male: II. Testosterone enhances gonadotrophin suppression induced by GnRH agonist. Clin Endocrinol (Oxf) 1984 Feb;20(2):119-28

Baum HB, et al. Effects of physiologic growth hormone therapy on bone density and body composition in patients with adult-onset of growth hormone deficiency. Ann Intern Med 1996;125:883 -90.

Blackman MR, et al. Growth hormone and sex steroid administration in healthy aged women and men: a randomized controlled trial. JAMA 2002;288:2282-92.

Belgorosky A, et al. High serum sex hormone-binding globulin (SHBG) and low serum non-SHBG-bound testosterone in boys with idiopathic hypopituitarism: effect of recombinant human growth hormone treatment. Journal of Clinical Endocrinology & Metabolism. 1987 Dec;65(6):1107-11

Carani C, et al. The effect of chronic treatment with GH on gonadal function in men with isolated GH deficiency. Eur J Endocrinology 1999 Mar;140(3):224-30

Carroll P, Christ E. Growth hormone deficiency in adulthood and the effects of growth hormone replacement: a review. Journal of Clinical Endocrinology & Metabolism. 1998;83:382 95.

Deijen JB. van der Veen EA. The influence of growth hormone (GH) deficiency and GH replacement on quality of life in GH-deficient patients. Journal of Endocrinological Investigation. 22(5):127-36, 1999.

Fazio S, Sabatini D, Capaldo B, et al A preliminary study of growth hormone in the treatment of dilated cardiomyopathy. New England J Medicine 1996;334:809 14.

Fisker S, Jorgensen JO, Christiansen JS. Variability in growth hormone stimulation tests. Growth Hormone, IGF Research 1998 Feb;8 (A):31-5

Fruchtman Sm Gift B, Howes B, Borski R.Insulin-like growth factor-I augments prolactin and inhibits growth hormone release through distinct as well as overlapping cellular signaling pathways. Comp Biochem Physiol B Biochem Mol Biol. 2001 Jun;129(2-3):237-42.

Gentili A, et al. Unequal impact of short-term testosterone repletion on the somatotropic axis of young and older men. Journal of Clinical Endocrinology & Metabolism. 2002 Feb;87(2):825-34.

Gibney J, et al. The effects of 10 years of recombinant human growth hormone (GH) in adult GH-deficient patients. Journal of Clinical Endocrinology & Metabolism. 1999 Aug; 84(8):2596-602.

Gomberg-Maitland M, Frishman WH. Recombinant growth hormone: a new cardiovascular drug therapy. Am Heart J 1996;132:1244 -62.

Grimberg A, Cohen P. Role of insulin-like growth factors and their binding proteins in growth control and carcinogenesis. J Cell Physiol. 2000 Apr;183(1):1-9.

Guistina A, Lorusso R, Borghetti V, Bugari G, Misitano V, Alfieri O. Impaired spontaneous growth hormone secretion in severe dilated cardiomyopathy. Am Heart J 1996;131:620 2.

Hoffman D, O'Sullivan AJ, Baxter RC, Ho KKY. Diagnosis of growth-hormone deficiency in adults. Lancet 1994;343:1064 8.

Johannsson G, et al. Two years of growth hormone (GH) treatment increases bone mineral content and density in hypopituitary patients with adult-onset GH deficiency. J Clin Endocrin and Metab 1996;81:2865 73.

Johnston DG, et al. Long-term effects of growth hormone therapy on intermediary metabolism and insulin sensitivity in hypopituitary adults. Journal of Endocrinological Investigation. 1999; 22(5 Suppl):37-40.

Kim KR, et al. Low-dose GH treatment with diet restriction accelerates body fat loss, exerts anabolic effect and improves growth hormone secretory dysfunction in obese adults. Hormone Research.1999; 51(2):78-84.

Lamberts S, van den Beld A, van der Lely A. The endocrinology of aging. Science. 1997;278:419-424.

Leifke et al. Age-related changes of serum sex hormones, IGF-1 and SHBG levels in men: cross-sectional data from a healthy male cohort. Clin Endocrinology (Oxf) 2000 Dec;53(6):689-95

Maison P, et al. Growth hormone as a risk for premature mortality in healthy subjects: data from the Paris prospective study. BMJ 1998 Apr 11;316(7138):1132-3

Merimee TJ, Zapf J, Hewlett B, Cavalli-Sforza LL. Insulin-like growth factors in pygmies. The role of puberty in determining final stature. New England Journal of Med. 1987 Apr 9;316(15):906-11.

Patek SM, 1998 - AACE Guidelines for clnical practice for the evaulation and treatment of hypgonadism in adult male patients. Hypogonadism Task Force. Endocr Pract. 1996; 2:440-453) at: www.acce.com/clin/guidelines/ hypogonadism.pdf

Papadakis MA, et al. Growth hormone replacement in older men improves body composition but not functional ability. Ann Intern Med 1996;124:708-716.

Rudman D, et al. Effects of human growth hormone in men over 60 years old. N Engl J Med 1990;323:1-6.

Taaffe DR, et al. Effect of recombinant human growth hormone on the muscle strength response to resistance exercise in elderly men. J Clin Endocrinol Metab 1994;79:1361-1366.

Savine R, Sonksen PH. Is the somatopause an indication for growth hormone replacement? J of Endocrinological Investigation. 22(5 Suppl):142-9, 1999.

Shim M. IGFs and Human Cancer: Implications Regarding the Risk of Growth Hormone Therapy. Horm Res 1999, Nov; (51) S3:42-51

Silva ME, et al. Effects of testosterone on growth hormone secretion and somatomedin-C generation in prepubertal growth hormone deficient male patients. Braz J Med Biol Res. 1992;25(11):1117-26.

Span JP, et al. Gender difference in insulin-like growth factor I response to growth hormone (GH) treatment in GH-deficient adults: role of sex hormone replacement. J Clin Endocrinol Metab 2000 Mar;85(3):1121-5

Su HY, Hickford JG, Bickerstaffe R, Palmer BR.Insulin-like growth factor 1 and hair growth. Dermatol Online J. 1999 Nov;5(2):1.

Waters DL, Yau CL, Montoya GD, Baumgartner RN. Serum Sex Hormones, IGF-1, and IGFBP3 Exert a Sexually Dimorphic Effect on Lean Body Mass in Aging. J Gerontol A Biol Sci Med Sci. 2003 Jul;58(7):648-52.

Vance, M. L. Can Growth Hormone Prevent Aging?. New England Journal of Medicine 2003; 348: 779-780

## Mankind's Poisons

Ashida H.Suppressive effects of flavonoids on dioxin toxicity. Biofactors 2000;12(1-4):201-6

Bagchi D, et al. Free radicals and grape seed proanthocyanidin extract: importance in human health and disease prevention. Toxicology 2000 Aug 7;148(2 3):187-97

Burton JE, Michalek JE, Rahe AJ. Serum dioxin, chloracne, and acne in veterans of Operation Ranch Hand. Arch Environ Health 1998 May;53(3):199-204

Cadbury D, The Estrogen Effect: How chemical pollution is threatening our survival. St. Martin's Press, NY. 1997

Colborn T, Dumanoski D, Myers JP, Our Stolen Future, Are We Threatening Our Fertility, Intelligence, and Survival? A Scientific Detective Story. Plum (Penguin) 1997.

Egeland GM, et al. Total Serum Testosterone and Gonadotropins in Workers Exposed to Dioxin. Am J Epidem 1994; 139 (3): 272-81.

Feeley M, Brouwer A. Health risks to infants from exposure to PCBs, PCDDs and PCDFs. Food Addit Contam 2000 Apr;17(4):325-33. mark-feeley@hc-sc.gc.ca

Fleming LE, Bean JA, Rudolph M, Hamilton K. Mortality in a cohort of licensed pesticide applicators in Florida. Occup Environ Med. 1999 Jan;56(1):14-21.

Gray LE Jr, Ostby J, Monosson E, Kelce WR. Environmental antiandrogens: low doses of the fungicide vinclozolin alter sexual differentiation of the male rat. Toxicol Ind Health 1999 Jan;15(1-2):48-64

Gray LE Jr. Xenoendocrine disrupters: laboratory studies on male reproductive effects. Toxicol Lett 1998 Dec 28;102-103:331-335

Harder B. Moms' POPs, sons' problems: Testicular cancer tied to a fetus' pollutant contact. Science News 2003; 163/2/22.

Johnson L, et al. Reduced Leydig cell volume and function in adult rats exposed to 2,3,7,8-TCDD without a significant effect on spermatogenesis. Toxicology 1992 Nov 30;76(2):103-18

Krimsky S, Hormonal Chaos: The Scientific and Social Origins of the Environmental Endocrine Hypothesis. The Johns Hopkins University Press, 2000.

Mehta J, et al.Maternal exposure to a low dose of 2,3,7,8- TCDD suppressed the development of reproductive organs of male rats: dose-dependent increase of mRNA levels of 5alpha-reductase type 2 in contrast to decrease of androgen receptor in the pubertal ventral prostate. Toxicol Sci 2001 Mar;60(1):132-43

Morgan K. Hormones: Here's the Beef. Environmental concerns reemerge over steroids given to livestock. Science News. Jan 5, 2002; 161, 10-11

Morgantaler A. Toxins in People. Journal of the American Medical Assoc. April 15, 1998

Murray TJ, et al.Endocrine disrupting chemicals: Effects on human male reproductive health. Early Pregnancy 2001 Apr;5(2):80-112

Roberts J. US scientists class dioxins as a 'health concern'. BMJ 1994 Sep 24; 309 (6957):759-760

Rowlands JC, Gustafsson JA. Aryl hydrocarbon receptor-mediated signal transduction. Critical Review of Toxicology 1997 Mar;27(2):109-34

Sweeney MH, Calvert GM, Egeland GA, Fingerhut MA, Halperin WE, Piacitelli LA. Review and update of the results of the NIOSH medical study of workers exposed to chemicals contaminated with 2,3,7,8-tetrachlorodibenzodioxin. (TTCD).Teratog Carcinog Mutagen 1997-98;17(4-5):241-7

Thornton J. Pandora's Poison : Chlorine, Health, and a New Environmental Strategy. MIT Press, 2000.

Watanabe S, et al. Effects of dioxins on human health: a review. J Epidemiol 1999 Feb;9(1):1-13

Whorton D, Krauss RM, Marshall S, Milby TH. Infertility in male pesticide workers. Lancet 1977 Dec 17;2(8051):1259-61

## Measuring Testosterone

Belgorosky A, Rivarola MA. Changes in serum sex hormone-binding globulin and in serum non-sex hormone-binding globulin-bound testosterone during prepuberty in boys. J Steroid Biochem 1987;27(1-3):291-5

Belgorosky A, Rivarola MA. Progressive increase in non-SHBG-bound testosterone and estradiol from infancy to late prepuberty in girls. J Clin Endocrinol Metab 1988 Aug;67(2):234-7

Christiansen KH. Serum and saliva sex hormone levels in Kung San men. Am J Phys Anthropol 1991;86(1):37-44

Cooke RR, McIntosh JE, McIntosh RP. Circadian variation in serum free and non-SHBG-bound testosterone in normal men: measurements, and simulation using a mass action model. Clin Endocrinol (Oxf) 1993 Aug;39(2):163-71

Corradi G, Szathmari M . Serum and salivary testosterone levels in erectile dysfunction.Orv Hetil 1998 Aug 23;139(34):2021-4

Fahrner CL, Hackney AC. Effects of endurance exercise on free testosterone concentration and the binding affinity of sex hormone binding globulin (SHBG). Int J Sports Med 1998 Jan;19(1):12-5

Govier FE, McClure RD, Kramer-Levien D. Endocrine screening for sexual dysfunction using free testosterone determinations. J Urol. 1996 Aug;156(2 Pt 1):405-8.

Hardy KJ, Seckl JR. Endocrine assessment of impotence—pitfalls of measuring serum testosterone without sex-hormone-binding globulin. Postgraduate Med Journal. 1994 Nov;70(829):836-7

Khan-Dawood FS, Choe JK, Dawood MY. Salivary and plasma bound and "free" testosterone in men and women. Am J Obstet Gynecol 1984 Feb 15;148(4):441-5.

Kuhn JM, et al. Studies on the treatment of idiopathic gynaecomastia with percutaneous DHT or dihydrotestosterone. Clin Endocrinol (Oxf) 1983 Oct;19(4):513-20

Michael A, Jenaway A, Paykel ES, Herbert J. Altered salivary dehydroepiandrosterone levels in major depression in adults. Biol Psychiatry 2000 Nov 15;48(10):989-95

Morley JE, et al. Longitudinal changes in testosterone, luteinizing hormone, and follicle-stimulating hormone in healthy men. Metabolism 1997 Apr;46(4):410-13

Nawata H, Kato K, Ibayashi H. Age-dependent change of serum 5alpha-dihydrotestosterone and its relation to testosterone in man. Endocrinology J. 1977 Feb;24(1):41-5

Pirke KM, Doerr P. Plasma dihydrotestosterone in normal adult males and its relation to testosterone. Acta Endocrinol (Copenh) 1975 Jun;79(2):357-65)

Rilling JK, et al. Ratios of plasma and salivary testosterone throughout puberty: production versus bioavailability. Steroids 1996 Jun;61(6):374-8

Tilakaratne A, Soory M. Androgen metabolism in response to oestradiol-17beta and progesterone in human gingival fibroblasts (HGF) in culture. J Clin Periodontol 1999 Nov;26(11):723-31

Vermeulen A, Verdonck L, Kaufman JM. A critical evaluation of simple methods for the estimation of free testosterone in serum. J Clin Endocrinol Metab 1999 Oct;84(10):3666-72 Comment in: J Clin Endocrinol Metab. 2001 Jun;86(6):2903.

## Melatonin, Prolactin and Biological Rhythms

Anderson RA, Lincoln GA, Wu FC. Melatonin potentiates testosterone-induced suppression of luteinizing hormone secretion in normal men. Hum Reprod 1993 Nov;8(11):1819-22

Cagnacci A. Melatonin in relation to physiology in adult humans. Pineal Res 1996 Nov;21(4):200-13

Czeisler C, Duffy J, Shanahan T, et al. Stability, precision, and near-24-hour period of the human circadian pacemaker. Science. 1999;284:2177-2181.

Dawson D, van den Heuvel CJ, Integrating the actions of melatonin on human physiology. Ann Med 1998 Feb;30(1):95-102

Drobnik J, Dabrowski R. Pinealectomy-induced elevation of collagen content in the intact skin is suppressed by melatonin application. Cytobios 1999;100(393):49-55

Fruchtman S, Jackson L, Borski R. Insulin-like growth factor I disparately regulates prolactin and growth hormone synthesis and secretion: studies using the teleost pituitary model. Endocrinology. 2000 Aug;141(8):2886-94.

Gilad E, Matzkin H, Zisapel N . Interplay between sex steroids and melatonin in regulation of human benign prostate epithelial cell growth. Clin Endocrinol Metab 1997 Aug;82(8):2535-41

Hanse L, Bedel lM. Psychotic Episode After Melatonin. Annals of Pharmacology. 1977;31:1408.

Kostoglou-Athanassiou I, Treacher DF, Wheeler MJ, Forsling ML. Bright light exposure and pituitary hormone secretion. Clin Endocrinol (Oxf) 1998 Jan;48(1):73-9

Kumar V. Melatonin: a master hormone and a candidate for universal panacea. Indian J Exp Biol 1996 May;34(5):391-402.

Nowak JZ, Zawilska JB. Melatonin and its physiological and therapeutic properties. Pharm World Sci 1998 Feb;20(1):18-27

Ohashi Y, et al. Differential pattern of the circadian rhythm of serum melatonin in young and elderly healthy subjects. Biol Signals 1997 Jul-Dec;6(4-6):301-

Okatani Y, Morioka N, Wakatsuki A . Changes in nocturnal melatonin secretion in perimenopausal women: correlation with endogenous estrogen concentrations. J Pineal Res 2000 Mar;28(2):111-8

Petterborg LJ, Thalen BE, Kjellman BF, Wetterberg L. Effect of melatonin replacement on serum hormone rhythms in a patient lacking endogenous melatonin. Brain Res Bull 1991 Aug;27(2):181-5

Pevet P. Melatonin and biological rhythms. Biol Signals Recept 2000 May-Aug;9(3-4):203-12

Rubin RT, Poland RE, Tower BB. Prolactin-related testosterone secretion in normal adult men. Clin Endocrinol Metab 1976 Jan;42(1):112-6

Van Cauter E, Plat L, Leproult R, Copinschi G. Alterations of circadian rhythmicity and sleep in aging: endocrine consequences. Horm Res. 1998;49:147-152.

Webley GE, Bohle A, Leidenberger FA. Positive relationship between the nocturnal concentrations of melatonin and prolactin, and a stimulation of prolactin after melatonin administration in young men. J Pineal Res 1988;5(1):19-33

Weitzman ED, et al. Studies of the 24 hour rhythm of melatonin in man. Neural Transm Suppl 1978;(13):325-3

Winters SJ. Diurnal rhythm of testosterone and luteinizing hormone in hypogonadal men. J Androl 1991 May-Jun;12(3):185-90

Zhdanova IV, Wurtman RJ, et al. Melatonin treatment for age-related insomnia. J Clin Endocrinol Metab 2001 Oct;86(10):4727-30

## Miscellaneous

Abrams, D. Use of Androgens in Patients Who Have HIV/AIDS: What We Know About the Effect of Androgens on Wasting and Lipodystrophy The AIDS Reader 2001; 11(3):149-156, 2001.

Allen NE, Appleby PN, Davey GK, Key TJ. Soy milk intake in relation to serum sex hormone levels in British men. Nutr Cancer. 2001;41(1-2):41-6.

Bowles JT. Sex, kings and serial killers and other group-selected human traits. Med Hypotheses. 2000 Jun;54(6):864-94. JeffBo@aol.com

Christiansen D, Weight Matters, Even in the Womb. Science News, Dec 9,2000;158:382-83

Dzugan SA, Arnold Smith R. Hypercholesterolemia treatment: a new hypothesis or just an accident? Med Hypotheses 2002 Nov;59(6):751-6

el-Awady MK, Salam MA, Gad YZ, el-Saban J. Dihydrotestosterone regulates plasma sex-hormone-binding globulin in prepubertal males: Clin Endocrinol (Oxf) 1989

Fink G, Sumner B, Rosie R, Wilson H, McQueen J. Androgen actions on central serotonin neurotransmission: relevance for mood, mental state and memory. Behav Brain Res 1999 Nov 1;105(1):53-68

Guay AT, Bansal S, Hodge MB. Possible hypothalamic impotence. Male counterpart to hypothalamic amenorrhea? Urology 1991 Oct;38(4):317-22

Guay, AT. Director, Center for Sexual Function/Endocrinology; Lahey Clinic Northshore, One Essex Center Drive, Peabody, MA. 01960. Personal Communication. November 14, 2003.

Hayashi T, et al. Dehydroepiandrosterone Retards Atherosclerosis FormationThrough Its Conversion to Estrogen: The Possible Role of Nitric Oxide. Arterioscler Thromb Vasc Biol 2000 Mar;20(3):782-792

Mokdad AH, Marks JS, Stroup, DF , Gerberding JL. Actual Causes of Death in the United States, 2000. JAMA, Mar10,2004;(291)10:1238-45

Ness, J, Sherman, F T, Pan CX. Alternative Medicine: What the data say about common herbal therapies. Geriatrics 1999;54 (10) 33-43

Seeman M. Psychopathology in women and men: focus on female hormones. Am J Psychiatry, 1997; Dec.154:12

Seppa N.Cetenarian Advantage. Science News 2003, October 18, 164; 243

Shively CA, et al.Soy and social stress affect serotonin neurotransmission in primates. Pharmacogenomics J. 2003;3(2):114-21.

Strain GW, et al. Effect of massive weight loss on hypothalamic-pituitary-gonadal function in obese men. J Clin Endocrinol Metab 1988 May;66(5):1019-23

Trichopoulou A, Costacou T, Bamia C, Trichopoulos D. Adherence to a Mediterranean diet and survival in a Greek population. NEJM 2003 Jun 26;348(26):2595-6 Weiner, Leslie. Vegetarianism and health. Special Report. *Nutrition Research Newsletter* 1988; 8:123-27.

van Niekerk JK, Huppert FA, Herbert J. Salivary cortisol and DHEA: association with measures of cognition and well-being in normal older men, and effects of three months of DHEA supplementation. Psychoneuroendocrinology 2001 Aug;26(6):591-612

Vojta CL, Fraga PD, Forciea MA, Lavizzo-Mourey R. anti-aging Therapy:An Overview. Hospital Practice. June15, 2001;43-49.

## Older Men, Memory and Testosterone

Arlt W, et al. Biotransformation of oral dehydroepiandrosterone in elderly men: significant increase in circulating estrogens. Clinical Journal of Endocrinology and Metabolism 1999 Jun;84(6):2170-6

Bain J. Andropause: Testosterone replacement therapy for aging men. Can Fam Physician 2001 Jan;47:91-7

Bhasin S, Buckwater JG. Testosterone supplementation in older men—A rational idea whose time has not yet come. J. Androl. 2001;22:718-31

Bowles J, The evolution of aging: A new approach to an old problem of biology. Med Hyptheses 1998; 51:179-221

Bowen RL, et al. Elevated luteinizing hormone expression colocalizes with neurons vulnerable to Alzheimer's disease pathology. J Neuroscience Research 2002 Nov 1;70(3):514-8

Cherrier MM, et al. Testosterone supplementation improves spatial and verbal memory in healthy older men. Neurology 2001 Jul 10;57(1):80-8

Gouchie C, Kimura D. The relationship between testosterone levels and cognitive ability patterns. Psychoneuroendocrinology 1991;16(4):323-34

Heaton JP, Morales A. Andropause a multisystem disease. Can J Urol 2001 Apr;8(2):1213-22

Friedrich MJ. Biological Secrets ofExceptional Old Age:Centenarian Study Seeks Insight into Aging Well. JAMA 11/2002;288:18:2247

Gambert S. Andropause and the Aging Male. Clinical Geriatrics 2003 Jan;11(1):12-13

Ly LP, et al.A double-blind, placebo-controlled, randomized clinical trial of transdermal dihydrotestosterone gel on muscular strength, mobility, and quality of life in older men with partial androgen deficiency. J Clin Endocrinol Metab 2001 Sep;86(9):4078-88

Nankin HR, Calkins JH. Decreased bioavailable testosterone in aging normal and impotent men. J Clin Endocrinol Metab 1986 Dec;63(6):1418-20

Morley JE, et al.Longitudinal changes in testosterone, luteinizing hormone, and follicle-stimulating hormone in healthy older men. Metabolism 1997 Apr;46(4):410-3

Morley JE. Andropause, testosterone therapy, and quality of life in aging men. Cleve Clin J Med 2000 Dec;67(12):880-2

Morley JE Testosterone replacement in older men and women. J Gend Specif Med 2001;4(2):49-53

Plymate SR, Tenover JS, Bremner WJ. Circadian variation in testosterone, sex hormone-binding globulin, and calculated non-sex hormone-binding globulin bound testosterone in healthy young and elderly men. J Androl 1989 Sep-Oct;10(5):366-71

Swartz, C. Low Serum Testosterone: a Cardiovascular Risk in Elderly Men. Geriatric Medicine Today. 1988, Dec; 7:12

Tenover JS, Matsumoto AM, Plymate SR, Bremner WJ. The effects of aging in normal men on bioavailable testosterone and luteinizing hormone secretion: response to clomiphene citrate. J Clin Endocrinol Metab 1987 Dec;65(6):1118-26

Urban RJ, et al. Testosterone administration to elderly men increases skeletal muscle strength and protein synthesis. Am J Physiol 1995 Nov;269(5 Pt 1):E820-6

Veldhuis JD, Iranmanesh A, Mulligan T, Pincus SM. Disruption of the young-adult synchrony between luteinizing hormone release and oscillations in follicle-stimulating hormone, prolactin, and nocturnal penile tumescence (NPT) in healthy older men. J Clin Endocrinol Metab. 1999 Oct;84(10):3498-505.

Winters SJ, Sherins RJ, Troen P. The gonadotropin-suppressive activity of androgen is increased in elderly men. Metabolism 1984 Nov;33(11):1052-9

## Oxytocin, the Love Hormone

Argiolas A, Melis MR, Murgia S, Schioth HB. ACTH- and alpha-MSH-induced grooming, stretching, yawning and penile erection in male rats: site of action in the brain and role of melanocortin receptors. Brain Res Bull. 2000 Mar 15;51(5):425-31. argiolas@unica.it

Anderson-Hunt M, Dennerstein L. Increased female sexual response after oxytocin. BMJ 1994;309:929.

Anderson-Hunt M, Dennerstein L. Oxytocin and female sexuality. Gynecol Obstet Invest 1995;40(4):217-21

Arletti R, Benelli A, Bertolini A. Oxytocin involvement in male and female sexual behavior. Ann NY Acad Sci 1992;652:180-93.

Blaicher W, et al.The role of oxytocin in relation to female sexual arousal. Gynecol Obstet Invest 1999;47(2):125-6.

Cantor JM, Binik YM, Pfaus JG. Chronic fluoxetine inhibits sexual behavior in the male rat: reversal with oxytocin. Psychopharmacology (Berl) 1999 Jun;144(4):355-62

Carter SC, et al. Oxytocin and social bonding. Ann NY Acad Sci 1992;652:204 11.

Carmichael MS, Warburton VL, Dixen J, Davidson JM. Relationships among cardiovascular, muscular, and oxytocin responses during human sexual activity. Arch Sex Behav 1994 Feb;23(1):59-79

Gimpl G, Fahrenholz F. The oxytocin receptor system: structure, function, and regulation. Physiological Reviews 2001 Apr;81(2):629-83

Insel TR. Post-partum increases in brain oxytocin binding. Neuroendocrinology 1986;44:515-8.

Ivell R, et al. Oxytocin and male reproductive function. Adv Exp Med Biol 1997;424:253-64

Kendrick KM, Keverne EB, Baldwin BA. Intracerebroventricular oxytocin stimulates maternal behaviour in the sheep. Neuroendocrinology 1987;46:56-61.

Kuhn JM, et al. Effects of 10 days administration of percutaneous dihydrotestosterone on the pituitary-testicular axis in normal men. Clin Endocrinol Metab 1984 Feb;58(2):231-5

McCarthy MM. Estrogen modulation of oxytocin and its relation to behavior. Adv Exp Med Biol 1995;395:235-45

Meuleman EJ, et al. A neuropeptide in human semen: oxytocin. Arch Androl 1998 Jul-Aug;41(1):17-22

Molinoff PB,et al. PT-141: a melanocortin agonist for the treatment of sexual dysfunction. Ann N Y Acad Sci. 2003 Jun;994:96-102.

Murphy MR, et al. Changes in oxytocin and vasopressin secretion during sexual activity in men. Journal of Clinical Endocrinology & Metabolism 1987 Oct;65(4):738-41

Murphy MR, Checkley SA, Seckl JR, Lightman SL. Naloxone inhibits oxytocin release at orgasm in man. J Clin Endocrinol Metab 1990 Oct;71(4):1056-8

Nicholson HD, Jenkin L. Oxytocin and prostatic function. Prostate 1999 Sep 1;40(4):211-7

Nicholson HD, Pickering BT. Oxytocin, a male intragonadal hormone. Regul Pept 1993 Apr 29;45(1-2):253-6

Ogawa S, Kudo S, Kitsunai Y, Fukuchi S. Increase in oxytocin secretion at ejaculation in male. Clin Endocrinol (Oxf) 1980 Jul;13(1):95-7

Pedersen CA, Ascher JA, Monroe YL, Prange AJ. Oxytocin induces maternal behavior in virgin female rats. Science 1982;216:649-84.

Sabatier N,et al. Oxytocin released from magnocellular dendrites: a potential modulator of alpha-melanocyte-stimulating hormone behavioral actions? Ann N Y Acad Sci. 2003 Jun;994:218-24.

Voisey J, Carroll L, van Daal A.Melanocortins and their receptors and antagonists. Curr Drug Targets. 2003 Oct;4(7):586-97.

Watson ED, Nikolakopoulos E, Gilbert C, Goode J. Oxytocin in the semen and gonads of the stallion. Theriogenology 1999 Mar;51(4):855-65

Young LJ, Lim MM, Gingrich B, Insel TR. Cellular mechanisms of social attachment. Hormonal Behavior 2001 Sep;40(2):133-8

## Penis Response to Topical Testosterone

Arisaka O,et al. Systemic effects of transdermal testosterone for the treatment of microphallus in children. Pediatr Int 2001 Apr;43(2):134-6

Baskin LS, et al. The effect of testosterone on androgen receptors and human penile growth. J Urol 1997 Sep;158(3 Pt 2):1113-8

Bin-Abbas B, et al. Congenital hypogonadotropic hypogonadism and micropenis: effect of testosterone treatment on adult penile size why sex reversal is not indicated. J Pediatr. 1999 May;134(5):579-83.

Chalapathi G, et al. Testosterone therapy in microphallic hypospadias: Topical or parenteral? J Pediatr Surg. 2003 Feb;38(2):221-3.

Charmandari E, et al. Kinetics and effect of percutaneous administration of dihydrotestosterone in children. Horm Res. 2001;56(5-6):177-81.

Danish RK, et al. Micropenis. II. Hypogonadotropic hypogonadism. Johns Hopkins Med J 1980 May;146(5):177-84

Franklin SL, Geffner ME. Precocious puberty secondary to topical testosterone exposure. J Pediatr Endocrinol Metab. 2003 Jan;16(1):107-10.

Godec CJ, Bates H, Labrosse K. Testosterone receptors in corpora cavernosa of penis. Urology 1985 Sep;26(3):237-9

Husmann DA, Cain MP. Microphallus: eventual phallic size is dependent on the timing of androgen administration. J Urol. 1994 Aug;152(2 Pt 2):734-9.

Jacobs SC, Kaplan GW, Gittes RF. Topical testosterone therapy for penile growth. Urology 1975 Dec;6(6):708-10

Kim KS, et al. Expression of the androgen receptor and 5 alpha-reductase type 2 in the developing human fetal penis and urethra. Cell Tissue Res. 2002 Feb;307(2):145-53. Epub 2001 Nov 27.

Klugo RC, Cerny JC . Response of micropenis to topical testosterone and gonadotropin. J Urol 1978 May;119(5):667-8

Kuhn JM,et al. Effects of 10 days administration of percutaneous dihydrotestosterone on the pituitary-testicular axis in normal men. Clin Endocrinol Metab 1984 Feb;58(2):231-5

Laron Z, Klinger B. Effect of IGF-I treatment on serum androgens and testicular and penile size in males with Laron syndrome (primary growth hormone resistance). Eur J Endocrinol 1998 Feb;138(2):176-80

Laron Z, Mimouni F, Pertzelan A. Effect of human growth hormone therapy on penile and testicular size in boys with isolated growth hormone deficiency: first year of treatment. Isr J Med Sci 1983 Apr;19(4):338-44

Shabsigh R, Raymond JF, Olsson CA, O'Toole K, Buttyan R. Androgen induction of DNA synthesis in the rat penis. Urology. 1998 Oct;52(4):723-8.

Spyropoulos E, et al. Size of external genital organs and somatometric parameters among physically normal men younger than 40 years old. Urology 2002 Sep;60(3):485-9; discussion 490-1

Teixeira J, et al. Mllerian Inhibiting Substance: An Instructive Developmental Hormone with Diagnostic and Possible Therapeutic Applications. Endocrine Reviews 22 (5): 657-674

Wessells H, Lue TF, McAninch JW. Penile length in the flaccid and erect states: guidelines for penile augmentation. J Urol 1996 Sep;156(3):995-7

## Progesterone, Sleep and Testosterone

Baulieu EE, Schumacher M. Progesterone as a neuroactive neurosteroid, with special reference to the effect of progesterone on myelination. Human Reproduction 2000 Jun;15 (1):1-13

Brady BM, Anderson RA, Kinniburgh D, Baird DT. Demonstration of progesterone receptor-mediated gonadotrophin suppression in the human male. Clin Endocrinol (Oxf) 2003 Apr;58(4):506-12

Barfield RJ. Glaser JH. Rubin BS. Etgen AM. Behavioral effects of progestin in the brain. [Review] Psychoneuroendocrinology. 9(3):217-31, 1984

Brown DV, Amann RP. Inhibition of testosterone metabolism in cultured rat epididymal principal cells by dihydrotestosterone and progesterone. Biol Reprod 1984 Feb;30(1):67-73

Cabeza M, et al. Antiandrogenic effect of new synthetic steroids. Proc West Pharmacol Soc. 2000;43:31-2.

Cabeza M, et al. Evaluation of new pregnane derivatives as 5alpha-reductase inhibitor. Chem Pharm Bull (Tokyo). 2001 May;49(5):525-30.

Carmody BJ, et al. Progesterone inhibits human infragenicular arterial smooth muscle cell proliferation induced by high glucose and insulin concentrations. J Vasc Surg 2002 Oct;36(4):833-8

Cistulli PA, Grunstein RR, Sullivan CE. Effect of testosterone administration on upper airway collapsibility during sleep. Am J Respir Crit Care Med 1994 Feb;149(2 Pt 1):530-2

Dewis P, Newman M, Anderson DC. The effect of endogenous progesterone on serum levels of 5 alpha-reduced androgens in hirsute women. Clin Endocrinol (Oxf) 1984 Oct;21(4):383-92

Finn MM, et al. The frequency of salivary progesterone sampling and the diagnosis of luteal phase insufficiency. Gynecol Endocrinol 1992 Jun;6(2):127-34

Fleischmann A. Etgen AM. Makman MH. Estradiol plus progesterone promote glutamate-induced release of gamma-aminobutyric acid from preoptic area synaptosomes. Neuropharmacology. 31(8):799-807, 1992

Fortune JE, Vincent SE. Progesterone inhibits the induction of aromatase activity in rat granulosa cells in vitro. Biol Reprod 1983 Jun;28(5):1078-89

Genazzani AR,et al. Effects of sex steroid hormones on the neuroendocrine system. Eur J Contracept Reprod Health Care 1997 Mar;2(1):63-9

Genazzani AR, et al. Progesterone, progestagens and the central nervous system. Hum Reprod 2000 Jun;15 Suppl 1:14-27

Grunstein RR, et al. Neuroendocrine dysfunction in sleep apnea: reversal by continuous positive airways pressure therapy. J Clin Endocrinol Metab 1989 Feb;68(2):352-8

Kapsimalis F, Kryger MH. Gender and obstructive sleep apnea syndrome, part 2: mechanisms. Sleep 2002 Aug 1;25(5):499-506

Koenig HL, et al. Progesterone synthesis and myelin formation by Schwan cells. Science 1995 Jun 9;268(5216):1500-3

Koenig HL, Gong WH, Pelissier P. Role of progesterone in peripheral nerve repair. Rev Reprod 2000 Sep;5(3):189-99

Kouchiyama S, et al. Prediction of the degree of nocturnal oxygen desaturation in sleep apnea syndrome by estimating the testosterone level. Nihon Kyobu Shikkan Gakkai Zasshi 1989 Aug;27(8):941-5

Leb CR, Hu FY, Murphy BE. Metabolism of progesterone by human lymphocytes: production of neuroactive steroids. J Clin Endocrinol Metab 1997 Dec;82(12):4064-8

Matsumoto AM, et al. Testosterone replacement in hypogonadal men: effects on obstructive sleep apnoea, respiratory drives, and sleep. Clin Endocrinol (Oxf) 1985 Jun;22(6):713-21

Mauvais-Jarvis P, Kuttenn F, Wright F. Progesterone administered by percutaneous route: an antiandrogen locally useful]. Ann Endocrinol (Paris) 1975 Mar-Apr;36(2):55-62

Manber R, Kuo TF, Cataldo N, Colrain IM. The effects of hormone replacement therapy on sleep-disordered breathing in postmenopausal women: a pilot study. Sleep

Meulenberg PM, Hofman JA. Salivary progesterone excellently reflects free and total progesterone in plasma during pregnancy. lin Chem 1989 Jan;35(1):168-72

Mohr PE, Wang DY, Gregory WM, Richards MA, Fentiman IS. Serum progesterone and prognosis in operable breast cancer. Br J Cancer 1996 Jun;73(12):1552-5

Muneyyirci-Delale O, et al. Serum ionized magnesium and calcium and sex hormones in healthy young men: importance of serum progesterone level. Fertil Steril 1999 Nov;72(5):817-22

Netzer NC, Eliasson AH, Strohl KP. Women with sleep apnea have lower levels of sex hormones. Sleep Breath 2003 Mar;7(1):25-30

Reid RL Progestins in hormone replacement therapy: Impact on endometrial and breast cancer. J. SOCGC.2000 Sep;22(9):677-681)

Saaresranta T, Polo O. Hormones and breathing. Chest 2002 Dec;122(6):2165-82

Santamaria JD, Prior JC, Fleetham JA. Reversible reproductive dysfunction in men with obstructive sleep apnoea. Clin Endocrinol (Oxf) 1988 May;28(5):461-70

Schairer C. Progesterone receptors - animal models and cell signalling in breast cancer: Implications for breast cancer of inclusion of progestins in hormone replacement therapies. Breast Cancer Res 2002;4(6):244-8

Schiavi RC, White D, Mandeli J. Pituitary-gonadal function during sleep in healthy aging men. Psychoneuroendocrinology 1992 Nov;17(6):599-609

Shahar E, et al. Hormone Replacement Therapy and Sleep-disordered Breathing. Am J Respir Crit Care Med 2003 May 1;167(9):1186-92

Sherwin BB. The impact of different doses of estrogen and progestin on mood and sexual behavior in postmenopausal women. J Clin Endocrinol Metab. 1991 Feb;72(2):336-43.

Steiner M, Dunn E, Born L. Hormones and mood: from menarche to menopause and beyond. J Affect Disord 2003 Mar;74(1):67-83

Tilakaratne A, Soory M. Androgen metabolism in response to oestradiol-17beta and progesterone in human gingival fibroblasts (HGF) in culture. J Clin Periodontol 1999 Nov;26(11):723-31

White DP,et al. Influence of testosterone on ventilation and chemosensitivity in male subjects. J Appl Physiol 1985 Nov;59(5):1452-7

## Prostate and Testosterone

Alavanja MC, et al. Use of agricultural pesticides and prostate cancer risk in the Agricultural Health Study cohort. Am J Epidemiol. 2003 May 1;157(9):800-14.

Barrett-Connor E, et al. A prospective, population-based study of androstenedione, estrogens, and prostatic cancer. Cancer Res 1990 Jan 1;50(1):169-73

Bartsch G, Rittmaster RS, Klocker H. Dihydrotestosterone and the concept of 5alpha-reductase inhibition in human benign prostatic hyperplasia. Eur Urol 2000 Apr;37(4):367-80

Berthaut I, et al. Pharmacological and molecular evidence for the expression of the two steroid 5 alpha-reductase isozymes in normal and hyperplastic human prostatic cells in culture. Prostate 1997 Aug 1;32(3):155-63

Bonkhoff H, Stein U, Aumuller G, Remberger K. Differential expression of 5 alpha-reductase isoenzymes in the human prostate and prostatic carcinomas. Prostate 1996 Oct;29(4):261-7

Carroll K et al. A link Between Diet and Cancer of the Prostate. Progressive Biochemical Pharmacology 1975; 10:308

Chan JM, Stampfer MJ, et al. Plasma insulin-like growth factor I and prostate cancer risk: a prospective study. Science 1998;279:563-566.

Guay AT, Perez JB, Fitaihi WA, Vereb M. Testosterone treatment in hypogonadal men: prostate-specific antigen level and risk of prostate cancer. Endocr Pract. 2000 Mar-Apr;6(2):132-8.

Gustafsson O, et al. Dihydrotestosterone and testosterone levels in men screened for prostate cancer: a study of a randomized population. Br J Urol 1996 Mar;77(3):433-40

Habib FK, et al. The localisation and expression of 5 alpha-reductase types I and II mRNAs in human hyperplastic prostate and in prostate primary cultures. J Endocrinol. 1998 Mar;156(3):509-17.

Habib FK, Ross M, Bayne CW. Factors controlling the expression of 5alpha-reductase in human prostate: A possible new approach for the treatment of prostate cancer. Eur Urol 1999;35(5-6):439-42

Hajjar RR. et al. Benign Prostatic Hypertropy. J Clin Endo Metab 1997;82:3793-96

Heikkila R, et al. Serum testosterone and sex hormone-binding globulin concentrations and the risk of prostate carcinoma: a longitudinal study. Cancer 1999 Jul 15;86(2):312-5

Iehle C, et al. Differences in steroid 5alpha-reductase iso-enzymes expression between normal and pathological human prostate tissue. J Steroid Biochem Mol Biol. 1999 Mar;68(5-6):189-95.

Krieg M, Schlenker A, Voigt KD. Inhibition of androgen metabolism in stroma and epithelium of the human benign prostatic hyperplasia by progesterone, estrone, and estradiol. Prostate 1985;6(3):233-40

Kyprianou N, Isaacs JT. Quantal relationship between prostatic dihydrotestosterone and prostatic cell content: critical threshold concept. Prostate 1987;11(1):41-50

Mahendroo MS, Russell DW. Male and female isoenzymes of steroid 5alpha-reductase. Rev Reprod 1999 Sep;4(3):179-83

McConnell J. et al. Medical Therapy of Prostatic Symptoms. Program Abstracts of the American Urological Association 2002. Annual Meeting (Abstract 1042, updatd}

Meikle AW, Smith JA, Stringham JD. Estradiol and testosterone metabolism and production in men with prostatic cancer. J Steroid Biochem 1989 Jul;33(1):19-24

Meikle AW, Smith JA, Stringham JD. Production, clearance, and metabolism of testosterone in men with prostatic cancer. Prostate 1987;10(1):25-31

Melcangi RC, et al. The 5alpha-reductase in the central nervous system: expression and modes of control. J Steroid Biochem Mol Biol 1998 Apr;65(1-6):295-9

Mills PK, Yang R. Prostate cancer risk in California farm workers. J Occup Environ Med. 2003 Mar;45(3):249-58.

Morgentaler A. Is low serum free testosterone a marker for high grade prostate cancer? J Urol 2000 Mar;163(3):824-7

Prehn RT. On the prevention and therapy of prostate cancer by androgen administration. Cancer Res 1999 Sep 1;59(17):4161-4

Randall VA. Role of 5 alpha-reductase in health and disease. Baillieres Clin Endocrinol Metab 1994 Apr;8(2):405-31

Radical Prostates. Female hormones may play a pivotal role in a distinctly male epidemic. Science News. Feb 22,1997; (151) 126127.

Rennie PS,et al. Kinetic analysis of 5 alpha-reductase isoenzymes in benign prostatic hyperplasia (BPH). J Steroid Biochem 1983 Jul;19(1A):169-73

Rimler A, Matzkin H, Zisapel N. Cross talk between melatonin and TGFbeta-1 in human benign prostate epithelial cells. J Clin Endocrinol Metab 2001;86:694-699.

Sciarra F. Effects of sex steroids and Epidermal Growth Factor (EGF) in benign prostatic hyperplasia (BPH). Ann N Y Acad Sci 1995;761: 66-78.

Shibata Y, et al. Changes in the endocrine environment of the human prostate transition zone with aging: simultaneous quantitative analysis of prostatic sex steroids and comparison with human prostatic histological composition. Prostate 2000 Jan;42(1):45-55

Steers WD. 5alpha-reductase activity in the prostate. Urology. 2001 Dec;58(6 Suppl 1):17-24; discussion 24.

Travis J. Do Arctic Diets protect prostates? Science News 2003, Oct. ;164: 253

Thompson I. et al. The Influence of Finasteride on the development of Prostate Cancer. New England Journal of Medicine 2003; 349:213

Weisser H, Krieg M. In vitro inhibition of androstenedione 5alpha-reduction by finasteride in epithelium and stroma of human benign prostatic hyperplasia. J Steroid Biochem Mol Biol. 1998 Oct;67(1):49-55.

Weisser H, Krieg M. Benign prostatic hyperplasia—the outcome of age-induced alteration of androgen-estrogen balance? Urologe A 1997 Jan;36(1):3-9

Winters SJ, et al. Testosterone, sex hormone-binding globulin, and body composition in young adult African American and Caucasian men. Metabolism. 2001 Oct;50(10):1242-7.

## Sexual Function and Testosterone

Adaikan PG, Srilatha B. Oestrogen-mediated hormonal imbalance precipitates erectile dysfunction. Int J Impot Res 2003 Feb;15(1):38-43

Alexander GM,et al. Mood and response to auditory sexual stimuli. Horm Behav 1997 Apr;31(2):110-9

Anderson RA, Bancroft J, Wu FC. The effects of exogenous testosterone on sexuality and mood of normal men. J Clin Endocrinol Metab 1992 Dec;75(6):1503-7

Arver S,et al. Improvement of sexual function in testosterone deficient men treated for 1 year with a permeation enhanced testosterone transdermal system. J Urol 1996 May;155(5):1604-

Bagatell CJ, Heiman JR, Rivier JE, Bremner WJ. Effects of endogenous testosterone and estradiol on sexual behavior in normal young men. J Clin Endocrinol Metab 1994 Mar;78(3):711-6 in: J Clin Endocrinol Metab 1994 Jun;78(6):1520

Bohlen JG, Held JP, Sanderson MO. The male orgasm: pelvic contractions measured by anal probe. Arch Sex Behav 1980 Dec;9(6):503-21

Brown WA, Monti PM, Corriveau DP. Serum testosterone and sexual activity and interest in men. Arch Sex Behav 1978 Mar;7(2):97-103

Carani C, et al. Effects of androgen treatment in impotent men with normal and low levels of free testosterone. Arch Sex Behav 1990 Jun;19(3):223-34

Carani C, Granata AR, Fustini MF, Marrama P. Prolactin and testosterone: their role in male sexual function. Int J Androl 1996 Feb;19(1):48-54

Carmichael MS, Warburton VL, Dixen J, Davidson JM. Relationships among cardiovascular, muscular, and oxytocin responses during human sexual activity. Arch Sex Behav 1994 Feb;23(1):59-79

Christiansen K, Knussmann R. Sex hormones and cognitive functioning in men. Neuropsychobiology 1987;18(1):27-36

Clopper RR,et al. Psychosexual behavior in hypopituitary men: a controlled comparison of gonadotropin and testosterone replacement. Psychoneuroendocrinology 1993;18(2):149-61

Davidson JM, Camargo CA, Smith ER. Effects of androgen on sexual behavior in hypogonadal men. Metab 1979 Jun;48(6):955-8

Exton MS, et al. Cardiovascular and endocrine alterations after masturbation-induced orgasm inwomen. Psychosom Med 1999 May-Jun;61(3):280-91

Exton NG, et al. Neuroendocrine response to film-induced sexual arousal in men and women. Psychoneuroendocrinology 2000 Feb;25(2):187-99

Fabbri A, Caprio M, Aversa A. Pathology of erection. J Endocrinol Invest. 2003;26(3 Suppl):87-90.

Gooren LJ. Androgen levels and sex functions in testosterone-treated hypogonadal men. Arch Sex Behav 1987 Dec;16(6):463-73

Jannini EA, et al. Lack of sexual activity from erectile dysfunction is associated with a reversible reduction in serum testosterone. Int J Androl 1999 Dec;22(6):385-92

Keefe DL. Sex hormones and neural mechanisms. Arch Sex Behav. 2002 Oct;31(5):401-3.

Knussmann R, Christiansen K, Couwenbergs C. Relations between sex hormone levels and sexual behavior in men. Arch Sex Behav 1986 Oct;15(5):429-45

Kruger T,et al.Neuroendocrine and cardiovascular response to sexual arousal and orgasm in men. Psychoneuroendocrinology 1998 May;23(4):401-11

Laumann EO, Paik A, Rosen RC. Sexual dysfunction in the United States: prevalence and predictors. JAMA 1999 Feb 10;281(6):537-44

Mantzoros CS, Georgiadis EI, Trichopoulos D. Contribution of dihydrotestosterone to male sexual behaviour. BMJ 1995, 310, 6990, pp 1289-91.

Meston CM, Frohlich PF. The Neurobiology of Sexual Function Arch Gen Psychiatry. 2000;57:1012-1030

Schwartz MF, Kolodny RC, Masters WH. Plasma testosterone levels of sexually functional and dysfunctional men. Arch Sex Behav 1980 Oct;9(5):355-66

Nicolosi A, et al. Epidemiology of erectile dysfunction in four countries: cross national study of the prevalence and correlates of erectile dysfunction. Urology 2003 Jan;61(1):201-6

Nusbaum MR. Erectile dysfunction: prevalence, etiology, and major risk factors. J Am Osteopath Assoc 2002 Dec;102(12 Suppl 4):S1-6

Rakic Z, Starcevic V, Starcevic VP, Marinkovic J . Testosterone treatment in men with erectile disorder and low levels of total testosterone in serum. Arch Sex Behav 1997 Oct;26(5):495-504

Riley A; Riley E. Controlled studies on women presenting with sexual drive disorder: I. Endocrine status. J Sex Marital Ther 2000 Jul;26(3):269-283

Schwartz MF, Kolodny RC, Masters WH. Plasma testosterone levels of sexually functional and dysfunctional men. Arch Sex Behav 1980 Oct;9(5):355-66

Turner BB. Influence of gonadal steroids on brain corticosteroid receptors: a minireview. Neurochem Res. 1997 Nov;22(11):1375-85.

## Sexual Preference, Handedness and Testosterone

Blanchard R, McConkey JG, Roper V, Steiner BW. Measuring physical aggressiveness in heterosexual, homosexual, and transsexual males. Arch Sex Behav 1983 Dec;12(6):511-24

Bem, DJ. Exotic Becomes Erotic: Interpreting the biological correlates of sexual orientation. Archives of Sexual Behavior. 2000; 29, 531-548.

Bogaert AF, Hershberger S. The Relation Between Sexual Orientation and Penile Size Arch. Sex. Behav. 1999; 28:213-221.

Elias AN, Valenta LJ. Are all males equal? Anatomic and functional basis for sexual orientation in males. Med Hypotheses 1992 Sep;39(1):85-7

Bogaert AF, Friesen C, Klentrou P. Age of puberty and sexual orientation in a national probability sample. Arch Sex Behav 2002 Feb;31(1):73-81

Bogaert AF, Blanchard, R. Handedness in homosexual and heterosexual men in the Kinsey interview data. Arch. Sex. Behav.1996; 25: 373-378.

Byne W, Parsons B. Human sexual orientation: The biologic theories reappraised. Arch.Gen.Psych. 1993; 50:228-39

Connolly P. Choate J. Resko J. Effects of endogenous androgen on brain androgen receptors of the fetal rhesus monkey. Neuroendocrinology. 59(3):27 1994 Mar.

Coolidge FL, Thede LL, Young SE. The heritability of gender identity disorder in a child and adolescent twin sample. Behav Genet 2002 Jul;32(4):251-7

Cohen KM. Relationships among childhood sex-atypical behavior, spatial ability, handedness, and sexual orientation in men. Archives of Sexual Behavior 2002 Feb;31(1):129-43

De Cecco JP, Parker DA. The biology of homosexuality: sexual orientation or sexual preference? Homosex. 1995;28(1-2):1-27.

Dorner G, et. Al. Prenatal stress as popssible aetiogenetic factor of homosexuality in human males. Endokrinologie. June 1980;75 (3):365-68.

Dorner G, Gotz F, Docke W. Prevention of demasculization and feminization of the brain in prenatally stressed male rats by perinatal androgen treatment. Experimental & Clinical Endocrinology. Jan. 1983; 81(1):88-90

Dunne MP, Bailey JM, Kirk KM, Martin NG. The subtlety of sex-atypicality. Arch Sex Behav 2000 Dec;29(6):549-65

Ellis L, Ames, M. A. Neurohormonal functioning and sexual orientation: A theory of homosexuality-heterosexuality. Psychol. Bull. 1987; 101: 233-258.

Friedman RC, Downey J.Neurobiology and sexual orientation: current relationships. J Neuropsychiatry Clin Neurosci 1993 Spring; 5(2):131-53

Gladue BA, Green R, Hellman RE. Neuroendocrine response to estrogen and sexual orientation. Science 1984 Sep 28;225(4669):1496-9

Hershberger SL, Bogaert AF. The Relation Between Nocturnal Penile Tumescence and Sexual Orientation. Correspondence. 2003. (unpublished) email:scotth@csulb.edu

Holtzen DW. Handedness and sexual orientation. J Clin Exp Neuropsychol 1994 Oct;16(5):702-12

Kinsey, A. C., Pomeroy, W. B., and Martin, C. E. (1948). Sexual behavior in the human male. W. B. Saunders, Philadelphia.

Lalumiere ML, Blanchard R, Zucker KJ. Sexual orientation and handedness in men and women: a meta-analysis. Psychol Bull 2000 Jul;126(4):575-92

LeVay, S. A difference in hypothalamic structure between heterosexual and homosexual men. Science. 1991; 253: 1034-1037.

Manning JT, Bundred PE. The Ratio of 2nd to 4th Digit Length: A New Predictor of Disease Predisposition? Medical Hypothesis 2000;54: 855-57

McCormick CM, Witelson SF, Kingstone E. Left-handedness in homosexual men and women: neuroendocrine implications. Psychoneuroendocrinology 1990;15(1):69-76

McFadden D, Pasanen EG, Callaway NL. Changes in otoacoustic emissions in transexual male during treatment with estrogen. J. Acoust. Soc. Am. 1998; 104:1555-58

McFadden D. Sex differences in the Auditory System. Dev. Neuropsychol. 1998;14:261-298

McFadden D, Champlin CA. Comparison of Auditory Evoked Potential in Heterosexual, Homosexual, and Bisexual Males and Females. JARO 2000: 01:89-99

Mortaud S, Degrelle H. Steroid control of higher brain function and behavior. Behav Genet 1996 Jul;26(4):367-72

Mustanski BS, Bailey JM, Kaspar S. Dermatoglyphics, handedness, sex, and sexual orientation. Arch Sex Behav 2002 Feb;31(1):113-22

Pirke KM, Doerr P Plasma dihydrotestosterone in normal adult males and its relation to testosterone. Acta Endocrinol (Copenh) 1975 Jun;79(2):357-65)

Popiendiville T, Nguyen T, Wisniewski A, Dobs AS. Changes in Brain Lateralization in Transsexuals Treated with Exogenous Hormones. 2001 Psychology; Medicine, Johns Hopkins University, Baltimore, MD

Sell R. Wells J. Wypij D. The prevalence of homosexual behavior and attraction in the United States, the United Kingdom, and France: results of national population-based samples. Archives of Sexual Behavior 24(3). 1995. 235-248.

Stahl F, Dorner G, Ahrens L, Graudenz W. Significantly decreased apparently free testosterone levels in plasma of male homosexuals. Endokrinologie 1976 Oct;68(1):115-7

Swaab, D. F., and Hofman, M. A. An enlarged suprachiasmatic nucleus in homosexual men. Brain Res. 1990; 537: 141-148.

Rahman Q, Wilson GD. Sexual orientation and the 2nd to 4th finger length ratio: evidence for organising effects of sex hormones or developmental instability? Psychoneuroendocrinology 2003 Apr;28(3):288-303

Robinson SJ, Manning JT. The raio of 2nd to 4th digit length and male homosexuality. Evolution and Human Behavior. 2000;21:333-345.

Spyropoulos E, et al. Size of external genital organs and somatometric parameters among physically normal men younger than 40 years old. Urology 2002 Sep;60(3):485-9; discussion 490-1

Pirke KM, Doerr P Plasma dihydrotestosterone in normal adult males and its relation to testosterone. Acta Endocrinol (Copenh) 1975 Jun;79(2):357-65

Pillard RC, Poumadere J, Carretta RA. A family study of sexual orientation. Arch Sex Behav 1982 Dec;11(6):511-20

Rahman Q, Silber K. Sexual orientation and the sleep-wake cycle: a preliminary investigation. Arch Sex Behav 2000 Apr;29(2):127-34

Swaab DF, Gooren LJ, Hofman MA. Brain research, gender and sexual orientation. J Homosex 1995;28(3-4):283-301

Van Wyk PH, Geist CS. Biology of bisexuality: critique and observations. J Homosex 1995;28(3-4):357-73

Voracek M, Manning JT. Length of Fingers and Penis Are Related Through Fetal *Hox* Gene Expression. Urology 2003:62(1);201

Zhou J, Hofman M. Gooren L. Swaab D. A sex difference in the human brain and its relation to transsexuality. Nature Nov. 1995; 378(6552):68-70

## Sperm Counts and Testosterone

Auger J, Kunstmann JM, Cazyglik F, Jouannet P. Decline in semen quality among fertile men in Paris during the past 20 years. N Engl J Med 1995; 332:281.

Hudson RW, et al. Seminal plasma testosterone and dihydrotestosterone levels in men with varicoceles. Int J Androl 1983 Apr;6(2):135-42

Irvine, S, et al. Evidence of deteriorating semen quality in the United Kingdom: Birth cohort study in 577 men in Scotland over 11 years. Br Med J 1996; 312:467.

Le Lannou D, et al. Testosterone and 5 alpha-dihydrotestosterone concentrations in human seminal plasma. Int J Androl 1980 Oct;3(5):502-6

Murray TJ, et al.Endocrine disrupting chemicals: Effects on human male reproductive health. Early Pregnancy 2001 Apr;5(2):80-112

Pavlovich CP, Goldstein M. Hormonal Regulation of Spermatogenesis J Urol 2001;165:837-841.

Sharpe RM, Skakkebaek NE. Are oestrogens involved in falling sperm counts and diosorders of the male reproductive tract? Lancet 1993;431:1392-95.

Yamamoto M, et al. In-vitro contractility of human seminiferous tubules in response to testosterone, dihydrotestosterone and estradiol. Urol Res 1989;17(4):265-8

## Transdermal Testosterones

Arver S et al, Improvement of sexual function in testosterone deficient men treated for 1 year with a permeation enhanced testosterone transdermal system, J Urololgy 1996;155:1604-1608.

Bals-Pratsch, M, Yoo YD, Knuth VA, Nieschlag E . Transdermal testosterone Substitution Therapy for male hypogonadism. Lancet 4/943-946.1986

Brocks DR, Meikle AW, Boike SC, Mazer NA, Zariffa N, Audet PR, Jorkasky DK.Pharmacokinetics of testosterone in hypogonadal men after transdermal delivery:influence of dose. J Clinical Pharmacology 1996 Aug;36(8):732-9)

Carey PO, Howards SS, Vance ML. Transdermal testosterone treatment of hypogonadal men. Urology 1988 Jul;140(1):76-9

Cutter CB. Compounded Percutaneous Testosterone Gel: Use And Effects in Hypogonadal Men . J American Board Family Practice 14(1):22-32, 2001.

English KM, et al. Low-dose transdermal testosterone therapy improves angina threshold in men with chronic stable angina. Circulation 2000;102:1906-11

Findlay JC, Place V, Snyder PJ. Transdermal delivery of Testosterone. J. Clinical Endocrinolology Metab. 64; 266-268. 1989

Howell S, Shalet S. Testosterone deficiency and replacement. Horm Res 2001;56 Suppl 1:86-92

Kenny AM, et al. Effects of transdermal testosterone on lipids and vascular reactivity in older men with low bioavailable testosterone levels. J Gerontol A Biol Sci Med Sci 2002 Jul;57(7):M460-5.

Mazer NA.New clinical applications of transdermal testosterone delivery in men and women. J Control Release 2000 Mar 1;65(1-2):303-15

McGriff-Lee NJ. Transdermal testosterone gel (Cellegy). Curr Opin Investig Drugs 2002 Nov;3(11):1629-32

McNicholas TA, et al. A novel testosterone gel formulation normalizes androgen levels in hypogonadal men, with improvements in body composition and sexual function. Brit J. Urology International. 2003 Jan;91(1):69-74.

Shifren JL, et al. Transdermal testosterone treatment in women with impaired sexual function after oophorectomy. N Engl J Med. 2000 Sep 7;343(10):682-8. janshifren@hotmail.com

Sitruk-Ware R. Transdermal delivery of steroids. Contraception 1989 Jan;39(1):1-20

Wang C, et al. Pharmacokinetics of a transdermal gel in hypogonadal men .application of gel at one sit versus four sites : a General Clinical Research Center Study. J Clin Endocrinol Metab 2000 Mar;85(3):964-9

Winters SJ, Atkinson L. Serum LH concentrations in hypogonadal men during transdermal testosterone replacement through scrotal skin: further evidence that ageing enhances testosterone negative feedback. Clin Endocrinol (Oxf). 1997 Sep;47(3):317-22.

Winters SJ. Current status of testosterone replacement therapy in men. Arch Fam Med. 2000 Mar;9(3):221. winters@med1.dept-med.pitt.edu

## Viagra, ED and Testosterone

Aversa A, Isidori AM, Spera G, Lenzi A, Fabbri A. Androgens improve cavernous vasodilation and response to sildenafil in patients with erectile dysfunction. Clin Endocrinol (Oxf). 2003 May;58(5):632-8.

Basar M, et al. The efficacy of sildenafil in different etiologies of erectile dysfunction (ED). International Urol Nephrol. 2001;32(3):403-7.

Becker AJ, et al. Cavernous and systemic testosterone levels in different phases of human penile erection. Urology. 2000 Jul;56(1):125-9.

Chatterjee R, et al. Management of ED by combination therapy with testosterone and sildenafil in recipients of high-dose therapy for haematological malignancies. Bone Marrow Transplant. 2002 Apr;29(7):607-10.

Gauthier A, et al. Relative Efficacy of Sildenafil Compared to Other Treatment Options for Erectile Dysfunction South Med J 93(10):962-965, 2000.

Guay AT, et al. Efficacy and safety of sildenafil citrate for treatment of erectile dysfunction in a population with associated organic risk factors. J Androl. 2001 Sep-Oct;22(5):793-7.

Lugg JA, Rajfer J, Gonzalez-Cadavid NF. Dihydrotestosterone is the active androgen in the maintenance of nitric oxide-mediated penile erection in the rat. Endocrinology 1995 Apr;136(4):1495-501

Lim PH, Moorthy P, Benton KG. The clinical safety of Viagra. Ann N Y Acad Sci. 2002 May;962:378-88.

Manecke RG, Mulhall JP. Medical treatment of erectile dysfunction. Ann Med. 1999 Dec;31(6):388-98.

McCullough AR, et al. Achieving treatment optimization with sildenafil citrate (Viagra) in patients with erectile dysfunction. Urology. 2002 Sep;60(2 Suppl 2):28-38.

Reiter WJ, et al. Dehydroepiandrosterone in the treatment of erectile dysfunction: a prospective, double-blind, randomized, placebo-controlled study. Urology 1999 Mar;53(3):590-4; discussion 594-5

Shabsigh R. Hypogonadism and erectile dysfunction: the role for testosterone therapy. Int J Impot Res. 2003 Aug;15 Suppl 4:S9-13.

Shabsigh R. The effects of testosterone on the cavernous tissue and erectile function. World J Urol. 1997;15(1):21-6.

Steers W, Guay AT, et al. Assessment of the efficacy and safety of Viagra (sildenafil citrate) in men with ED. Int J Impotence Res. 2001 Oct;13(5):261-7.

Svetec DA, et al. The effect of parenteral testosterone replacement on prostate specific antigen in hypogonadal men with erectile dysfunction. J Urol 1997 Nov;158(5):1775-7

# About the Author

Born in Lodz, Poland, Abraham H. Kryger graduated from Canada's University of Manitoba in 1969 as a dentist. After a year of dental practice, the doctor returned to earn his medical degree from the same university in 1973.

Dr. Kryger is a board-certified Family Practitioner and Preventive Medicine specialist with a full-time private practice in Monterey, California. His practice includes treatment for hormone imbalances and sexual dysfunction, nutritional evaluations, depression, anxiety and appetite disorders.

In the 1980s he filed an INDA (Investigational New Drug Application) with the FDA to investigate the use of Lentian (an extract of Letinula edodes or Shitake) in cancer care. The doctor has been studying the effects of mushrooms on the immune system for the past two decades. He uses nutritional evaluations, which measure vitamin and mineral levels in the blood serum and treats patients by prescribing organically grown fruit and vegetable supplements.

Dr. Kryger has been a sports medicine advisor for Monterey athlete, Chad Hawker, world famous triathlete and winner of the Kona Half Ironman for six years in a row (1998 to 2004). Chad has been using MRL mushroom nutraceutical products to improve his stamina for the five grueling triathlons he races in each year.

Dr. Kryger is a past member of the International Academy of Preventive Medicine, the International Association of Metabolic Medicine and has served on the board of the Monterey County Aids Project. Dr. Kryger is also an associate of the American Society of Pain Management and the Endocrine Society of America.

For over twenty-five years Dr. Kryger has pioneered research in the field of male and female hormone replacement, with special focus on anti-aging and wellness medicine. His book developed from his research into hormones and depression.

## A Startling Discovery About Libido and Aging

Early in his training Dr. Kryger encountered many men who, although only in their early thirties, complained of a reduced or non-existent sex drive. They often described themselves as feeling old. Laboratory tests revealed that the testosterone levels in many of these men had dropped prematurely. Dr. Kryger further observed that those men and women who maintained normal hormone levels throughout their lives looked, felt, and functioned significantly better than those with abnormal hormone levels. It was unclear why some people were able to maintain normal levels while others were not.

During his search for the cause of the phenomenon, Dr. Kryger studied possible environmental factors. After the revelation, in January, 2001, that dioxin, a chemical used in the manufacture of vinyl products, and the pesticide DDT had been identified as carcinogenic, Dr. Kryger began searching for other possible problems related to dioxin. He discovered that, in healthy men, exposure to government approved levels of dioxin could reduce testosterone production to abnormal levels. Further study demonstrated that low levels of testosterone were responsible for a much wider range of symptoms than previously realized, and encompassed not only sex-related problems, but also depression, memory problems, osteoporosis, loss of muscle mass, fatigue and loss of the enjoyment of life.

Since that time, Dr. Kryger has devoted much of his time and energy to educating other physicians and the public about this growing problem, and successfully treating patients with hormonal imbalances.

Dr. Abraham Kryger is world-renowned in the medical community for his extensive training and more than twenty-five years of experience in conventional, holistic and complementary medicine. He is a frequent source of expert commentary in the USA Today.com column, *Spotlight Health,* the world's most widely read daily medical, health and wellness column. He is the originator and author of *Hormone News,* a newsletter for physicians and endocrinologists. He was medical consultant for the Monterey, California television program, *The Morning Show,* and hosted a call-in radio program on medical issues for Monterey radio station KMBY. Dr. Kryger has been interviewed on television and radio and has published numerous newspaper articles on health issues.

In 1997 Dr. Kryger pioneered a uniquely personal approach to medical education, **Wellness MD** (www.wellnessmd.com). Combining Internet technology with private telephone consultation, the service offers general health information online and personalized non-medical consultation by telephone.

To contact the doctor or make comments about the book, please write to Dr. Kryger, 1084 Cass Street, Suite B, Monterey, CA 93940, or email DRK@WellnessMD.com.

# Index

## N



## O



## P

# R



# S

# Z

# Coming soon...

Have you ever wondered why the thyroid gland stores iodine?

Why do most people only know about the form of thyroid called T4?

What about the "quick acting" form of thyroid hormone called T3?

A new book by Dr. Kryger is on its way—

## The Butterfly Gland
### How the Thyroid Gland Controls Your Weight

Ask to be placed on the waiting list to know when this book is available—

Abraham Kryger, MD, DMD

WellnessMD Publications

1084 Cass Street, Monterey, California 93940